Biobehavioral
Measures
of
Dyslexia

Biobehavioral
Measures
of
Dyslexia

edited by

David B. Gray
James F. Kavanagh

This book was manufactured in the United States of America. Typography by Brushwood Graphics Studio, Baltimore, Maryland. Printing by Collins Lithographing and Printing Company, Inc., Baltimore, Maryland. Cover design by Joseph Dieter, Jr.

Library of Congress Catalog Card Number 85-052392.

ISBN 0-912752-10-6

Contents

This book is dedicated to the memory of
Norman Geschwind, M.D.

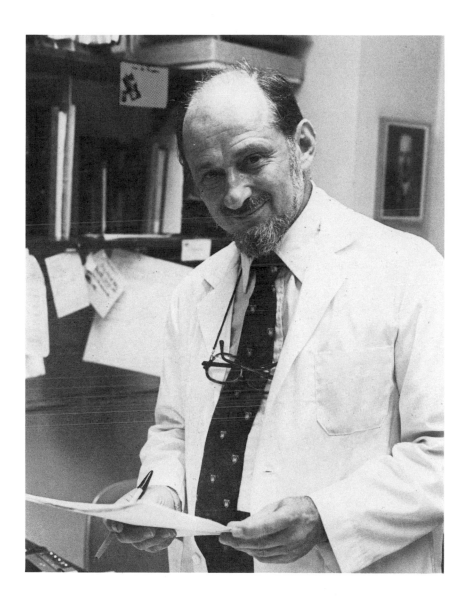

January 8, 1926—November 4, 1984

Preface

$\mathcal{L}$ earning to read is a major problem for a significant portion of children who, except for the inability to read, appear to have normal cognitive and behavioral abilities. The emotional and economic costs paid by dyslexics, their parents, and society are great. Numerous congressional reports have called for additional Federal support for research that would clarify the variables influencing the development and acquisition of the ability to read. As a result of this interest, several Federal agencies have become heavily involved in sponsoring research on dyslexia. Most notable are the National Institute of Child Health and Human Development (NICHD), National Institute of Mental Health (NIMH), National Institute of Neurological, Communicative Disorders, and Stroke (NINCDS), the National Institute of Education (NIE), and the Office of Special Education and Rehabilitative Services of the Department of Education, specifically the National Institute of Handicapped Research (NIHR).

During the past two decades there has been an explosion of research on the topic of reading. Psychologists and linguists, as well as a variety of other behavioral and biological scientists have become fascinated and many times frustrated by the fact that, although reading and listening may have some linguistic similarities, they are, in a very real sense, quite different. Some American children fail to learn to read even though they apparently can listen to and comprehend the spoken language of their parents. There remains today a widespread public interest and educational controversy over why many Johnnys and, at least some, Marys can not read. Are these children otherwise really normal? Do they really handle the spoken language well and only fail when presented with written material? Or do they, in fact, have certain more central language processing problems which make them at risk for reading failure? Are they, in fact, dyslexic before they manifest a reading disorder?

While significant progress has been achieved in describing some of the fundamental linguistic and cognitive deficits that characterize poor readers, few studies have been made that test the convergent and divergent validity of the research findings in relation to these general theories. One reason for this may be that cross-sample validation of findings is difficult. Subjects for the empirical studies are often drawn from unique clinical populations or from schools based upon the scientifically inadequate criteria contained in Public Law 94-142. In addition, most of the research is carried out by scientists who focus on only one aspect of dyslexia from a single theoretical vantage point. Although these researchers have excellent credentials in their own field of science, they are often not aware of recent discoveries in other scientific disciplines that might be applied to the study of dyslexia.

To help solve this problem, a conference entitled "Biobehavioral Measures of Dyslexia" was held in Bethesda, Maryland from September 10 through 12, 1984. The goal was to provide an opportunity for the exchange of research findings by scientists with an interest in dyslexia and a background in reading, linguistics, psychometrics, computer science, cognition, genetics, and neurology. Drs. David B. Gray and James F. Kavanagh of the NICHD had the major responsibility for planning the conference. Dr. David Pearl (NIMH), Drs. Sarah Broman and Martha Denckla (NINCDS), and Dr. Douglas Fenderson (NIHR) each assisted in important ways in planning the conference. This meeting was the ninth in a series of conferences sponsored by the NICHD on "Communicating by Language." Other books in this series include *Language by Ear and by Eye, Child Phonology,* and *Orthography, Reading, and Dyslexia.*

Because the NICHD is currently supporting one collaborative interdisciplinary research project with a focus on reading, the Colorado Reading Project, this project served as one of the cornerstones for the development of the conference. The other major influence in formulating the conference was Dr. Norman Geschwind. The importance of Dr. Geschwind to the conference was aptly expressed by Dr. Alexander, Director of NICHD, in his introduction of Dr. Geschwind, "Given this topic (dyslexia) and our emphasis on linking neurobiology and behavior, Dr. Geschwind was the first name to come to mind . . . and as I recall, availability wasn't even an issue because we said we'd have it when he could come." Dr. Geschwind died shortly after his participation in this conference. This book is dedicated to Dr. Geschwind.

The first chapter, "The Biology of Dyslexia," represents Dr. Norman Geschwind's after dinner reflections on the study of dyslexia from the perspective of his long and productive career. In this edited narrative, Dr. Geschwind explicates and interrelates within a broad theoretical context many of the empirical findings from a diverse array of scientific domains including neurology, neuroanatomy, neurochemistry, developmental neurology, immunology, neuropsychology, quantitative and qualitative genetics, and epidemiology. The responsibility of editing his oral presentation was assumed, in large part, by Dr. James F. Kavanagh. Every effort was made to preserve the distinctive oral style of the speaker.

In succeeding chapters, conference participants discuss the variety of scientific methods that have been applied to refining the samples of reading disabled individuals being studied. Paul Satz, Robin Morris, and Jack Fletcher provide an overview of the controversies surrounding the theoretical and methodological issues in the field of learning disability. Dr. Martha Denckla's chapter "Issues of Overlap and Heterogeneity in Dyslexia" covers several specific behavioral and biological research strategies currently being applied to address the boundaries between individuals categorized as "pure" dyslexic and those described as reading disabled with attention deficit disorders. In their chapter, Drs. Dykman, Ackerman, and Holcomb present their findings from electrophysiological recordings and psychopharmacological responsiveness studies of children with reading disability, with attention deficits, and with reading disability and attention disorders. In the next chapter, Dr. Richard

Coppola provides an overview of recent developments in neuroimaging techniques. Dr. John R. Hughes provides a historical framework for understanding the current electrophysiological methods being used to subtype learning disabled children. Dr. David Shucard describes his longitudinal, electrophysiological studies of the good and poor readers who are participating in the Colorado Reading Project.

The next four chapters of the book reflect the growing interest in the scientific community in studies that assess the interactive influences of genetics and environment on the development of reading skills. Dr. John R. DeFries describes a large scale longitudinal study, the Colorado Reading Project (CRP), which has examined the same sample of subjects using a variety of behavioral and biological measures. The preliminary results of the reading characteristics of identical and fraternal twins in the CRP are presented by Dr. Sadie Decker. Dr. Joan Finucci reviews the advantages of using family data to systematically characterize subtypes of dyslexia. Drs. David Housman, Shelley Smith, and David Pauls provide a review of how the new molecular genetics is being applied to behavioral disorders.

The remaining portion of this book includes chapters that describe theoretical issues and empirical findings essential for a deeper understanding of the development of the reading process in normal and reading disabled children. Dr. Isabelle Liberman, in her chapter with Drs. Rubin, Duquès, and Carlisle, reviews evidence supporting the fundamental importance of a child's linguistic sophistication for the development of normal reading skills and its relationship to spelling skills. Drs. Frank Vellutino and Donna Scanlon trace a series of intricate studies conducted over the past twenty years which offer empirical evidence for often reported age dependent linguistic deficits exhibited by poor readers. Dr. Richard K. Olson describes the results of his examination of the eye movements and phonetic abilities of normal and poor readers and the within group differences of disabled readers who are part of the Colorado Reading Project. The importance of using eye movements to gain access to changes in the temporal and sequential mental processes taking place as children develop the ability to read are described by Drs. George McConkie and David Zola in their chapter. In the next chapter, Dr. Marion Blank reviews her work on the importance of the type of words that are difficult for inexperienced and disabled readers. Dr. Ellis Richardson's chapter gives the rationale for a new measurement tool, the Decoding Skills Test (DST), which can be used to assess the phonetic deficiencies of dyslexic children. The development of this test was supported by a NICHD contract. The final chapter of the book by Dr. Dillon Inouye reviews the diversity of methods that have been applied to the study of dyslexia and describes how four different generations of computers can be used to collect qualitatively different types of information on reading disabled children.

The editors would like to express their appreciation to Elinor Hartwig of York Press for the dedication, patience, and care she provided in the preparation of this book. Mr. Gary Carter's work in planning and Ms. Victoria Bolton's work in arranging the conference are also gratefully acknowledged.

Participants

Duane F. Alexander, M.D.
Acting Director
National Institute of Child Health and
  Human Development
Building 31, Room 2A04
9000 Rockville Pike
Bethesda, MD 20892

Marion Blank, Ph.D.
171 Van Nostrand
Englewood, NJ 07631

Sarah H. Broman, Ph.D.
Chief
Mental Retardation and Learning
  Disorders Section
Developmental Neurology Branch
National Institute of Neurological and
  Communicative Disorders and
  Stroke
Federal Building, Room 8C06
9000 Rockville Pike
Bethesda, MD 20892

Monte S. Buchsbaum, M.D.
Professor of Psychiatry and Human
  Behavior
Department of Psychiatry
University of California
Irvine, CA 92717

Sadie Neef Decker, Ph.D.
Faculty Fellow
University of Colorado
300 Gaylord Street
Denver, CO 80206

John C. DeFries, Ph.D.
Director
Institute for Behavioral Genetics
University of Colorado
Campus Box 447
Boulder, CO 80309

Martha B. Denckla, M.D.
Chief
Autism and Behavioral Disorders
  Section
Developmental Neurology Branch
National Institute of Neurological and
  Communicative Disorders and
  Stroke
Federal Building, Room 820
9000 Rockville Pike
Bethesda, MD 20892

Roscoe A. Dykman, Ph.D.
Professor
Slot #588
University of Arkansas for Medical
  Sciences
4301 West Markham
Little Rock, AR 72205

Douglas A. Fenderson, Ph.D.
Director
National Institute of Handicapped
  Research
Switzer Building, Room 3060
330 "C" Street, S.W.
Washington, DC 20202

Joan M. Finucci, Ph.D.
Assistant Professor
Department of Pediatrics
Johns Hopkins University
550 Bldg. Suite 508
Baltimore, MD 21205

Norman Geschwind, M.D.*
Neurologist-in-Chief
Beth Israel Hospital
330 Brookline Avenue
Boston, MA 02215

David B. Gray, Ph.D.
Health Scientist Administrator
Human Learning and Behavior
  Branch
Center for Research for Mothers and
  Children
National Institute of Child Health and
  Human Develoment
Landow Building, Room 7C18
9000 Rockville Pike
Bethesda, MD 20892

David E. Housman, Ph.D.
Associate Professor of Biology
Center for Cancer Research
E17-541
Massachusetts Institute of
  Technology
Cambridge, MA 02139

John R. Hughes, M.D.
Professor of Neurology
University of Illinois
Medical Center
912 Southwood Street
Chicago, IL 60612

Dillon K. Inouye, Ph.D.
Professor
Department of Curriculum and
  Instructional Science
Brigham Young University
Provo, UT 84601

James F. Kavanagh, Ph.D.
Associate Director
Center for Research for Mothers and
  Children
National Institute of Child Health and
  Human Development
Landow Building, Room 7C04
9000 Rockville Pike
Bethesda, MD 20892

Norman A. Krasnegor, Ph.D.
Chief, Human Learning and Behavior
  Branch
Center for Research for Mothers and
  Children
National Institute of Child Health and
  Human Development
Landow Building, Room 7C18
9000 Rockville Pike
Bethesda, MD 20892

Isabelle Y. Liberman, Ph.D.
Professor of Education
University of Connecticut
School of Education
Box U 64
Storrs, CT 06268

Mortimer B. Lipsett, M.D.**
Director
National Institute of Child Health and
  Human Development
Building 31, Room 2A03
9000 Rockville Pike
Bethesda, MD 20892

George W. McConkie, M.D.
Professor
Center for the Study of Reading
51 Gerty Drive
Champaign, IL 61820

* Dr. Geschwind passed away on November 4, 1984.
** Dr. Lipsett passed away on November 10, 1985.

Richard K. Olson, Ph.D.
Professor of Psychology
Department of Psychology
University of Colorado
Boulder, CO 80309

Betty Osman, Ph.D.
Educational Therapist
36 Fenimore Road
Scarsdale, NY 10583

David Pearl, Ph.D.
Chief
Behavioral Sciences Research Branch
National Institute of Mental Health
Parklawn Building, Room 10C09
5600 Fishers Lane
Rockville, MD 20857

Ellis Richardson, Ph.D.
Research Scientist
Nathan Kline Institute for Psychiatric
    Research
Orangebury, NY 10962

Paul Satz, Ph.D.
Professor in Chief
Neuropsychology Department
University of California
Los Angeles, CA 90024

David W. Shucard, Ph.D.
Professor
Department of Psychiatry
University of Colorado
School of Medicine
Director, Brain Sciences Laboratories
Department of Pediatrics
National Jewish Hospital and
    Research Center
3800 East Colfax Avenue
Denver, CO 80206

Frank R. Vellutino, Ph.D.
Director, Child Research and Study
    Center
1400 Washington Avenue
State University of New York
Albany, NY 12222

Mary S. Wilson, Ph.D.
Allen House
Department of Communication
    Science and Disorders
University of Vermont
Burlington, VT 05405

The Biology of Dyslexia: The After-Dinner Speech

Norman Geschwind

*G*t is safe to say that, if someone had been asked to talk about the biology of childhood dyslexia in 1978, there would have been very little hard data that showed a biological underpinning. Some of the data available at that time include the striking male predominance of childhood dyslexia and the elevated rate of non-righthandedness. (As many of you know, the latter has been disputed, however, we have some data which, I think, show convincingly an overwhelming relationship to non-righthandedness.)

In 1978, there was also suggestive older data—I say "suggestive" because I don't know how good the studies were. For example, certain people had suggested an elevated rate of dyslexia among twins. There was also the fact of familial aggregations. In addition, there were some older impressions that suggested biological features. I say "impressions" because there are areas that still haven't been studied, but which deserve to be; for example, the belief that there are differences between ethnic groups, and although I've never seen hard data on it, the claim that there are elevated rates in adopted children.

However, if we go back to the story of when the biology starts, it actually begins in the 19th century with the description of the acquired alexias. By 1890, it was well known among the German, French, and British neurologists that there were patients who had brain lesions, and who lost reading ability in an isolated fashion. In fact, it was so well known that nobody bothered to ask the question, "Does this alexia really exist?"

Then a very strange thing happened. When I went to medical school and trained in neurology I was taught that although such conditions had been described in the 19th century, they must have been mythology because nobody saw such cases.

This is an edited version of the after-dinner speech Dr. Geschwind gave on September 11, 1984 at the conference "Biobehavioral Measures of Dyslexia." Dr. Kavanagh has lightly edited the transcript while keeping the flavor of Dr. Geschwind's style.

Later, I had the pleasure of showing a case of acquired alexia to a very distinguished professor who had made that statement. In fact, since then I've seen many, many cases. It is clear that people had a better understanding of that topic in 1890 than they had in the early 1960's.

But the real step forward came when, in the years 1891 and 1892, the French neurologist, Déjérine described the first post mortems on patients with acquired alexia. Several conditions occur in which patients who have previously been able to read lose the ability to do so in the presence of preserved visual abilities.

One of these conditions is called alexia without agraphia. These patients lose the ability to read but they see perfectly well as demonstrated by the fact that they can copy with great ease words they can't read. They can write, but they can't read what they have written. The fact that the lesion is not involving the part of the brain critical for reading is proved by the fact that they preserve knowledge possessed only by someone who knows how to read.

Although these patients cannot read the simplest word, if you say, "How do you spell clock?" they will spell it immediately. If you spell a word to them, they will name it. If you give them letters in their hands, they immediately identify them. They can read through the ear. They can read through the hand. They cannot read through the eye. Except for their ability to copy, what they resemble most is a normal person with his eyes closed.

In the condition known as hemi-alexia, patients can read in the right visual field, but cannot read in the left visual field, even though they can see perfectly in both visual fields. This condition was first described in 1937, the first patient being one in whom it was shown that a surgical lesion of the corpus callosum produced disconnection of the hemispheres. The work was done in Baltimore, Maryland at the Johns Hopkins Hospital by John Tresher and Frank Ford.

Returning to the condition called alexia without agraphia, some of you may think that if there is a condition of alexia without agraphia and a condition of alexia with agraphia, the second one must have the same lesion as the first, but with something added. That is not true. The lesion for alexia with agraphia has no overlap with the lesion for alexia without agraphia. They are in two completely different locations.

Alexia with agraphia is a rather remarkable condition because the patient loses the ability to read, although he can name objects with no difficulty whatsoever. He loses the ability to read; he can no longer write, although he has nothing wrong with his hands (he can do anything else with his hands that he could do formerly); he can no longer spell. So, if you ask him, "How do you spell clock?" he will say, "I have no idea." If you say, "What is h-o-u-s-e?" he will say, "H-o-u-s-e? I don't know. I think I should know that." In other words, these people have been reduced to the state of illiteracy because they do exactly the same things an illiterate would do.

The lesion in this condition was described by Jules Déjérine a year before he described alexia without agraphia. Since then it has been confirmed many times.

Alexia with agraphia is a rarer condition than alexia without agraphia, but

I have seen half a dozen; on the other hand I have seen probably 50 cases of alexia without agraphia.

You can also acquire alexia as a component of Wernicke's aphasia. There is a lesion in Wernicke's area further forward, but that alexia is part of a syndrome in which the patient has difficulty with every aspect of language, including comprehension of spoken language. The patient speaks badly; he doesn't comprehend written language; he writes badly.

By the way, it is interesting that in Broca's aphasia, patients may have a very curious type of problem with reading. They may comprehend written material rather well, but they cannot read aloud the names of letters.

In the late 1890's Pringle Morgan described the first case of congenital "word blindness" and later a British ophthalmologist named Hinshelwood took this up and described many further cases.

The interesting thing was that at that point in the 1890's, investigators wondered where the anomaly in the brain that's going to cause this condition might be located. They theorized that the most reasonable place to put it was where Déjérine showed them as special for reading. In fact, they were right.

It took from 1896, when they made that observation, until 1979 for somebody to look. Why didn't anybody look for 83 years? There is an important lesson in this. They didn't look for 83 years because, first of all, people thought that "all that old stuff was nonsense" so why pay attention to it and they never thought of going back to read the papers to see that it wasn't nonsense after all.

The second reason was that there were people who said it was naive to assume that the anomaly in the brain would be anything like that in the adult acquired disorders—therefore, it was unnecessary to look. In fact, there are still papers being written in 1984 stating that it is naive, when there are already five post-mortem cases showing that these people were right. (One should cultivate naiveté with great care. The sophisticated don't make important discoveries. They always know they are going to be wrong about everything.)

In 1925, Orton, at the age of 46, saw his first dyslexic and wrote his first paper on the subject. In that paper he said this is where the anomaly in the brain ought to be, although for some reason he thought there should be no structural disorder.

In 1968, Walter Levitsky and I decided that we were going to look for anatomical asymmetries in the cortex and we found them. In fact, we found that they were readily visible to the naked eye. These asymmetries could have been discovered in the 1600's, if someone had looked.

If you pass a knife through the Sylvian fissure, you will uncover the upper surface of the temporal lobe and then, if you cut into the white matter, what you see first is a big structure that is Heschl's gyrus, the primary auditory cortex, and on the left behind it, a big triangular, flat area and on the right, a much smaller area.

There were 100 brains in the original series that Levitsky and I published that showed this very large triangular area on the left side. This has been confirmed in at least five other series in many hundreds of brains. The statistics for our original series show that the area was larger on the left in 65 percent of the total, roughly equal in 24 percent and larger on the right in 11 percent.

Another asymmetry was the one that was discovered by Marjorie Lemay, but previously described by the great Irish anatomist, Cunningham, in the 1890's. On the left side, the Sylvian fissure remains horizontal as it reaches the back end, but on the right side it turns up. Essentially the same statistics I have just mentioned hold for this asymmetry also.

I will give an example of another asymmetry to show you that the phrenologists were right when they said that the shape of skulls mirrors the underlying brain and is also related to psychological characteristics. It turns out to be true, as Dr. Lemay discovered, that in the human brain as seen in computerized x-rays, the left occipital region is wider than the right in about 70 percent of brains. The right frontal region is wider than the left with the corresponding asymmetry mirrored in the shape of the skull. Moreover, this asymmetry, at least in her data, is related to handedness. This asymmetry, by the way, is present in the fetus, just as is the asymmetry I described in the upper surface of the temporal lobe and planum temporale. That asymmetry is visible in the brain of the fetus at 31 weeks of gestation.

Dr. Galaburda and I decided that we should go beyond this business of knowing that there is a gross asymmetry; we wanted to get down to a finer level. It was high time we used a microscope.

We took brains which were cut into serial sections and mapped out the sizes of areas of particular cellular architecture. Dr. Galaburda was able to show that what made the enlargement of this region of the left cortex was the enlargement of an area of particular cellular architecture. In one brain, it was 750 percent larger on the left. There is nothing subtle about these changes. It was clear that this was reflecting some underlying structure that wasn't just an accident of the manufacturer folding this thing carelessly.

In addition, this is part of the language cortex. It is an extension of the upper surface of the temporal lobe of Wernicke's area which is the same microscopic structure.

We look now at the question of whether there is an anomaly in the brain in childhood alexia. There was a paper published some years ago by a group in Boston who claimed that dyslexics with poor verbal abilities showed a reversal of that asymmetry in the occipital region.

However, those data simply have not been confirmed and so remain up in the air. The first claim that there was an abnormality in the brain of childhood dyslexics was published in California in 1968 by W. E. Drake, a physician. He reported on a 12-year-old boy with a strong history of dyslexia. He had some kind of intestinal immune disease, asthma, a strong family history of left-handedness, migraine, and he died of a cerebral hemorrhage. Drake described microscopically that underneath the temporal lobe there were large numbers of neurons which were not in their proper locations. Unfortunately, that paper was totally neglected. Even at his own institution the neuropathologists did not believe him.

After Galaburda and I had looked at the cellular architecture in normal humans, we thought it would be very interesting to look at the brain of a child who was dyslexic. It turned out there was a childhood dyslexic who was killed in an automobile accident. He was a 20-year-old man whose brain had been cut in serial sections and kept in Boston for about 10 years.

At the time of death, he had severe difficulties. He read very badly and he had two brothers and a father who were slow readers. He had seizures which were controlled very easily by drug therapy. He was a metalsmith and made superb silver jewelry. He was highly skilled visually and spatially.

When Dr. Galaburda and Dr. Kemper looked at that brain, they had a great surprise. The first thing Dr. Galaburda found was that the planum temporale was about the same size on the two sides. That alone wouldn't be surprising; we find that in about a quarter of the brains we see. However, when he looked microscopically, he found something curious. He had no trouble mapping the areas of particular cellular architecture on the right, but when he tried to map the left he couldn't do it. They were distinctly abnormal in architecture. They had nothing like a normal appearance.

The right hemisphere, not just in the temporal lobe, but everywhere else, was perfectly normal. The only abnormalities were on the left and were most prominent in the language area on the left, at the junction of the temporal and parietal lobes.

In the abnormal brain you may notice that a ball of cells is jutting up. They are clearly out of place. There are lots of other abnormalities which would take much more trouble to describe.

In other abnormal brains the upper temporal region of the cortex will have a pretty normal thickness. Then all of a sudden there is an extra piece of cortex which is out of place.

Lesions of this kind have been well known and certainly it is plain that the patient had seizures and a lot of people said that it is a coincidence that it is in the speech area on the left and in the same location where Pringle Morgan and Hinshelwood and others predicted that these things would be and anyway he's an epileptic and everyone knows that dyslexics don't have seizures. The fact that there were two or three other people in the family that were dyslexic certainly doesn't matter.

We will discuss that point later. At any rate, here was this clear-cut anomaly and, as I said, confined to the left side of the brain.

There are certain features about this case that deserve comment. First of all, the lesions were predominantly on the left side, very marked in the temporal speech region.

I have said that the planum temporale was roughly equal on both sides and that has been true now in all of the dyslexic brains that we have looked at. We have seven brains. We have looked at four all together. They all have similar abnormalities. We have not had a negative case.

If you wanted to figure out, at the one percent level of confidence, how many dyslexics would have to be represented, it is obvious that this must represent the pathology of a large number of dyslexics. We clearly do not say *all* because you can never make that prediction, but you can certainly put some confidence limits on the figures. Clearly, you couldn't be as low as ten percent because this would then be four successive cases and would be too unlikely.

There are a lot of people who say that this microscopic thing is very nice, but you don't need microscopes anymore because since the invention of the CAT scan, the PET scan and so on all you have to do is look at the pictures. But, that's not true.

This abnormality will not show up in a CAT scan. Furthermore, when you do a CAT scan on a brain like this, you find that it "has normal asymmetries" because the left posterior region is wider than the right.

But it is not normal. The left temporal lobe is bigger because it is abnormal. This is a mild condition of what is called megalencephaly, a condition in which you have a huge brain because the neurons migrating up to the cortex have been delayed. So, they are spread out over large distances and fill up all that space with a lot of extra glial tissue and so on. So, this is abnormally enlarged and there would be no way for the CAT scan to distinguish it from the normal one. Only when you look at it microscopically can you begin to see this.

We have some other cases. Incidentally, one of the ways we get these brains is through the help of The Orton Dyslexia Society. We were able to set up a brain bank and we've received brains that have been willed to us. The second case that we got was a 12-year-old boy who was found dead in bed. He was a severe dyslexic and had, I believe, two dyslexic brothers. He also had immune disease in the family. His mother had juvenile rheumatoid arthritis. I am going to return later to his sudden death for which we believe we have an explanation that is related to his being dyslexic. This is the first case we had seen where the abnormality extended into the temporal-parietal region and the speech area. In this case, the abnormalities were bilateral. Of the four cases we have looked at so far, two have been strictly unilateral, two have been bilateral, but they all involved the language region on the left.

Some of you may know about a patient described in *Neurology* some years ago by Landow, Goldstein, and Klefner. This is a case of a boy with severely delayed speech and described as a case with failure of proper development of the medial geniculate body. Dr. Galaburda has been over that paper in great detail and it is clear that in that case of severely delayed speech there is a pathology similar to what we have seen in the dyslexic.

In other words, there are neuronal migration defects. There is also immune disease in the family. Of course, that case was not studied by the standards that we would now employ for such a case, but that is the only other learning disability studied besides dyslexia; we suspect the brain would be rather similar.

What about these cases in life? Sometime after we had seen this second post-mortem case, we had a 35-year-old man who had been a significant childhood dyslexic come into our service. He had done quite well and had gone to law school. He had a first seizure at the age of 35. When he came in, we did a computerized x-ray and found, right in the same region you saw those anomalies, something in the CAT scan that was clearly blood. An arteriogram was done and what he had was an arterial venous malformation sitting right in the cortex of the same region. Now, an arterial venous malformation is like a strawberry mark on the surface of the skin. This was in the cortex and the tissue around it was malformed.

So, we know that this man had a malformation in that same location. Subsequently, my co-worker, Peter Behan in Glasgow, hearing about that case, called me and said that he had seen a 17-year-old dyslexic girl with a ruptured arterial venous malformation and her arterial venous malformation was in the same piece of cortex!

Soon thereafter a paper was published from the Massachusetts General Hospital describing a boy who was said to have become dyslexic because at the age of six he had a left temporal lobectomy. We read that paper and wondered why someone would take out the left temporal lobe of a six-year-old boy. He had an arterial venous malformation in his left temporal lobe as well. In fact, we are convinced that the boy was not dyslexic because they removed his left temporal lobe. We're convinced he would have been dyslexic whether or not they had taken out his left temporal lobe. In other words, this was a boy who obviously had a malformation in the same location.

We have one further piece of information to fit in here. A French neurosurgeon wrote about 17 cases of people who had arterial venous malformation in the primary speech areas on the left, Wernicke's area or Broca's area. Many of you know that it is hardly commonplace in medicine to ask if patients were dyslexics or stutterers or had other problems in childhood. So, we don't have any data on that; however, 13 of those 17 arterial venous malformations in the speech area on the left were in males. There was a four-to-one ratio of male versus female which we think fits in with the notion of male predominance of these conditions and we suspect that most of these cases were dyslexic.

Obviously the question comes up of how we account for this, now that we say this anomaly is there. Let me make a comment about that.

I've had people say to me that this is the worst thing that could have happened to dyslexia—that there are many people who are against dyslexics anyway and if we now say they are brain-damaged it will only reinforce them. My answer is that the reverse is true. Let me offer the following example.

I was having coffee with a professor of pediatric neurology who, after we had been discussing these cases, said that he guessed he was going to have to change his tune. He said that he had always had the private view that dyslexia was a fancy diagnosis invented by the parents of wealthy children to justify their lazy, stupid children. I told him that there is no way that he can hold that view now. In fact, it's pediatric neurology and he had been missing it.

Secondly, many people say that, if this is true, what good does it do to treat these children. The whole history of medicine has shown that discovery of structural basis has not stopped treatment. After all, it was the discovery that the pancreas was responsible for diabetes that lead to the successful treatment of diabetes. I mention that because I think it is very important.

Well, what is the cause of this abnormal brain? The first question is whether or not it can be purely genetic. We have no doubt that there is a genetic component. I want to stress that point; however, I don't think that it is genetic in the sense that Huntington's chorea is, i.e., it has a gene with 100 percent penetrance. I think this is an instance in which there are large effects determined exterior to the genes of the bearers and that is not in conflict with any of the data we heard today at this conference.

However, we got a new clue from another source. In November of 1980, I was involved with a meeting of The Orton Dyslexia Society; Dick Masland had asked me to help him organize a meeting on sex differences in dyslexia.

At that meeting Joan Finucci presented a paper on the genetics of dyslexia and I said that I thought it would be a good idea to look for conditions other than dyslexia in the families of dyslexics. We know that there are many conditions like myasthenia gravis in which we know that you rarely see an effected relative, but yet it is clear that there is something genetic because when you look at the relatives you discover there is another group of diseases that share something in common. Why don't we look at everything in the family of dyslexics.

After that session a lot of people came up to me and asked me if I really meant what I had said—was I really interested in knowing about these other things. I replied that I was, indeed, interested. This is true, by the way—I'm quite serious about this.

The first woman who came to me told me about her family and she had a dramatic family history in which she had many dyslexic relatives and several people who had various forms of immune diseases, either allergies or much more serious immune diseases, such as, ulcerative colitis and myasthenia gravis.

I thought at the time that that was odd but felt that I couldn't take it too seriously because, after all, somebody with a family history like that would tell me about it; however, the rest of the day people kept coming up and I heard the same story again and again and again. I finally said to myself that this was very strange. I have been in medicine long enough to know that when you take histories from patients who say they have a brother with ulcerative colitis and an uncle with Hoshimoto thyroiditis this is not your standard history. These family histories were really exceptional.

The interesting thing is, by the way, when I went to an Orton meeting three years later, the very first person who had come up to speak to me at that meeting in Boston, came up to me again, using a cane. She, in the interim, had developed an immune disease which she had not had at the time that she first spoke to me.

Those data seemed so striking and I began to look around and ask people and all along what struck me was that it was not merely dyslexics and stutterers in whom one was finding this. In fact, I discovered that a former professor of mine was a severe stutterer, was left-handed, and had written about this extensively. I then realized that he had severe rheumatoid arthritis which is an immune disease and that many members of his family had immune diseases also.

So, the first thing I thought was that the immune diseases theory was in relation to the learning disablities and then it struck me that the relationship was a broader one, that it was actually a relationship to left-handedness. It was in families of left handers.

The issue of left-handedness, by the way, is one I can not go into now because it is complicated. If any of you think you know how to measure handedness, I will disagree with you. There is no good test for handedness.

I got hold of Dr. Peter Behan, who is a distinguished neuroimmunologist and a former resident student of mine. I told him that I had a strange proposition for him which would seem odd. I told him that there is more immune disease in left-handers. And Peter, being a semi-manic Irishman, took this without saying anything, although a year later he told me that he had thought I was crazy. But since I was his teacher he figured we would do this study, see if I was wrong and forget about it unless I had really gone round the bend. Indeed, it may have sounded very odd when I proposed this to him. At any rate, we decided to do the study. What we did was to collect large numbers of people in Glasgow. These were not patients. We had medical students administer a questionnaire to this large group of subjects. There were questions about disease, but there was also a handedness battery.

We decided at this point to look only at the extremes. We used only people who scored minus 100 on the handedness battery (these were extreme left-handers) or plus 100 (extreme right-handers). We removed all those in the middle where there was a major amount of noise in the measurement.

In these studies, what we have found so far—and this is only a partial list—is that among non-right-handers, autoimmune diseases are increased, not necessarily all autoimmune diseases, but many, particularly the ones involving the gut (ulcerative colitis, regional ileitis, celiac disease) and the thyroid. Those are the particularly frequent ones. Some of the others we are still studying.

The childhood developmental learning disorders are increased, migraine headaches are increased as in fact are skeletal anomalies and congenital heart disease.

Some of you may say that this is terrible. It must be awful to be left-handed or dyslexic. I want to call to your attention that I see in this room some people who are not nervous about their selective tendency to disease. For example, there is a group of people in this room who will get diseases that I can never get, diseases that could be fatal. I'm referring to the women in the room. I am not going to die in childbirth; I'm not going to get cancer of the ovary. Now, the interesting point, although women have this long list of diseases which only they get or they get overwhelmingly, at every age they have a lower death rate than men.

The point is, I believe the dyslexic group exists because it confers an important advantage to society. We do not have data on this yet. There is only one thing we do know which is that left-handers have lower rates of senile dementia; these are results of a study done by one of my residents. They have higher rates of pre-senile Alzheimer's, but senile dementia is a much more common disease. So, they have at least one advantage and I suspect that there are many others. They just have not been studied yet.

I'm not going to go into these studies in detail, but suffice it to say in the first series we had 253 extreme left-handers, 250 extreme right-handers—we found immune disorders present in 11 percent of our extreme left-handers and in four percent of our extreme right-handers. That probability was less than .005 and furthermore immune disorders were more common in their first degree relatives.

We looked at learning disorders. Now, there is an issue because anybody who reads the literature on handedness in relation to childhood dyslexia would say that everybody knows there are some series that claim there is an increase in left-handedness in childhood dyslexia, but there are other series that say there is none.

Let me give you our data on this. We looked at our 253 extreme left-handers. Ten percent of them had reported dyslexia or stuttering; of our extreme right-handers, less than one percent. In this particular case, it was a twelve-to-one ratio; the p was less than .05 and furthermore learning disorders were markedly elevated in the first degree relatives.

Let me stress that the first degree relatives who have learning disorders or immune disease need not be left-handed. I am not going to go into the reason why the right-handed relatives of left-handers have a higher susceptibility to these things because that would be too much to deal with here.

In the second study we accepted immune disease only if it had been diagnosed in the teaching hospital in Glasgow. Again, although the numbers were smaller, we found two and a half times the rate of right-handers with 900 people in the study. So, between these two series, we are talking about 1,400 people. This is not a small series.

Again, we looked at the rate of learning disorders—nearly eleven percent in the extreme left-handers, 1.2 percent in the extreme right-handers. Since that time, we have run another series with another 1,400 people and we got again the exact same results.

Now, some of you might ask, if that is true, why are there such disagreements in the literature? Why is it said that we have series of dyslexics and do not find any increase in left-handedness? In fact, some people say it with such contempt—the idea that anybody ever dared to say that.

I think I can give you the reasons for that. In the first place, you sometimes see papers in which there are 23 individuals. Consider that the rate of left-handedness, by whatever measure you want to use, might be, let's say, ten percent. That is 2.3 left-handed subjects. There is nothing you could do statistically in that.

The second thing is that people have used all sorts of different criteria for handedness and one of the problems is that there is a huge group in the middle who get called right-handed who are not, those who get misclassified for reasons for which we believe we have data.

In addition, what we have done is to look at a whole group of people with particular diseases. We've looked at those with immune disorders of the gut and people with celiac disease. Thirty percent of them are left-handed, defined by criteria I will not go into now, versus eight percent in the general population and 65 percent of the right-handers have left-handed relatives. So, practically all of them are either personally or familially sinistral. That is the highest ratio, but we have high rates for ulcerative colitis and regional ileitis. We have high rates for asthma and for many other conditions.

Now, we have some further confirmations. A study that was done by Schachter, a member of my department, and myself included sending questionnaires to 1,000 individuals. These people are all professionals and what we found was this. Instead of looking at the extremes, we now looked at the entire distribution of handedness scores from minus 100 to plus 100.

Your chance of being dyslexic runs about nine percent, the same figure we got in our other series. On the continuum from being an extreme left-hander, all the way to being mildly left-handed (performing three out of the ten things on our list with your left hand), the probability of dyslexia remains roughly at nine percent, up to scores of plus 70.

Above plus 70, it drops precipitously to three percent. In other words, anybody who does two or fewer things with the left hand has a three percent chance of being dyslexic. Anybody who does three or more has a nine percent chance. There is a very clear cut-off and, in fact, we did not choose arbitrary cut-off points. We made as many cells as we could in the square. We let the data show us where it was going, the main point being that clearly a very large group would have been called right-handed in most series because people have made arbitrary decisions as to whom to call left-handed—I'm not going to go into that here, but those data make it again very clear that the rate of dyslexia remains high.

In that study, by the way, we also showed—this was something that had been predicted—that blondes have a much higher rate of non-right-handedness and I mean a significantly higher rate. Forty-four percent of 131 blonds scored less than plus 70 as against 24 percent of 986 non-blonds, not a small series, and that p value is very high as well.

I had several reasons for making the prediction, one being that northern Europeans have more immune disease than southern Europeans and all blonds are of northern European descent. If you are blond, there are a whole lot of other diseases that you have got on your list. For example, hairlip and spina bifida are much more common in blonds; the rate of spina bifida in the northern European countries is ten times what it is in China or Japan or the Philippines. There are clear relationships.

The reason the Siamese cat is cross-eyed is that melanin is needed in the system in order to get proper migration of neurons to their final locations and, blondes, like the Siamese cat, are semi-albinos. We think that this is the mechanism. But they have certain advantages—they are not going to get rickets!

Confirmations have come from other sources. Marcel Kinsbourne and Ben Brandon in Boston have been looking at children from the Landmark

School and have studied left-handed dyslexics or those dyslexics who had first degree left-handed relatives and what they have shown is that this group has a much higher rate of immune disease than the right-handed dyslexics without sinistral relatives.

Another study carried out by Larry Ward, who runs the thyroid clinic at the Mass. General, showed that in patients with immune thyroid disease the rate of left-handedness is much higher than it is in patients with nonimmune thyroid disease, which is exactly the same results that Behan and I got.

Another confirmation which is extremely interesting is the one of Benbow and Stanley from Johns Hopkins University. They asked for our questionnaire and they studied mathematically-gifted children and found that in mathematically-precocious children the rate of left-handedness is significantly raised. It is at least double that of kids who get average scores on the SAT. In fact, the best use of the SAT might be to figure out how left-handed the population is.

The rate of allergies in kids who score over 700 on the math SAT is over 50 percent, dramatically elevated compared to control groups. There is again an association of immune disease and left-handedness in that population (also myopia—that I can't explain but we're thinking about it).

I can't present the theory for all of this in detail. I'm just going to tell you part of it very rapidly because there are two further points I want to make.

If you are going to have a theory to account for left-handedness and for learning disabilities, you have to account for the fact that in both of those there is a male predominance. Our study clearly showed that males are more likely to be non-right-handed and overwhelmingly likely to have learning disabilities.

Obviously, that is an interesting issue from a genetic theory. Dr. DeFries pointed out that left-handers cannot possibly be X-linked recessives because fathers don't give X chromosomes to their sons and fathers clearly give their sons left-handedness, stuttering, and dyslexia, or at least they contribute to these disorders.

So, it obviously can't be that. Y-linked chromosomes, Y-linked genes are very unusual, most people agree. If you've got hairy ears, that may work, but there aren't many others that would fit in with that. The other possibility is that there may be genes on other chromosomes which affect the sex chromosomes, but you have got to account for that. In fact, our hypothesis is that male hormone slows the development of the left hemisphere preferentially and, in fact, leads to increased left-handedness.

We think in the cases of extreme slowing you get those lesions mentioned earlier and you get the learning disabilities. This is not pure speculation. There is now positive evidence for this mechanism in rats. In normal male rats who are castrated the right hemisphere cortex is thicker than the left. The rats are castrated at birth so there is no testosterone. They have the female pattern which is that the cortex is thicker on the left. So, we have some direct evidence. Rats have cerebral dominance, by the way, but that's another story.

Where does genetics come in? Well, one thing that is very interesting about chromosome 15, mentioned today by several people, is that obviously we don't know the exact locus on chromosome 15 that would be involved in dyslexia, assuming those data are correct. However, I found the chromosome 15 data fascinating for the reason that chromosome 15 has on it a locus—and there are not loci like this on every chromosome—which is essential to the formation of the testes and the same location is also essential for production of something called beta-2-microglobulin which is a substance necessary for immune reactions. Again, that may not be the locus, but at any rate the immunity, the sex hormone story, the dyslexia, seem to fit in.

The next part of the story was that we said, if humans with learning disabilities have neuronal migration defects in the cortex and they have immune disease, then perhaps we should look at some other conditions. For instance, Down syndrome patients have a high rate of immune disease. They have neuronal migration defects in the cortex. There are many of those diseases—dystrophia myotona is a very common one.

However, we said we would like to have an animal model for dyslexia. Animals can't read; therefore, they're already dyslexics. All we have to do is show that they have neuronal migration defects and we're in!

Nichols and Chen's work on the effect of sex hormones in increasing the rate of attention deficit disorder showed that sex hormones were the most important variable. If the mother took sex hormones, that was more likely to increase the rate of attention deficit disorder in the offspring than any other kind of substance.

We obtained brains of a strain of mouse that gets spontaneous immune disease. We wondered: if they get spontaneous immune disease, are they going to have nice unilateral migration defects—and there it is in the brain of that mouse. That is a neuronal migration effect like I showed you in that dyslexic.

As we were looking at the dyslexics, we also collected some large groups of kids with specific disabilities. For example, we collected a large number of kids with attention deficit disorders in Glasgow, looked at those children again and found very high rates of non-right-handedness in them and their families, high rates of immune disorders, allergies, and so on.

Peter Behan collected 132 families in which there were 183 dyslexic children. When we looked at those families, one of the things that turned up was what we already thought, i.e., that skeletal anomalies were increased in these families, things like scoliosis, as well as herpes, and other diseases. But the thing that intrigued us was (this was not something we expected at first) a very high rate of cardiac anomalies, including some interesting asymmetrical ones such as, transposition of the great vessels.

In fact, what we found was that in these 132 families there were nine children who had major cardiac congenital anomalies. Two of them were dyslexics. In fact, they were identical dyslexic twin sisters, a rather unusual pair, but the other seven were siblings of dyslexics.

As soon as we looked into that, it was obvious that the figure of nine major congenital anomalies was ridiculously high. Peter Behan very quickly realized something interesting about this involving a substance called rho.

A French doctor investigated a woman named Madame Robert and found that she was carrying an antibody against the ribonuclear protein, rho. It was subsequently discovered that antibodies against rho are commonly found in certain immune disorders such as lupus erythematosus, Sjorgran syndrome and a few others.

But this is where the plot thickened. Somebody noticed that women with lupus erythematosus rarely get pregnant, but if they get pregnant the children have a very high rate of congenital anomalies—cardiac congenital anomalies.

Somebody thought that perhaps it was anti-rho that was causing this. A large group of children who had congenital heart block were studied and it was found that nearly all of the mothers of such children were carrying antibody against this rho antigen. Babies with congenital heart block at birth also carry it, but it disappears in three months. That means it is coming from the mother through the placenta—a non-genetic effect, by the way, although obviously there will be a greater tendency for those kids to produce that antibody themselves also.

It seemed pretty clear that this anti-rho antibody was being passed from the mothers to the fetus, damaging the hearts (it is known that the rho antigen is present in very high concentration in the conducting system of the heart).

If this antibody is producing cardiac congenital anomalies and we are now finding these cardiac congenital anomalies at high rates in the families of dyslexic children, the question then is, do the mothers of dyslexic children carry this antibody? So, 45 women (mothers of dyslexics) were studied and the antibody was found in four of them. I want to make clear the magnitude of that. In a series in Leeds, England, they studied 700 normal women, that is, women without immune disease, without a history of congenital anomalies in their offspring. Not one of them carried the antibody. We had 262 control women, one of whom carried it and even one in 262 versus four in 45 is significant at less than a .01 level. But the important point is that even that one woman in 262 turned out to be epileptic and had given birth to children with congenital anomalies. She probably did not even belong in the control group.

There is an interesting thing about the rho antigen. It is present in a high concentration in the heart. It is found in one other tissue at equally high concentrations and that is the brain. We suspect that what may be going on in fact, is that malformations in the brain are also being produced in a certain number of cases.

We do not think that anti-rho antibody alone could account for this. We still have to account for the male predominance because the daughters are not dyslexic just like congenital heart block is more common in males. We think there is a complicated interaction of certain genetic susceptibilities, probably male hormone and anti-rho, which is governing these things.

Obviously, this is a new idea, but I think it raises a very interesting point, not only that there are non-genetic effects. I think it is worth stressing though because that doesn't diminish the importance of the genetic effects, but because it means that now you have got something that you conceivably could control and prevent and that, secondly, you have a mechanism by which you might be able to identify now the beginnings of a mechanism for identifying those people who are at greater risk for having children with these conditions. Thank you. (Question and answer session follows)

QUESTION: Time Magazine and The Orton Society say that we have about 25 million dyslexics in this country, about ten percent of the population, and the problem for the field is that it looks, on the best evidence we have now, that there's a normal distribution of reading ability in the population. So, where you cut this distribution, let's say, and all the guys over here are dyslexics and all of you are normals, is pretty arbitrary.

I wondered what your feeling was about that kind of a problem. One of the things I'm wondering about is that some of the cases you look at, real severe abnormalities, are really very far on the tail end of that distribution, really extreme.

DR. GESCHWIND: Let me say that I would formulate the problem quite differently. I think that one of the things you learn in the history of medicine is that many people think that the way to study a problem is to define the problem and then study it. That turns out again and again to be wrong because you discover the only way to define the problem properly is to know the answer. Since you don't know the answer, you then get a committee together and what the committee does then, in fact, is often to hold up research.

So, you then have the problem of saying, okay, we're studying dyslexia. I agree with you. You have to cut the line somewhere. That's all you can do, by the way. No amount of arguing is going to make the people who are tough necessarily righter than the people who aren't tough because maybe it is a continuum, maybe it isn't.

But what happens again and again in research is that the question comes out of the research. In other words, my argument would be at a certain point, if, let's say, you look at this brain thing and you begin to look at large numbers and you have good data on people. Now, you may have looked at, not the seven brains we have so far, but at 200 and by the time you've looked at 200 you have some good data. You look at this and beside the ones that have abnormality, the interesting thing is that the ones who had normal brains, show certain things that you wouldn't have thought of.

So, my answer to you is you can't say in advance that that's what the problem is going to be. My guess is it will be as though someone had said at a certain point that if you take people's hemoglobin level, you'll find a continuum. Of course, you'll find a continuum, but nobody questions the existence of anemias. There will always be a gray area.

My view is that I don't think that will be the problem but all we can do is wait and see.

QUESTION: What do you think are the forces, possibly physical, that account for the counterclockwise torque of the brain that allows us to talk about, as you did, the differences between left and right hemisphere? Isn't it really a counterclockwise torque? Do you think there are physical forces in utero or what?

DR. GESCHWIND: The issue of what makes asymmetry in the first place is rather fascinating. For instance, I can tell you what makes one claw of a lobster bigger and the answer is that the lobster comes out with two pinchers, both small. If you tie one pincher and give it some oyster shells to crush with the other one, the first one to crush sometimes becomes bigger and the other one is inhibited. There's a neural mechanism for inhibiting the other side. That's a nice mechanism.

Lesley Rogers in Australia has shown that chicks have cerebral dominance. There is beautiful data from Gabriel Horne at Cambridge that two hemispheres quite regularly are doing different things in the chick.

There are many, many mechanisms that are taking place. I think the major one in the human is that there is asymmetry actually in the ovum. That may seem strange to you because how can you have asymmetry in a single cell. In the 1920's somebody took 162 paramecia and showed that 100 of them, when they swim forward, rotate to the right, the other 62 rotate in the other direction. They are single cells.

I think there is asymmetry at a very early stage and that then you get into chemical asymmetries and this is why chemicals are acting differently on the two sides. The chemical asymmetry has already been documented. I think there are lots of asymmetries. I don't think physical forces are playing a big role in humans.

QUESTION: The early characterization of left-handedness in dyslexics was associated quite commonly with spatial disorder, such things as spatial confusion and such anomalies as reversal errors that seem to have been somehow intrinsically related to handedness. If I understand the way you're characterizing the problem, it's perhaps something different.

DR. GESCHWIND: In fact, I think there's another whole story in this. I just don't really have time to go into it. I'll give you only the briefest picture.

You see, one of the interesting issues is there are 25 million dyslexics in the United States. So, dyslexia is not rare. We will all admit that in the United States at least five percent of male school children are dyslexic and it may well be much higher.

COMMENT: It depends on where you cut the curve.

DR. GESCHWIND: No, no, I'm sorry, I don't agree with you on that. When you're saying it depends on where you cut the curve, the number of people who have pernicious anemia is not determined by where you cut the curve. We know these people are different because they have identifiable differences in certain ways.

In other words, the decision is not made by us and I'm trying to argue that when you get further information you then discover that there are differences between the groups that you've missed. It is like cluster headache and migraine—when someone finally separated them it became apparent that cluster headaches are 90 percent male and migraines, 60 percent female.

All I'm saying to you is that I just don't think there is any example in history in which the thing you're suggesting has happened.

QUESTION: Supposing that your autoimmune influences on brain development are also on a continuum.

DR. GESCHWIND: Look, I'm not questioning the possibilities. All I can say at this time is that based on previous experience the way to go is simply to say that no amount of arguing will permit you to make that decision.

There are classic examples of arguments about certain diseases. Von Recklinghausen disease, for instance. Two of the three original cases he described didn't have the disease to which his name is attached. Luckily the third one did, otherwise he'd have his name attached to a disease he never saw. Now, the point is, Von Recklinghausen was a very smart man. How come, when he described three cases of a disease, only one turned out to have it? How could he have been wrong about the majority? But the answer is he had his finger on something, but it was only later, when more was known about calcium metabolism and all sorts of other things that the differentials came out.

My argument is, in other words, that this is the kind of thing that people are doing in the study of dyslexia. Someone may come along and suddenly say, my god, now I see that this fits in. This group that you've been describing really are turning out to be a different group from the others.

We can't make that a priori decision and say that things will come out this way. That's the only point I'm making. For example, look at Michael Rutter's material on identical twins with autism. If one identical twin is autistic, the concordance rate was 36 percent (for non-identical twins the rate is zero) however, of the remaining 64 percent, 54 were either dyslexics or stutterers.

Obviously, that group are not just simply on some continuum. There's clearly a relationship between those conditions and one of the questions is why are these conditions common. You always have to ask the question, "Is there an advantage?" My own belief happens to be that the reason for the high frequency of dyslexia is that those genetic predispositions which lead to the susceptibility of certain environmental influences, in fact, are of net advantage to society.

In other words, I think that the main reason is because there's a mechanism for producing people with high visual-spatial skills and that that mechanism goes wrong in a small number and that is what this whole meeting is about, the small number that goes wrong.

That, by the way, raises an interesting problem because what it means is this: if you have a simple method of preventing the existence of dyslexia, if we just put that into play tomorrow, society might be worse off because we might get rid of five million dyslexics and we might get rid of ten million highly talented people who are superb artists, metalsmiths, engineers and so on. We are dealing with a rather tricky problem here in which there is an advantage and a disadvantage.

QUESTION: So, in effect, you're suggesting that this group of children many have actually high visual-spatial abilities?

DR. GESCHWIND: Oh! I think several people have argued that. Harold Gordon in Pittsburgh has argued that and I think there is a lot of interesting data on the subject.

QUESTION: You referred to the neural migration. Why should it be more often in one hemisphere than the other?

DR. GESCHWIND: I think this is because the two hemispheres are chemically asymmetrical. That may surprise you but we already have evidence for that. For example, two groups of investigators gave an experimental psychodelic agent similar to LSD to subjects in Hungary and Italy. Both investigators found that during the period that the people were psychotic many of them had delusions about their bodies. They were always delusions about the left side of the body being enlarged. Many of them had tremors on the left.

Stanley Glick has shown that in rats, if you give injections of amphetamines, 55 percent of female rats start rotating to the right. That is an excess that go to the right.

By the way, there are almost certainly immune differences. There are certain immune diseases that hit one side of the body over the other. The neuritis you get from horse serum (which is not used very often anymore) affects the right brachial plexus in males.

I think that this kind of selectivity of right and left is no more surprising than would be selectivity of any other structure in the body.

QUESTION: One thing I was kind of puzzling over—in the NZBW mice it's known that the female mice died from autoimmune disease and the males didn't. Does that conflict with this?

DR. GESCHWIND: No, it doesn't, in fact. I'm glad you said that. I meant to include that. Autoimmune disease in humans is in general much more common in females. If we say that testosterone is doing it, then why don't we see a predominance of males with autoimmune disease?

The point is that we have evidence that testosterone delays the development of the thymus and the bursa Fabricius. In fact, MacFarland Burnette, the famous immunologist, used testosterone to destroy the bursa Fabricius. The thymus is definitely slowed.

However, I think the case is this: Males have a higher susceptibility to immune disease. They are protected, however, by the fact that after puberty they begin to produce testosterone and then the effect of it is to reduce immune disease. Now, the evidence in direct favor of that is the fact that in the New Zealand mouse the females get much more autoimmune disease than the males. If the males are castrated, they get the disease as fast as the females. If the females are given testosterone, they slow down.

So, in other words, in utero, you are getting a slowing of development in the thymus which is setting the scale for later immune disease, but after puberty you (males) are being protected and there's a specific thing in favor of this.

That should mean that the highest rate of immune disease should be against males exposed in utero to high testosterone, but then hypergonadal in puberty and that's what happens in Klinefelter syndrome, the XX-Y's. They have very high testosterone in cord bloods at birth, but by the time they are pubertal they are severely hypergonadal.

Most people I know who are working in areas such as lupus say there is a huge increase in autoimmune disease. So, it fits in with this protective effect.

QUESTION: Has anybody collected enough cases in CAH to test this hypothesis?

DR. GESCHWIND: Okay, congenital adrenal hypertrophy is the condition in which the females are more masculinized than the males.

In fact, there is a group at Cornell that is now looking at this congenital adrenal hypertrophy. There are other data, by the way, fitting in with this.

There are data, for instance, on testicular feminization. This is the curious condition of females or XY who come out as pretty girls, grow up and get married and then discover they are sterile and they have testes inside their abdomen. They have a blind uterus and they produced enormous amounts of testosterone. They do not get masculinized at all because they are completely resistant to it.

QUESTION: How about the DES daughters?

DR. GESCHWIND: Oh, the diethylstilbesterol daughters. This is interesting because diethystilbesterol in the rat acts in certain locations of the brains like testosterone. So, it will masculinize certain kinds of behavior at the right critical stage.

We have collected a large number of diethylstilbesterol daughters and given them handedness studies. They have a tremendous increase in left-handedness.

COMMENT: Melissa Hines data on DES daughters show that on all the sort of standard sex difference tests they look like males.

COMMENT: Some people may not know this. The rat masculinizes with estrogen; the primate does not. Estrogen is necessary for masculine behavior in the rat, not in the primate.

DR. GESCHWIND: We do have some data, by the way, from monkeys which show that there are testosterone receptors. Patricia Goldman has shown this in the young monkey's cortex, but not in the rat. That fits in with your points very nicely.

Thank you again

The Biology of Dyslexia: The Unfinished Manuscript

Norman Geschwind

*T*he understanding of childhood dyslexia begins with study in the last century of the losses of reading ability after localized brain lesions. Several such syndromes were described (Benson and Geschwind 1969) but the one most clearly relevant to the problem of childhood dyslexia is the syndrome of pure alexia with agraphia, in which a previously literate person is in effect reduced to the state of illiteracy. The patient cannot comprehend written language nor read aloud yet he has normal visual acuity and can name objects and respond normally to other visual stimuli. Like the illiterate he cannot spell words spoken to him; cannot identify words spelled aloud to him; he cannot identify words formed by block letters he is permitted to palpate. In the first post mortem Déjérine (1891) found a lesion of cortex at the left temporo-parieto-occipital junction (the angular gyrus); a finding confirmed in later studies.

Within a few years of Déjérine's publication Pringle Morgan (1896) and Hinshelwood (1904) described the first cases of congenital word-blindness, later renamed specific reading disability or developmental dyslexia. The suggestion was made that the locus of the impairment would be in essentially the same site as the lesion of alexia with agraphia, i.e., in the left angular gyrus. Orton (1925) in his classic first paper on developmental dyslexia made the same suggestion, although he thought that the defect would be purely functional and that there would be no structural deviation from normal.

The hypothesis that a unilateral structural anomaly might be a cause of at least some cases of dyslexia was criticized on several grounds: a) that there was no reason to expect structural anomaly in dyslexia; b) that it was naive to believe that a developmental disorder would have pathology similar to that of an acquired disorder; c) that since there was good recovery from language disorder after early left lesions there was no reason to expect permanent dyslexia after such a lesion.

In the weeks prior to his death on November 4, 1984, Dr. Geschwind was preparing a manuscript for this book. This is the incomplete draft of that manuscript.

Since we know that a unilateral developmental lesion can lead to developmental dyslexia it is clear that these arguments were not correct. It is worth, however, commenting on why the third criticism is incorrect since a priori it appeared to be reasonable. The reason for the error is that there had been an incorrect extrapolation from the effects of childhood lesions to the effects of prenatal abnormalities. If a language area is damaged in infancy before language develops there is later good if not perfect development of language. If a unilateral lesion produces aphasia in childhood there is good if not perfect recovery. It was, therefore, assumed tacitly that if these "early" lesions did not lead to severe permanent language difficulty then an even earlier unilateral lesion, i.e., in the prenatal period, would have even fewer unfavorable consequences. This extrapolation is not correct. As we shall see later at least in many cases a prenatal unilateral lesion leads to permanent problems. Such a lesion may, however, lead to enhanced development and possibly superior function of other areas, an effect probably not seen after birth.

If there were structural anomalies in dyslexia, where might they be located? I have already noted the suggestion that they might be in the same region as that in which the lesion of alexia with agraphia is found. Another possibility is suggested by the finding that many dyslexics also have some delay in the acquisition of spoken language and some persistent difficulties in spoken language. As is well known lesions of Wernicke's area in the posterior superior temporal region produce a disturbance of all modalities of language. Hence it also appears rational to consider the possibility that this region might be at fault. One might ask why a congenital lesion in this region would lead to so much greater an impairment of written than spoken language. This is an interesting problem that I hope to address at another time but I will not deal with here.

Although the suggestion that there might be a focal unilateral anomaly in childhood dyslexia was made almost a century ago it was not until 1969 that the first description of the brain of a dyslexic appeared (Drake 1969). Drake claimed that there were an excessive number of subcortical neurons particularly in the temporal lobes and a thin posterior corpus callosum. Unfortunately the published material makes it difficult to assess these claims. I suspect that there was developmental abnormality in the cortex on the basis of the fact that there was clear developmental anomaly in the cerebellum, also a late developing structure. Indeed, the cause of death was hemorrhage from an arteriovenous malformation in the cerebellum.

The first definite demonstration of developmental anomaly in dyslexia was described by Galaburda and Kemper (1979). The patient was a 20 year old man still severely dyslexic at the time of death in an accident. The patient was left-handed, a highly skilled metalsmith and had two dyslexic brothers, as well as a mother with rheumatoid arthritis.

In this case, the cortical anomalies were found only on the left. There were *heterotopias*, i.e., groups of nerve cells in anomalous locations, e.g., clusters of nerve cells in layer 1 of the cortex which is normally cell-free, or a large island of infolded cortex in the white matter and fused to the lower layers of cortex. There were in addition dysplasias, anomalies in the organization of the cortex, i.e., abnormal spatial patterns of nerve cells at the microscopic level, or of gyri at the macroscopic level. On the basis of what we know about development of the cortex this anomaly would have to be produced before the seventh month of gestation.

The anomalies in the cortex were most prominent in the upper and posterior portion of the temporal lobe, and its junction with the parietal lobe, i.e., the anomaly was maximal in Wernicke's area and to a smaller extent involved the angular gyrus. Although the cortical anomalies were present only on the left, there were bilateral anomalies in the thalamus.

Since that time Galaburda has studied the brains removed at autopsy from three other dyslexics. Three more brains are in preparation. Of the total of seven brains that have been available to him several have been obtained from the brain bank set up with the help of The Orton Dyslexia Society.

In all three of the additional brains studied anomalies have been found similar to those in the first case, i.e., there have been no negative cases. In these cases there have been bilateral anomalies but in all three cases more marked on the left. In two of the cases there is definite anomaly in the posterior temporal region. This region is not directly involved in the last case but anomalies are present in cortex a short distance away.

One might raise the question as to whether these anomalies are found in normals and if therefore the findings in these cases could only be chance. Although such anomalies are well known (especially as a cause of epilepsy) they are often in regions quite remote from the locations found in the dyslexics. The frequency of these anomalies might be as high as 10%, but even this could not be accepted as the figure in "normals," since the usual definition of normal is a patient who dies without a "neurological" history. Most dyslexics would clearly have been classified as normal. Furthermore even if one accepted 10% as the normal level the probability of finding four consecutive cases by chance is <.0001. Another way of looking at the data is to ask what is the likely frequency of such anomalies in dyslexia. A conservative estimate is that such anomalies will be present in at least 38% of severe male dyslexics. One of the brains yet to be studied is that of a severe female dyslexic which will obviously be very interesting.

There are, in addition, several cases in which studies in life have made it clear that there must be similar developmental structural anomalies in the posterior language region or nearby. One case was that of a childhood dyslexic who in adult life had a first epileptic seizure. He was found to have an arteriovenous malformation (AVM) in the posterior superior temporal gyrus, so that the surrounding cortex must have an anomalous pattern. We know of two other cases in which such a malformation has been found in the temporal lobe. It is interesting that Caron (1982) found that AVM's in the speech areas are more common in males than females.

References

Benson, D. F., and Geschwind, N. 1969. The alexias. *In* P. J. Vinken and G. W. Bruyn (eds.). *Handbook of Clinical Neurology*, Vol 4. Amsterdam: North Holland Pub. Co.

Caron Reference not located.

Dejerine, J. 1891. Sur un cas de cécité verbale avec agraphie, suivi de autopsie. *Mém. Soc. Biol.* 3:197-201.

Drake, W. E. 1968. Clinical and pathological findings in a child with a developmental learning disability. *Journal of Learning Disabilities,* 1:9-25.

Galaburda, A. M., and Kemper, T. L. 1979. Cytoarchitectonic abnormalities in developmental dyslexia: A case study. *Annals of Neurology,* 6:94-100.

Hinshelwood, J., and Macphail, A. 1904. A case of word blindness with right homonymous hemianopsia. *British Medical Journal,* 2:1304-1307.

Morgan, W. P. 1896. A case of congenital word-blindness. *British Medical Journal,* 2:1378.

Orton, S. T. 1925. "Word blindness" in school children. *Archives of Neurology and Psychiatry,* 14:581.

2

Hypotheses, Subtypes, and Individual Differences in Dyslexia: Some Reflections

Paul Satz, Robin Morris, and Jack M. Fletcher

𝒥 n the past decade much research has been devoted to the field of learning
disabilities. Numerous conferences, symposia, books and journal articles
have resulted from these efforts. Despite significant progress in our understanding of these disabilities, considerable controversy (see below) continues to exist
at both theoretical and methodological levels. The controversy is of sufficient
magnitude at this time to retard further progress in the field and to compromise
future extramural funding. It is for this reason that the current chapter is written.

Why the controversy? The controversy, in our opinion, seems to relate in
part to the diverse number of disciplines that have historically investigated the
problem of reading/learning disabilities. The list includes education, reading,
psychology, child development, rehabilitation, pediatrics, neurology, psychiatry, speech and hearing, and most recently, linguistics and neurolinguistics.
Despite its historical roots in education, the field of learning disabilities belongs
to no primary discipline. Researchers from many disciplines have made unique
contributions to the learning process and its disabilities. Unfortunately, each of
these disciplines has its own special orientation in conceptualizing and investigating problems. Because of these theoretical and methodological differences,
each discipline is potentially susceptible to biases that could blind one to
advances in other disciplines. We feel that this has happened with sufficient
frequency in recent years to compromise the cross-fertilization of information
and knowledge that is so desperately needed for an integrated theory of normal
and disordered learning.

The theoretical and methodological consequences of cross-disciplinary
rivalry and its influence on research on learning disabilities were described by
Doehring (1978) and Satz and Fletcher (1980). Of the various issues discussed
in these papers, one stands out as a continued problem impeding progress in our
understanding of learning disabilities, namely the emphasis on *single syndrome*
(Doehring 1978) or *unitary deficit* (Satz and Fletcher 1980) explanations of

reading/learning disabilities. In brief, many investigators hypothesize that learning disabilities result from a single type of deficiency that presumably explains all forms of the disability. Examples of unitary deficit hypotheses include Bryan's (1977) nonverbal communication hypothesis, Hagen's (1972) strategy/deficiency hypothesis of short-term memory, Satz and Van Nostrand's (1973) maturational lag hypothesis, Liberman's linguistic deficit hypothesis (this volume), Vellutino's verbal mediation hypothesis (this volume), Cruickshank's (1972) perceptual deficit hypothesis, Dykman, Ackerman, Clements, and Peter's (1971) motor impulsivity hypothesis, E. R. John's (1977) neurometrics hypothesis and Levinson's (1980) cerebellar-vestibular hypothesis.

Despite the attractiveness and simplicity of these hypotheses, they essentially represent a *unitary* view of learning disabilities that categorizes all disabled learners within a single classification group. In other words, learning problems are homogeneous entities with little intersubject variability. At a descriptive level, these positions are rather straightforward and parsimonious, but at an explanatory level the argument seems less than compelling. In addition to variability across subjects, such theories also fail to deal with the complex cognitive operations and neural substrates that are also known to correlate with, if not underlie, the child's ability to read/learn. By adopting a more molecular and criterion-referenced framework in which to describe the learning process and its disabilities, such an approach excludes the influence of other cognitive and/or information processing variables in the learning process. A salient criticism of these unitary deficit approaches has been voiced by Applebee (1971):

> Research has been successful only in showing that these simplest models do not fit the problem with which we are dealing; and that if we hope in the future to add anything of significance to our understanding of the problems, we must concentrate on new models which correspond more closely to the heterogeneity of the disorder. Such a shift will require more sophisticated methods of analysis than have been employed in the past, and will probably bring with them a whole new set of problems of interpretation and design. Nevertheless, to continue any longer with models which have outlived their usefulness seems as foolish as to abandon any attempts at resolution of the problems whatsoever. (p. 112)

Heterogeneity in Reading Disabilities: Fact or Myth? One of the more insightful reports on this phenomenon was presented recently by Weener (1981). He reviewed all studies reported in the *Journal of Learning Disabilities* and *Psychological Abstracts* between 1973 and 1981 which compared regular classroom ("normal") children with learning disabled (LD) children who were receiving special educational services. Weener found that the variability across all of these studies within the learning-disabled and normal control groups was similar and representative of about 75% of the variance within a randomly selected subject sample on the measures used. Probably more disconcerting was the finding that the average difference between the two groups was less than .75 Standard Deviation, which he described as about 1/6 the range of performance within either group. He also showed that approximately 23% of the LD group scored above the mean of the control groups and a corresponding percentage of control children fell below the mean of the learning-disabled group. As Weener points out, there would have to be a 2.5 SD difference between the means of the groups across all these studies in order for all LD subjects to fall below the mean of the control groups, but more than a 5 SD difference for the two distributions to be non-overlapping. As Weener concludes:

> . . . it is clear that there are many LD children who do not have problems in vigilance, impulsivity, visual-perception, memory, auditory-visual integration, or any of the other specific traits which are often associated with LD children. This can be accurately communicated only if research studies emphasize *within* group variability as well as *between* group differences. The facts are that LD groups represent a wide range of ability on every cognitive process variable and the mean difference between an LD group and normal group is relatively small compared with the range of ability present within each group. (p. 231)

In fact, Weener observed that for almost every cognitive process variable investigated, there were LD children who were performing better than the regular classroom children and there were regular classroom children who were scoring below the average of the LD group. This degree of variability, both within and between diagnostic groups across 47 studies, has some obvious implications about the current state of knowledge about reading and learning disabilities. First, *heterogeneity* is a fact that has to be recognized in any theory or hypothesis that attempts to explain the behavioral performance deficiency or strength of these children. Second, that this heterogeneity may be expressed not only in terms of *etiology*, where multiple putative determinants have already been suggested, including, for example, genotype (DeFries and Decker 1982; Finucci and Childs 1981), environment (Eisenberg, 1966), and lesion substrate (Benson 1976; Galaburda and Kemper 1979), but also in terms of *prognosis* where significant variability in achievement outcome has recently been reported (Bruck 1985; Schonhaut and Satz 1983). Third, that this variability, at least within the reading-disabled population, may reflect the expression of individual differences or the presence of discrete underlying subtypes who differ in terms of etiology, task performance, and/or prognosis.

In the past few years, investigators have increasingly recognized the fact that this variability exists. Some have also suggested that it reflects the presence of relatively homogeneous underlying subtypes. A critical review of this literature can be found in Satz and Morris (1981). Although historically the concept of heterogeneity was noted by some educators and clinicians working with reading disabled children, its importance was conveniently dismissed by the use of exclusionary criteria to define a smaller, and presumably more homogeneous, subset of the reading-disabled population. A classic example is the World Federation definition of specific developmental dyslexia (Waites 1968). This diagnosis, which excludes disabled readers with low intelligence, poor motivation, disadvantaged social status, motor/sensory handicap, brain-injury, or emotional dysfunction, is used to identify children whose reading problems are presumed to be neurological or constitutional in origin. Despite the appeal of this type of definition, it represents a diagnosis by exclusion and the presumption of a neurological or constitutional basis is just that—a presumption (Benton 1975). One could also question the logic behind a diagnostic formulation that attempts to define the condition by what is not (Ross 1976). Rutter (1978) is more to the point. Such a definition ". . . suggests that if all the known causes of reading disability can be ruled out, the unknown (in the form of dyslexia) should be invoked. A counsel of despair indeed" (p. 42). William Yule (1978) is equally critical of the use of exclusionary criteria, especially as it relates to the term MBD:

> . . . I agree with Ingram (1973) when he says that . . . 'Minimal brain damage is not a diagnosis; it is an escape from making one.' It seems to me that MBD is a concept rather like dyslexia—it may have been valuable in drawing attention to a heterogeneous group of developmental disorders, but its continuing usage is probably more harmful than helpful since (a) it assumes a homogeneous symptomatology, and (b) it implies a known aetiology—namely some form of brain damage or dysfunction. Neither of these implications is in line with research findings. (p. 51)

Recent studies have questioned the validity of the preceding assumptions (a, b) as it relates to the concept of developmental dyslexia. The total sample (two cohorts) of severely disabled readers in the Florida Longitudinal Project (Taylor, Satz, and Friel 1979) was divided into two subgroups, one of which met the World Federation definition of developmental dyslexia (Waites 1968). The two groups were then compared on a number of test variables that were not used in the classification of the groups. The results showed that the dyslexic subgroup could not be distinguished from the non-dyslexic poor readers along any of several dimensions including the initial severity and progression of the reading impairment, frequency of reversal errors, familial reading and spelling competencies, math skills, neuro-behavioral performance, or personality functioning. Since these represent most of the dimensions along which dyslexics have been traditionally viewed as distinctive, the results raised serious doubts as to the clinical or research value of this exclusionary diagnosis.

In recent years, investigators have begun to abandon the use of exclusionary criteria in the search for homogeneous subtypes of reading/learning disabled children. Although much of this effort was influenced by pioneering clinical-inferential studies (Kinsbourne and Warrington 1966; Bannatyne 1971; Denckla 1972; 1979; Boder 1973; Mattis, French, and Rapin 1975), recent studies have largely used multivariate statistical methods (Q-technique and cluster analysis) in their attempts to identify homogeneous subtypes of disabled readers. Since the last review by Satz and Morris (1981), a number of new studies have been reported using fairly sophisticated Q-technique and cluster analytic methods on a broad range of cognitive and linguistic variables (see Rourke 1985). Although a critical review of these studies is not called for at this time, the results do warrant a brief commentary as they relate to some of the methodological and theoretical controversies that continue to exist in this field. Our comments will focus on two critical issues in this research: subtype stability and subtype interpretation.

Subtype Stability.   Despite increasing recognition of the heterogeneity in disabled readers/learners, Andrew Ellis (personal communication) has pointed out that:

> . . . sheer repetition does not make any claim any more (or any less) true. The strength of the belief in heterogeneity must carry some weight, but it has to be set against the obvious reluctance of several experienced researchers to adopt the new orthodoxy. Further, it is one thing to assert that dyslexics form a heterogeneous population, and quite another thing to agree on how that heterogeneity should be measured and mapped.

A critical point to remember is that the presence of heterogeneity in a multidimensional data set need not imply the presence of homogeneous underlying subtypes. Subtypes may exist—even stable ones—which may be due to minor, possibly random, deviations from a contiguous spread of points in the psychometric measurement space. Therefore, a major challenge for classification researchers is first to establish that emergent subtypes are replicable (i.e., internally valid). A variety of techniques exist for establishing internal validity, including split-sample cross-validating, replication across statistical algorithms, various data manipulation techniques, and comparison of observed subtypes with Monte Carlo simulations of the data (see Fletcher and Satz 1985; Morris, Blashfield, and Satz 1981). In addition, the heterogeneity of the subtypes, i.e., whether the clusters are compact and well-separated mathematically (Generelli 1963), must be established. This latter issue has rarely been investigated. If subtypes of reading disabled children exist, but are shown to be poorly separated and heterogeneous, then the classification approach, whether clinical or statistical, may merely reflect methodological limitations or the effects of individual differences that are distributed continuously rather than in discrete, well-separated categories. Although a critical discussion of these problems was presented in an earlier review by Morris et al. (1981), the reader is referred to two recent studies that have questioned the existence of homogeneous subtypes of reading-disabled children, i.e., Watson, Goldgar, and Ryschon 1983; Vogler, Baker, Decker, and DeFries, personal communication. The study by Watson and associates (1983) deserves closer attention because it identifies three clusters in a cohort of 65 reading-disabled children that were subsequently found to be stable and reproducible using appropriate clustering and partitioning methods. The clusters revealed a generalized language-disorder subtype, a visual-processing deficit subtype, and a minimal deficit subtype. Of greater concern was the fact that the clusters failed to meet some of the quantitative criteria for compactness and homogeneity that would have increased their utility as clinical subtypes. The study by Volger and associates (personal communication), while identifying two of four subtypes previously described on the same cohort using a clinical classification (Decker and DeFries 1981), also failed to demonstrate the compactness and homogeneity of these clusters using appropriate data manipulation techniques. Although the latter results may in part be due to the use of factor scores as clustering variables—which can inadvertently normalize the distribution (Morris, et al.

1981)—both studies are of sufficient merit to warrant caution in a premature rejection of the Null Hypothesis in the search for reading-disabled subtypes. Regardless of the method used for the assignment of children to a putative subtype (i.e., clinical or statistical), one must not presume that the matter of subtype homogeneity has been demonstrated. Ironically, clinical approaches have largely been spared this level of internal validation. Should one presume, for example, that children identified, using clinically derived approaches, as dysphonetic by Boder (1973), as language disordered by Mattis, French and Rapin (1975), or as 'genetic' dyslexic by Bannatyne (1971) represent relatively homogeneous subtypes? Obviously the answer to this question depends, in part, on the number of variables or cues employed in the classification schemes. If multiple variables are used, then the potential for subtype heterogeneity increases, signaling the need for internal data manipulation techniques that have already been recommended for statistical approaches (Morris et al. 1981). If, on the other hand, one asks whether children assigned to these clinically derived subtypes are homogeneous with respect to the construct they purport to represent (i.e., linguistic or genetic), then one is dealing with issues that involve the interpretation and, ultimately, the validity of the hypothesized subtypes.

Subtype Interpretation. This is the area that has been given the least critical attention in the subtype literature. The reasons for this lack are not hard to understand when one realizes the complex theoretical and methodological problems involved in the interpretation and validation of hypothesized subtypes. The task is not merely to determine whether the subtypes differ on variables external to those used in the clustering procedure (Fletcher and Satz 1985; Skinner 1981), but ultimately to determine whether the subtypes tell us anything useful about etiology: its neural or cognitive substrates, treatment response mode, and/or prognosis, for example. Furthermore, it is essential that the selection of variables used in the validation of the hypothesized subtypes be made on both empirical and theoretical levels. Investigators should have a conceptual framework that guides the formulation and test of the subtypes. At present, we are far from satisfying any of these criteria. However, to abandon these pursuits is nearly as foolish as is the traditional use of exclusionary criteria in the identification of presumably homogeneous etiological subgroups (Waites 1968; Critchley 1970).

The following section reviews briefly some recent developments in subtype research that relate to issues of subtype validation, interpretation, and clinical utility. We hope to show that these developments might help to resolve some of the controversy that continues to exist in the field of reading/learning disabilities.

Unexpected (UNX) Subtype. One of the more interesting, if not puzzling, subtypes that has emerged in many of the recent studies is the "unexpected subtype" (Satz and Morris 1981). This term was used to describe one of the five learning-disabled subtypes derived from the Florida Longitudinal Project at the end of Grade 5 (Satz and Morris 1983). What was especially noteworthy about this group of reading/learning disabled boys (UNX, 14%)

was their relatively higher performance on all of the language and visuo-spatial variables used in the clustering analysis (PPVT, WISC Similarities, Verbal Fluency, Recognition-Discrimination, Beery VMI). In contrast, the remaining subtypes were characterized by different levels and/or patterns of cognitive deficit as follows: (a) a generalized verbal-deficit subtype (GV, 31%), (b) a specific verbal-deficit subtype (SV, 16%); (c) a global-deficit subtype (GD, 12%) and (d) a visuo-perceptual-motor deficit subtype (VPM, 27%).

The fact that the unexpected subtype was not anticipated prompted several analyses to determine whether the subtype was a statistical artifact or whether it identified a subset of children with motivational or emotional problems. Neither hypothesis was supported by several other methodological replications, nor by the results of the Children's Personality Questionnaire (Porter and Cattell 1972). Since that initial report, several other investigators have identified a subset of their reading/learning-disabled children who are relatively free of any cognitive or linguistic deficits (DeFries and Decker 1982; Lyon 1982; Lyon, Stewart, and Freedman 1982). The incidence of this subtype has ranged from a low of 14% (Satz and Morris 1981) to a high of 43% in the Watson et al. study (1983) and 46% in the DeFries and Decker study (1982). Averaging across studies reveals an incidence of approximately 25%.

What might account for this subtype? Although no adequate explanation has yet been advanced, the answer may rest in part on the concept of heterogencity discussed earlier in this chapter. Note that Weener (1981) found significant variability both within LD and normal control groups across studies and considerable overlap between distributions. In fact, the average incidence of the unexpected subtype (approximately 25%) closely matches the frequency of higher performance (overlap) on cognitive tasks in the LD groups reported by Weener (1981). In other words, a subgroup of LD children may exist whose problems in reading and spelling may not be associated with deficiencies in higher-order cognitive or language processes. Hence, there may be no compelling evidence to postulate a cognitive or neural substrate for the learning difficulties of this subset of disabled children. If this formulation is true, including the rejection of a motivational disturbance, then what might explain this apparent dissociation between reading achievement and performance on other non-reading cognitive/linguistic tasks? One clue is the observation that this subset of disabled learners was not as severely impaired in reading and spelling in the Lyon and Watson study (1981). A second and more revealing clue is found in the results of a recent retrospective analysis of subtypes in the Florida Longitudinal Project. Separate cluster analyses, using the same cognitive measures, were computed on the same children when they were in Kindergarten, Grade 2, and Grade 5. In other words, these analyses were computed on the same children at three different age periods (approximately, ages five, eight, and eleven) in order to determine whether the five subtype profiles changed or remained the same during this developmental period. Note that this question requires the use of a longitudinal prospective design which, incidentally, has seldom been used in dyslexia research and virtually never in subtype research. The results were as follows: three of the subtypes remained essentially unchanged (general verbal, global deficit, and visual-perceptual-motor) and two revealed selective, though significant, changes relative to the population of controls and learning-disabled subjects (specific verbal and unexpected). For brevity, only three of the subtypes (VPM, SV, UNX) are presented below in Figure 1.

Although the visual-perceptual-motor subtype remained virtually unchanged from Grades K to 5, the specific verbal and unexpected subtypes changed dramatically during this same interval. The change, however, was characterized by a pattern of increasing improvement in cognitive performance in both subtypes, except for the persistent defect in verbal fluency in the specific verbal subtype. In terms of external validation, it was earlier reported (Satz and Morris 1981) that these two subtypes had a lower incidence of soft neurological signs; they also came from families with higher educational and occupational attainment who had higher reading achievement scores relative to the total population (when adjusted for socioeconomic status).

What clue might be inferred from these results? We suggest that the pattern of increasing improvement in cognitive information processing abilities—especially the dramatic spurt in the unexpected subtype between Grades 2 and 5, coupled with their more advantageous neurological, SES and familial reading status—may represent a genotypic precursor to later recovery in reading and writing at the phenotypic level. In other words, although at eleven

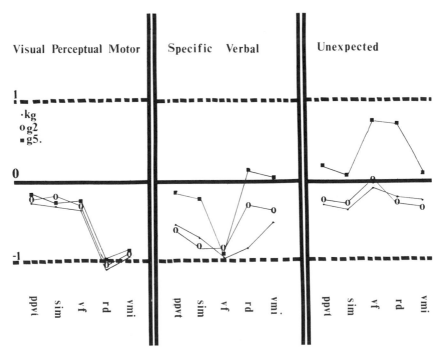

Figure 1. Subtype patterns at kindergarten (kg), second grade (g2), and fifth grade (g5) of children followed longitudinally.

years of age children in the unexpected subtype have clear achievement deficiencies, we hypothesize that changes in cognitive abilities may signal early prognostic signs of improvement in some reading-disabled subjects when tested as adolescents. Unfortunately, no efforts have yet been made to determine whether prognosis can be predicted in some subgroups of reading-disabled children. In fact, the general question of prognosis has seldom been investigated in the review of this literature (Schonhaut and Satz 1983). Although most of these studies revealed unfavorable outcomes in academic skills, including reading deficits that persisted into early adolescence, a few studies have reported favorable outcomes in some individuals (see also chapter by Olsen, this volume). One of the more favorable reports concerns the recent long-term follow-up study by Bruck (1985). She found a subgroup of individuals whose childhood reading problems improved substantially by late adolescence or young adulthood. Most of these individuals were currently enrolled in colleges or universities that placed increasing demands on literacy skills. The author, however, did not attempt to predict which variables might be related to long-term outcome. This is rather unfortunate because the examinations of their *childhood* education and psychological assessments revealed that,

> specific learning difficulties were associated with poor visual processing and/or spatial skills for 45% of the cases, with poor auditory processing and/or language skills for 6% of the cases, and with both poor visual/spatial and poor auditory language skills in 48% of the cases . . . In addition, 75% were experiencing difficulties in the area of mathematics (p. 21).

It would have been interesting to know whether long-term outcome (improvement vs. persistence) was related to any of the preceding subgroups. Also, this rather informal approach to subtyping provides no information on whether a subgroup of disabled learners existed who were free of significant cognitive impairment. Despite these concerns, the Bruck study (1985) provides some evidence that the long-term outcome in reading (at least by late adolescence to young adulthood) may be better for an unspecified subset of learning-disabled children. Based on our results, we hypothesize that this subset probably is composed of those individuals who showed more dramatic rates of change in cognitive development during late childhood or early adolescence. We suggest that the unexpected subtype—and probably the specific verbal-disorder subtype—comprise a number of those children. It is interesting to note that if a more favorable prognosis is eventually demonstrated for children in either of these two subtypes, then one might reintroduce the hypothesis of a maturational lag as a putative mechanism in at least a subset of the learning disordered population. Until confirmed by longitudinal methods, however, this hypothesis should be viewed with appropriate caution.

Visual-Perceptual-Motor Subtype. This is the subtype that has engendered much of the controversy in the literature, especially among proponents who view the reading process and its disabilities within a linguistic framework (see chapters by Liberman, Blank, Olson, Vellutino, this volume). Despite claims to the contrary virtually all of the subtype studies have revealed a subgroup of learning-disabled children who have relatively intact language processing ability but impaired performance on visual-perceptual-motor tasks (Satz and Morris 1981). The incidence of children in this subtype has also ranged from a low of 4–8% (Mattis et al. 1975) to a high of 45% (Lyon and Watson 1981). What is the basis for this subtype? Some investigators have shown that early phases of the acquisition of word recognition skills require visual analysis of graphemic attributes of words, which in turn may be related to visual and spatial abilities (Satz and Fletcher 1980). Lyon et al. (1982) provide the following interpretation:

> The visual perceptual difficulties manifested by youngsters in Subgroup 1 appear to impede their oral reading of single words more than their ability to read orally in context and to comprehend word meanings and the information presented in passages. As Myklebust (1978) has noted, the oral reading deficits observed in this type of LDR could be due to difficulties in attaining consistent meaning from letters and phonetically irregular single words because of deficits in visual discrimination, imagery, and visual-spatial analysis. (p. 358)

The hypothesis that children in this subtype have relatively spared semantic and morpho-syntactic skills might explain their positive and differential response to phonetics training in two recent studies. In the first study (Lyon 1982), a random sample of five learning-disabled children were selected from each of six empirically derived subtypes (e.g., language, global, visual-perceptual, unexpected). The children were then provided one hour of reading instruction per week, in addition to their LD and regular classroom work, for 26 weeks. A synthetic phonic program (Traub and Bloom 1975) was selected because it is well sequenced, provides for systematic skill and introduces phonics concepts. Following training, all Subjects were post-tested with the Peabody Individual Achievement Test (PIAT). Two groups showed significant gain in reading (recognition/comprehension), the unexpected subtype (x = 11.2 months) and the visual-perceptual subtype (x = 7.8 months). It was suggested that the significant auditory memory, auditory comprehension, and sound blending deficits observed in the different language-impaired subtypes may have impeded their response to phonics instruction. This interpretation was recently supported in a study by Aaron, Grantham, and Campbell (1982). The authors compared two different treatment methods of teaching reading (phonics and look-say) to two subgroups of reading-disabled children (dysphonetic and dyseidetic) classified by Boder's method (1973). Although sample size was small in each group, the results revealed a treatment method by subtype interaction. Briefly, the dyseidetic children benefited more from the phonics method (analytic-sequential), while the dysphonetic children benefited more from the look-say method (gestalt-holistic). These results, although in need of replication, suggest that reading-disabled children are likely to improve when taught by methods that utilize their strengths rather than those that attempt to strengthen their weaknesses. Lyon (1985) presents data to support this hypothesis, and provides additional evidence for subtypes by teaching method interactions.

The preceding results provide some preliminary external validation for the utility of the visual-perceptual subtype in terms of treatment response, but they do not tell us much concerning etiology or subtype interpretation. A possible clue to interpretation is the association between impaired visual-spatial processing and mathematics as suggested by Bruck's (1985) description of her subjects during childhood. The fact that 75% of her children were deficient in math, 45% were deficient in visual-spatial processing, and 48% were deficient in visual-spatial processing and auditory language, strongly buttresses this putative relationship. In fact, Rourke (1975) had earlier suggested that children who exhibited outstandingly poor arithmetic performance and adequate reading and spelling performances would be relatively deficient in visual-perceptual and visual-spatial abilities. Although the Bruck study (1985) did not permit determination of the relative status of reading, spelling, and math in her subjects, some recent studies have shown that these achievement patterns, which vary markedly in learning-disabled samples, may be used to classify subgroups who differ in terms of cognitive information processing ability (Rourke and Finlayson 1978; Rourke and Strang 1978; Fletcher 1985). Each of these studies has shown that a subgroup of learning-disabled children exists whose primary deficiency is in arithmetic achievement. This arithmetic subgroup, when compared to children with primary deficiencies in reading and spelling, has revealed consistent deficits on visual-spatial tasks and contrasting strengths on verbal-cognitive tasks. In the Fletcher study (1985), four subgroups of learning-disabled children were identified using patterns of Wide Range Achievement Test (WRAT) Scores as recommended by Rourke et al. (1978): (1) Reading-Spelling Disabled (R-S); (2) Reading-Spelling Arithmetic Disabled (R-S-A); (3) Spelling-Arithmetic Disabled (S-A); and Arithmetic Disabled (A). Two analogous memory tasks were employed, one verbal (animal names) and one non-verbal (random dot patterns) using selective reminding procedures that permit separation of storage and retrieval aspects of memory. Results revealed that, relative to controls, the A and S-A children had significantly lower storage and retrieval scores on the nonverbal task, but did not differ on the verbal task; the R-S children differed only on retrieval scores from the verbal task, and the R-S-A children on retrieval scores on the verbal task and storage and retrieval scores on the nonverbal task.

The preceding results are rather instructive. They suggest that in an unselected cohort of learning-disabled children, different patterns of achievement may exist which in turn may correlate with different types of cognitive information processing ability. If true, these findings have major implications for some of the research controversy in reading and learning disabilities. One implication involves the method of subject ascertainment. If only a measure of spelling or word recognition is used in the selection process, one cannot be certain about the status of other relevant achievement skills such as reading comprehension or mathematics, each of which may have different cognition correlates or substrates. As such, the selected sample of disabled readers may be quite heterogeneous both in terms of achievement and performance skill, regardless of the dependent variable under study. The only way to reduce much of the heterogeneity would be to include only those children in the study sample who demonstrated a specific type of achievement defect (e.g., word recognition, spelling, or arithmetic). Unfortunately, few investigators utilize or report this method of selection on the criterion variable. Rarely do studies of disabled readers report arithmetic scores. In fact, we are often led to believe that children with reading difficulties do not have arithmetic problems. Of the 236 children to whom the WRAT was administered at the end of Grade 5 in the Florida Longitudinal Project, only one child met the criteria for the Reading-Spelling disabled group; 20 children had poor arithmetic and average reading, while 62 children met the criteria for the reading-, spelling-, and arithmetic-impaired group. Other laboratories (Rourke and Siegel, personal communications) report similar findings, even when other measures of achievement are used.

An illustrative example of this problem was observed in the initial cluster analytic search for subgroups in the Florida Longitudinal Project (Satz and Morris 1981). This was accomplished by means of a cluster analysis of the WRAT Subtests (Word Recognition, Spelling, Arithmetic) on all of the boys who continued to reside in Alachua County at the end of Grade 5 (six years later). The sample included children (N = 236) at all levels of achievement. This approach represented the first attempt to use cluster analysis to identify the learning-disability subgroup(s) and comparison subgroups prior to the search for subtypes. Nine relatively homogeneous subgroups emerged with different patterns of reading, spelling, and arithmetic skill. Six of these subgroups had at least average to superior achievement levels on the WRAT, while three subgroups had impaired achievement. The three LD subgroups showed patterns similar to those described by Rourke and Finlayson (1978), Rourke and Strang (1978) and Fletcher (1985): one subgroup demonstrated specific problems in arithmetic, and two showed generally depressed performance on all three WRAT subtests.

It should be noted that these same subgroups were recently observed in a cross-cultured replication using the same instrument (WRAT) on a similar sample (N = 236) of eleven year old boys from normal and special schools in Holland (Van der Vlugt and Satz 1985). The results, while lending credence to some of the different patterns of achievement reported by Rourke et al. (1978) and Fletcher (1985) for learning-disabled samples, also buttress the variability and overlap reported by Weener (1981) in his insightful review of studies on learning-disabled and "normal" control children. The arithmetic-disability subtype is particularly instructive in this regard. An unspecified subset of the learning-disabled population exists whose primary deficiency is in arithmetic; however, if only a word recognition measure is used in subject selection, an unknown proportion of both disabled readers (probably a majority) and "normal" controls may have an arithmetic disability and—more importantly—a selective impairment in visuo-spatial ability. This is precisely what was observed in a recent study of the internal and external validation of the Florida subtypes (Satz and Morris 1983). Subjects in the arithmetic disability subgroups were added to the other two LD subgroups which constituted the cohort from which the five subtypes described on page 31 were obtained. A cluster analysis was then computed. Interestingly, the same five subtypes emerged with no additional clusters. What happened to children in the arithmetic-disability subgroup? They divided into two subtypes with the majority (50%) falling in the visual-perceptual-motor subtype, and a minority (33%) falling in the unexpected subtype. None of these children fell within the language-disorder subtypes. This internal data manipulation procedure not only lends support to the stability of the original clustering solution, but also provides further support for the role of visual-spatial processing in arithmetic disability.

Summary

Some summary comments are in order. As long as investigators choose to ignore these findings, heterogeneity will continue to exist in both learning-disabled and "normal" control groups. Moreover, where results lead to rejection of the Null Hypothesis, one cannot by any means reject the presence of individual differences or underlying subtypes in the data set. Weener (1981) has already made this point. The between-group difference, which traditionally constitutes the evidence in support of one's special hypothesis, most often a unitary deficit formulation, may account for only a small, though significant, amount of the variance between groups. However, substantial variability may still exist within groups, which if not addressed, may produce premature, if not misleading, claims about the putative cause of reading or learning disabilities. It is unlikely that any unitary deficit hypothesis, whether in faulty phonetic or orthographic coding, short-term memory, symbolization, visual-spatial processing, eye movements, evoked potentials, or neuroanatomical substrate, will account for the majority of these children who fall in reading and writing. To think otherwise is reminiscent of Samuel Pepys' reflections on accomplishments: "Indeed it is good, but wronged by one's overgreat expectations."

It is hoped that the concerns and findings presented in this chapter will lessen the intense inter- and intra-disciplinary rivalry that has prevailed in the field of reading and learning disabilities. We have tried to account for some of this controversy but do not expect that the issues will be resolved in the near future. The field is quite diverse from a disciplinary standpoint—as it should be—with each discipline bringing its own unique methods and theories to bear on the problem of the learning process and its disabilities. While much of the current controversy springs from this diversity, progress will depend ultimately on the resolution of the classification issues (Morris and Satz 1984). Doehring (1978) and Satz and Fletcher (1980) described the methodological problems underlying the continued emphasis on a unitary deficit hypotheses of learning disabilities. These concerns have been repeatedly echoed (Applebee 1971; Rourke 1985). In this chapter we have tried to provide additional theoretical rationale, along with empirical data, for a multivariate and multidisciplinary approach to research on learning disabilities. In fact, the available evidence, while not providing an adequate typology of learning disabilities, clearly shows that LD children (and their so-called controls) are heterogeneous. This heterogeneity implies that subject selection methods—not hypotheses or differences on various dependent variables—may explain in part the contrasting results across studies. The classification issues will not be resolved in the near future. In fact, it may be necessary to develop different classifications for different research problems (e.g., etiology versus treatment). Increased collaboration across disciplines and tolerance of alternative theoretical viewpoints would represent a major step in our understanding of disabled learners. No one homogeneous orientation can account for the heterogeneity of these data.

References

Aaron, P. G., Grantham, S. L., and Campbell, N. 1982. Differential treatment of reading disability of diverse etiologies. *In* R. N. Malatesha and P. G. Aaron (eds.). *Reading Disorders: Varieties and Treatments*. New York: Academic Press.

Applebee, A. N. 1971. Research in reading retardation: Two critical problems. *Journal of Child Psychology and Psychiatry*, 12:91–113.

Bannatyne, A. *Language, Reading and Learning Disabilities*. 1971. Springfield, IL: Charles C Thomas.

Benson, D. F. Alexia. 1976. *In* J. T. Guthrie (ed.). *Aspects of Reading Acquisition*. Baltimore: Johns Hopkins Press.

Benton, A. L. 1975. Development dyslexia: Neurological aspects. *In* W. J. Friedlander (ed.). *Advances in Neurology* 7:1–47. New York: Raven Press.

Boder, E. 1973. Developmental dyslexia: A diagnostic approach based on three atypical reading patterns. *Developmental Medicine and Child Neurology* 15:663–387.

Bryan, H. 1977. Learning disabled children's comprehension of non-verbal communication. *Journal of Learning Disabilities* 10(8):501–506.

Bruck, M. The adult functioning of children with specific learning disabilities: A follow-up study. *In* L. Siegel (ed.). *Advances in Applied Developmental Psychology*. NY: Oxford University Press. in press (1985).

Critchley, M. 1970. *The Dyslexic Child*. Springfield, IL: Charles C Thomas.

Cruickshank, W. M. 1972. Some issues facing the field of learning disability. *Journal of Learning Disabilities* 5:380–383.

Decker, S. N., and DeFries, J. C. 1981. Cognitive ability profiles in families of reading disabled children. *Developmental Medicine and Child Neurology* 23:217–227.

DeFries, J., and Decker, S. 1982. Genetic Aspects of Reading Disability: Family Study. *In* R. N. Malatesha and P. G. Aaron. (eds.). *Reading Disorders: Varieties and Treatments*. New York: Academic Press.

Denckla, M. B. 1972. Clinical syndromes in learning disabilities: The case for ''splitting'' vs. ''lumping''. *Journal of Learning Disabilities* 5:401–406.

Denckla, M. B. 1979. Childhood learning disabilities. *In* K. Heliman and E. Valenstein (eds.). *Clinical Neuropsychology*. New York: Oxford University Press.

Doehring, D. G. 1978. The tangled web of behavioral research on developmental dyslexia. *In* A. L. Benton and D. Pearl (eds.). *Dyslexia: An Appraisal of Current Knowledge*. New York: Oxford University Press.

Dykman, R. A., Ackerman, P. T., Clements, S. D., and Peters, J. E. 1971. Specific learning disabilities: An attentional deficit syndrome. *In* H. R. Myklebust (ed.). *Progress in Learning Disabilities, Vol. II*. New York: Grune and Stratton.

Eisenberg, L. 1966. The epidemiology of reading retardation and a program for preventive intervention. *In* J. Money (ed.). *The Disabled Reader: Education of the Dyslexic Child*. Baltimore: Johns Hopkins Press.

Finucci, J., and Childs, B. 1981. Are there really more dyslexic boys than girls? *In* A. Ansara, N. Geschwind, A. Galaburda, M. Albert, and N. Gartrell (eds.). *Sex Differences in Dyslexia*, Baltimore: The Orton Dyslexia Society.

Fletcher, J. 1985. External validation of learning disability typologies. *In* B. P. Rourke (ed.), *Learning Disabilities: Advances in Subtypal Analysis*. New York: Guilford Press.

Fletcher, J., and Satz, P. 1985. Cluster analysis and the search for learning disability subtypes. *In* B. P. Rourke (ed.). *Learning Disabilities: Advances in Subtypal Analysis.* New York: Guilford Press.

Galaburda, A. M., and Kemper, T. L. 1979. Cytoarchitectonic abnormalities in developmental dyslexia: A case study. *Annals of Neurology* 6:94–100.

Generelli, J. A. 1963. A method for detecting subgroups in a population and specifying their membership. *Journal of Psychology* 55(2):457–468.

Hagen, J. W. 1972. Some thoughts on how children learn to remember. *Human Development* 14(4):262–271.

John, E. R. 1977. Neurometrics: Numerical taxonomy identifies different profiles of brain function within groups of behaviorally similar people. *Science* 196:1393–1410.

Kinsbourne, M., and Warrington, E. K. 1966. Developmental factors in reading and writing backwardness. *In* J. Money (ed.). *The Disabled Reader: Education of the Dyslexic Child.* Baltimore: Johns Hopkins Press.

Lyon, R. 1982. Subgroups of LD readers: Clinical and empirical indentification. *In* H. R. Myklebust (ed.). *Progress in Learning Disabilities, Vol. 5.* New York: Grune and Stratton.

Lyon, R. 1985. Educational validation studies of learning disability subtypes. *In* B. P. Rourke (ed.). *Neuropsychology of Learning Disabilities: Essentials of Subtype Analysis.* New York: Guilford Press.

Lyon, R., Stewart, N., and Freedman, D. 1982. Neuropsychological characteristics of empirically derived subgroups of learning disabled readers. *Journal of Clinical Neuropsychology* 7: 343–366.

Lyon, R., and Watson, B. 1981. Empirically derived subgroups of learning disabled readers: Diagnostic considerations. *Journal of Learning Disabilities* 14:256–261.

Mattis, S., French, J. H., and Rapin, I. 1975. Dyslexia in children and adults. Three independent neuropsychological syndromes. *Developmental Medicine and Child Neurology* 17:150–163.

Morris, R., Blashfield, R., and Satz, P. 1981. Neuropsychology and cluster analysis: Potentials and problems. *Journal of Clinical Neuropsychology* 3:79–99.

Morris, R., and Satz, P. 1984. Classification issues in subtype research: An application of some methods and concepts. *In* R. N. Malatesha and H. A. Whitaker (eds.). *Dyslexia: A Global Issue,* Holland: Martinum Mijhoff Publishers.

Porter, R. D., and Catell, R. B. 1972. *Handbook for the Children's Personality Questionnaire (the CPQ).* Champaign, IL: Institute for Personality and Ability Testing.

Ross, A. O. 1976. *Psychological Aspects of Learning Disabilities and Reading Disorders.* New York: McGraw-Hill.

Rourke, B. P. 1975. Brain-behavior relationships in children with learning disabilities. A research program. *American Psychologist* 30:911–920.

Rourke, B. P. 1985. *Learning Disabilities in Children: Advances in Subtypal Analysis,* New York: Guilford Press.

Rourke, B. P., and Finlayson, M. A. J. 1978. Neuropsychological significance of variations in patterns of academic performances, verbal and visual-spatial abilities. *Journal of Abnormal Child Psychology* 6:121–133.

Rourke, B. P., and Strang, J. D. 1978. Neuropsychological significance of variations in patterns of academic performances: Motor psychomotor, and tactile-perceptual abilities. *Journal of Pediatric Psychology* 3:62–66.

Rutter, M. 1978. Prevalence and types of dyslexia. *In* A. L. Benton and D. Pearl (eds.). Dyslexia: *An Appraisal of Current Knowledge,* New York, Oxford University Press.

Satz, P., and Fletcher, J. M. 1980. Minimal brain dysfunctions, an appraisal of research, concepts and methods. *In* H. Rie and E. Rie (eds.). *Handbook of Minimal Brain Dysfunction.* New York: Wiley Interscience.

Satz, P., and Morris, R. 1981. Learning disability subtypes: A review. *In* F. S. Pirozzolo and M. A. Wittrock (eds.). *Neuropsychological and Cognitive Processes in Reading.* New York: Academic Press.

Satz, P., and Morris, R. 1983. The search for subtype classification in learning disabled children. *In* R. E. Tarter (ed.). *The Child at Psychiatric Risk.* New York: Oxford University Press.

Satz, P., and Van Nostrand, G. K. 1973. Developmental dyslexia: An evaluation of a theory. *In* P. Satz and J. Ross (eds.). *The Disabled Learner: Early Detection and Intervention.* Rotterdam: Rotterdam University Press.

Schonhaut, S., and Satz, P. 1983. Prognosis for children with learning disabilities: A review of follow-up studies. *In* M. Rutter (ed.). *Developmental Neuropsychiatry.* New York: Guilford Press.

Skinner, H. A. 1981. Toward the integration of classification theory and methods. *Journal of Abnormal Psychology* 90(1):68–87.

Taylor, H. G., Satz, P., and Friel, J. 1979. Developmental dyslexia in relation to other childhood reading disorders: Significance and utility. *Reading Research Quarterly* 15:84–101.

Traub, N., and Bloom, G. 1975. *A Recipe for Reading*. Cambridge: Educator's Publishing Service.

Van der Vlugt, H., and Satz, P. 1985. Reading disability subtypes: A cross-cultural validation. *In* B. P. Rourke (ed.). *Learning Disabilities in Children: Advances in Subtypical Analysis*. New York: Guilford Press.

Waites, L. 1968. World federation of neurology: Research group on developmental dyslexia and world illiteracy. *Report of Proceedings 22*. Washington, D.C.

Watson, B. U., Goldgar, D. E., and Ryschon, K. L. 1983. Subtypes of reading disabilities. *Journal of Clinical Neuropsychology* 5(4):377–399.

Weener, P. 1981. On comparing learning disabled and regular classroom children. *Journal of Learning Disabilities* 14:227–232.

Yule, W. 1978. Diagnosis: Developmental psychological assessment. *In* A. F. Kalverboer, H. M. Van Praag, and J. Mendlewicz (eds.). *Advances in Biological Psychiatry: Vol. 1 Minimal Brain Dysfunction: Fact or Fiction?* Basel: S. Karger.

3

Issues of Overlap and Heterogeneity in Dyslexia

Martha Bridge Denckla

*H*istorically, the term learning disability has been used to describe individuals who have a significant discrepancy between measured intelligence that is normal or superior and academic achievement that is lower than expected for that IQ. The exclusion of social-cultural, psychoemotional and neurological etiologies for the underachievement of apparently normal children has been an important second step in clarifying a diagnosis of learning disability. Recently, however, the exclusion of subtle neurological factors has become less clear for a type of learning disability, i.e., dyslexia or specific reading disability. The importance of distinguishing between individuals who are dyslexic with additional neurologic involvement and those without such involvements has resulted in several scientific investigations that focus on the etiology or etiologies of reading disability. Replacing earlier assurances about "an intact nervous system," modifiers such as "gross," "obvious," or "classical" have appeared before the term "neurological" in the exclusionary list qualifying subjects as fit for a study of dyslexia (Rudel 1980; Wilsher, Atkins, and Manfield 1985). Even within those populations of "pure" dyslexics, scientists have discovered left-hemisphere-based neurological deficits which, although subtle, cannot be dismissed (Denckla, Rudel, and Broman 1981; Rudel 1980; Wilsher et al. 1985). Much of the current research in the field of reading disability is directed toward reducing the heterogeneity of the samples of reading disabled children being studied. This chapter describes the use of neuropsychological tests, psychopharmacological probes, and electrophysiological measures to characterize children who have great difficulty in learning to read as demonstrably different from those children who exhibit attentional problems in addition to their reading disabilities.

Dyslexia and Attention Deficit Disorder

Psychological Measures

An official diagnosis of "Attention Deficit Disorder" (ADD) among the developmental disorders (DSM III 1980) resulted in increased scrutiny of the

41

behavioral and neurological overlap between reading and attention deficits. Wechsler, himself, noted that some subtests of the WISC such as Digit Span, seem to test an ability of which a certain absolute basal or minimum endowment is relevant to academic success (Rudel 1980).

One of the earliest studies on the attention component of reading disability was that of Symmes and Rapoport in 1972. They selected a group of unexpectedly dyslexic boys, that is, with no predictors of reading difficulty; and found only three WISC IQ subtest scaled scores low—the "attentional triad" of Digit Span, Arithmetic and Coding. Both they and subsequent authors have been left with the dilemma: is it attention deficit or sequencing dysfunction that lowers this triad of subtest scaled scores? Other research since 1972 has examined verbal list learning abilities of reading disabled children. The general findings are that the metalinguistic or metamnemonic deficits are in the domains of "selective attending" or "intentional coding." These direct learning studies suggest an impairment of the ability to attend or concentrate mental effort at the highest level. This deficiency may be as prevalent among the reading-disabled as are their distinctive core linguistic impairments (Denckla 1977; Rudel 1980; Denckla et al. 1981). In sum, these studies have led many clinicians to use the double diagnosis of learning disability (LD) and ADD for some children with reading disabilities.

Psychopharmacological Probes

The use of psychopharmacologically active drugs to treat children diagnosed as having attention deficit disorder (ADD) has provided another approach to studying the relationships between reading disability and attention deficits. Several central nervous systems (CNS) stimulants (d-amphetamine sulfate and methylphenidate) have been shown to improve cognitive performance involving attentional components. For children whose performance is both learning disabled and hyperactive (with attention deficits) CNS stimulants are known to alter the hyperactive component but not the academic performance (i.e., reading scores). The value of bringing about attention-promoting effects of stimulants has been questioned when there is no commensurate reading gain. Piracetam, a putative "left hemisphere drug," was shown to have significant effects upon verbal learning in normal volunteers and a variety of patient populations. These results have inspired research studies of Piracetam in dyslexic boys, ages 8–14 years (Wilsher et al. 1985). The intent of the study was to address the differential effect of Piracetam on "left-hemisphere skills" as distinct from the attention/concentration dimension. However, there is no published record of an attempt to exclude ADD-positive dyslexic subjects or, if overlap exists, to analyze data by subgroups (Wilscher et al. 1985). Thus, the negative findings from this study are suspect and need to be confirmed for samples of children screened for ADD.

Rudel, participating in a similarly-designed multicenter trial of Piracetam, initiated a comparison of two groups of children with reading problems to test the specificity of Piracetam's effects on reading disabled children with or without attentional difficulties. Her New York dyslexia sample consisted of individuals diagnosed as reading disabled who had not been screened for ADD. The heterogeneity of behavioral and possibly etiological subtypes of reading disability in this sample, the "mixed" ADD and dyslexia group, was probably quite high. The second sample of reading disabled individuals had been screened previously for ADD by means of the Conners Rating Scales and clinical observations (Denckla, Rudel, Chapman, and Krieger 1985). Thus, this group of "pure" dyslexics was clearly more homogeneous with regard to reading disability than the "mixed" ADD and dyslexia group. Since previous research has established that motoric developmental anomalies are powerful discriminators between normal-reading ADD boys and controls (Denckla and Rudel 1978), developmental motor status was used to compare the "mixed" dyslexia group with the "pure" dyslexia group. It did turn out, as hypothesized, that motor developmental status was quantitatively (speed of movement) and qualitatively (overflow, rhythmicity) more suspect in the "mixed" ADD and dyslexia group than in the "pure" dyslexia group. This, in turn, has a practical bearing upon what conclusions can be drawn from the negative results, i.e., lack of significant benefit, with respect to Piracetam treatment of an "unpurified" dyslexic sample (Denckla et al. 1985).

Electrophysiological Measures

Even when great rigor is exercised in "purifying" a dyslexic sample, physiological measures hint at an attentional component to the problems of reading. Previous research using the regional cerebral blood flow method has suggested that the frontal supplementary motor areas are bilaterally activated during speech and reading. The preliminary findings of the BEAM studies (Duffy, Denckla, Bartels, and Sandini 1980) suggest that these areas of activation are the correlates of a higher order selective attention or intention mechanism which are inefficiently operating in dyslexics (Duffy et al. 1980). The unearthing in the "pure" dyslexic group of a frontal patch of under-activation surprised even the researchers.

Work in progress at the National Institutes of Health (involving Drs. Currie and Goldberg of the National Eye Institute, Dr. Rumsey of the National Institute of Mental Health, and Dr. Denckla of the National Institute of Neurological Communicative Disease and Stroke) is adding further physiological evidence of the overlap of attentional phenomena with the dyslexia puzzle. Behaviorally unimpaired, non-hyperactive, self-referred adults with mild dyslexia, mainly of the very slow/inefficient, or "rate-disabled" variety (Lovett 1984) have been shown to suffer from saccadic intrusions in their oculomotor scanning of text as measured by infrared oculography. Preliminary results from this study indicate that these dyslexics respond positively to methylphenidate. Literature suggests that saccadic intrusions are sensitive indicators of high-level selective attention (Lipton, Levy, Holzman, and Levin 1983). Thus we are, at present, left with a complex interrelationship between attentional and reading skills/deficits, an overlap that appears to be taking on increasing importance for future research into dyslexia.

Heterogeneity within "Pure" Dyslexia Samples

The physiological studies measuring brain electrical activity and saccadic eye movements in carefully screened dyslexic persons, i.e., those who would not be diagnosed by DSM III standards as "ADD-positive," raises the issue (beyond overlap) of heterogeneity *within* dyslexic populations.

Furthermore, these findings suggest that past approaches to subgrouping have not gone far enough (Denckla 1977; Rudel 1980). It is of interest, from an historical perspective, to reflect that in past debates about subgroups of dyslexic persons the major focus has been on evidence in support or in refutation of a visual-perceptual (or visual-spatial) subgroup (Vellutino 1977; Rudel 1980). As the general consensus of research has swung toward the language disorder concept of dyslexia, psycholinguistic analyses have claimed the major share of subgrouping approaches. The evidence suggesting that attentional deficit, while perhaps too subtle and selective to be at or above the threshold for an "ADD" diagnosis, contributes to some dyslexia, also suggests that some cases, perhaps milder, e.g., purely rate-disabled (Lovett 1984), may be treated with attention-promoting psychopharmacologic therapeutic agents. Other dyslexic persons may have a combination of attentional and linguistic information-processing problems, each implying a separate therapeutic attack.

Delineating a variety of dyslexia subtypes is important not only for treatment but for recognizing natural history, estimating prognosis, and performing genetic analysis. A word of caution, however, is necessary when dealing with heterogeneity in the context of genetic research: it is advisable to maintain an open mind with respect to the possible occurrence of a spectrum of phenotypically similar subtypes with the same underlying genetic mechanism (Geschwind 1984).

Research on dyslexia subgrouping by means of brain electrical activity mapping (BEAM) is still in the process of data analysis. Preliminary results, however, involving brain maps of forty-four "dyslexia-pure" boys, are consistent in discriminating previous subgroupings based upon language disorder concepts (Denckla 1977). There are regions of activity in dyslexics that are different from normal controls; in addition, regions of activity differ among the three dyslexic subgroups. These brain maps suggest a surprising number of right-sided regions distinguishing the dysphonemic sequencing subgroup from normal controls. Bilateral frontal regions of difference characterize all the dyslexic subgroups compared to controls. The globally language-disordered subgroups differed most markedly from all the others, both in the number of brain regions and the magnitude of these regional effects, while the dysphonemic-sequencing-disordered subgroup, was closest to normal controls. The anomic dyslexic subgroup appeared to be intermediate in the extent and magnitude of regional deviations (Duffy, Denckla, Holmes, Bartels, and McAnulty 1985).

The biological interpretation of these significance probability maps must be approached with caution. The existence of a difference does not indicate which group is more or less normal, i.e., it does not localize or even imply processing deficit, much less a "lesion" in the usual neurodiagnostic sense. For example, the regions on the right side of the brain wherein electrical activity differs most between the dysphonemic-sequencing dyslexic subgroup and the normal controls may be utilized by these particular dyslexics during the phonemic discrimination evoked response condition, or during the reading recognition condition, because of *superiority* of such regions on the right in the dyslexic subgroup. The absence of the left temporal auditory association (or speech-processing) regions from the significance probability maps marking inter-subgroup or total dyslexic/control differences may simply mean that anybody and everybody is activated in this region to the same degree regardless of how normal or abnormal this crucial region may be. The most interesting outcomes of the BEAM data analysis thus far are 1) the bilateral distribution of regions of interest distinguishing subgroups; and 2) the condition of auditory phonetic discrimination evoked response as consistently yielding the single best subgroup discriminating feature (Duffy et al. 1985).

Finally, it should be emphasized that physiologic measures of heterogeneity are no more "hard" or anatomical than are pencil-and paper behavioral tests. Physiologic measures are assumed to be more culture-free than are behavioral tests of language and cognition. They may serve as pattern markers for relatives at risk for reading disability. For example, they may be used in genetic studies to identify children prior to school age and/or older relatives remediated or compensated too well to show certain test deficits. The alliance between scientists studying the behavioral characterizations, psychopharmacological responsiveness, electrophysiologic and cerebral blood flow imaging of brain activity, molecular genetics, and infrared oculography may go far to clarify issues of overlap and heterogeneity which exists in the current nosology of learning disability and dyslexia.

References

Denckla, M. B. 1977. Minimal brain dysfunction and dyslexia: Beyond diagnosis by exclusion. *In* M. E. Blaw, I. Rapin, and M. Kinsbourne (eds.). *Child Neurology*. New York Spectrum Publications.

Denckla, M. B., and Rudel, R. G. 1978. Anomalies of motor development in active boys without learning disabilities. *Annals of Neurology* 3:231–233.

Denckla, M. B., Rudel, R. G., and Broman, M. 1981. Tests that discriminate between dyslexic and other learning-disabled boys. *Brain and Language* 13:118–129.

Denckla, M. B., Rudel, R. G., Chapman, C., and Krieger, J. 1985. Motor proficiency in dyslexic children with and without attentional disorders. *Archives of Neurology* 42:228–231.

Diagnostic and Statistical Manual III. 1980. Washington, D.C. American Psychiatric Association.

Duffy, F. H., Denckla, M. B., Bartels, R. H., and Sandini, G. 1980. Dyslexia: Regional differences in brain electrical activity by topographic mapping. *Annals of Neurology* 7:412–420.

Duffy, F. H., Denckla, M. B., Holmes, J., Bartels, R. H., and McAnulty, G. 1985 (work in progress). Subgrouping dyslexic boys by BEAM characteristics.

Geschwind, N. Personal communication. September 11, 1984.

Goldberg, M., Currie, J., Rumsey, J., and Denckla M. B. 1985. Work in progress.

Lipton, R. B., Levy, D. L., Holzman, P. S., and Levin, S. 1983. Eye movement dysfunctions in psychiatric patients: A review. *Schizophrenia Bulletin* 9:13–71.

Lovett, M. 1984. A developmental perspective on reading dysfunction: Accuracy and rate criteria in the subtyping of dyslexia children. *Brain and Language* 22:67–91.

Rudel, R. G. 1980. Learning disability: Diagnosis by exclusion and discrepancy. *Journal of the American Academy of Child Psychiatry* 19:547–569.

Symmes, J. S., and Rapoport, J. L. 1972. Unexpected reading failure. *American Journal of Orthopsychiatry* 42(1):82–91.

Vellutino, R. 1977. Alternative conceptualizations of dyslexia. *Harvard Educational Review* 47:334–354.

Wilsher, C., Atkins, G., and Manfield, P. 1985. Effect of Piracetam on dyslexics' reading ability. *Journal of Learning Disabilities* 18(1):19–25.

4

Reading Disabled and ADD Children: Similarities and Differences

Roscoe A. Dykman, Peggy T. Ackerman, and Phillip J. Holcomb

$\mathcal{T}$his paper will cover selected findings from three studies comparing different diagnostic groups of educationally troublesome boys: those having attention deficit disorder (ADD) with or without hyperactivity (HY) but normal reading ability, those with reading disability (RD) but not HY, and a mixed type who are both RD and HY (see Table 1). We are one of the few groups to contrast two or more clinical groups with each other and normal achievers. Such a contrast is a necessity if one wishes to claim diagnostic specificity for findings inasmuch as normal achieving controls are superior to clinical groups on most measures obtained in the laboratory (Chapman and Chapman 1973).

All diagnoses were made by a veteran child guidance team using DSM-III guidelines. Additional research criteria were also employed. Thus, for a diagnosis of RD, a child had to have a combined average spelling and reading standard score on the Wide Range Achievement Test (WRAT) ≤ 90. Additionally, this mean score was 10 points or more below the child's Verbal or Performance WISC IQ in virtually all of the RD children. A child accepted into the HY study groups had to have a score of ≥ 15 on Conners' 10-item teacher rating scale. All subjects had WISC-R full scale IQs ≥ 90. There were 15–25 subjects per group in all studies reviewed, although one earlier electro-physiological analysis reported below (under Study I) involved only 10 subjects per group.

The studies reviewed below were quite complex, and the reader will have to consult the original sources for complete descriptions of samples and documentation of the results capsulized here. One theme bridges all the studies reviewed: both severe attentional and learning disorders of normally intelligent children appear to be rooted in subtle dysfunctions of the brain, particularly in the frontal and temporal areas.

Key to Abbreviations

ADD -Attention Deficit Disorder

B -The signal detection measure theorized to measure response bias or risk-taking

CNS -Central Nervous System

CPT -Continuous Performance Task

d' -The signal detection measure theorized to measure response sensitivity to an infrequently occurring stimulus

db -Decibel

ERP -Event Related Potential, the electrophysiological waveform elicited to a discrete stimulus

HR -Heart Rate

HY -Hyperactive

LD -Learning Disabled

N1–P2 -The slope of the first negative and second positive peaks of averaged event-related potentials

P3 -The third positive peak of averaged event related potentials

RAN -Rapid Automatized Naming Task

RD -Reading Disabled

RT -Reaction Time

SC -Skin Conductance

Study I

Some years ago, we (Dykman, Ackerman, Clements, and Peters 1971) proposed, on the basis of our earlier work and that of others (Conners 1969; Conners, Rothschild, Eisenberg, Schwartz, and Robinson 1969; Conners, Eisenberg, and Barcai 1967; Sprague, Barnes, and Werry 1970), that attention deficits characterize learning disabled (LD) as well as HY children. Since this 1971 theoretical paper was entitled *Specific Learning Disabilities: An Attentional Deficit Syndrome,* it was not always quoted in the rapidly growing hyperactivity literature. But, like Douglas (1972), in her classic paper *Stop, Look and Listen,* we argued that attentional deficits rather than motoric restlessness should be of central research interest.

Even though the majority of LD children exhibit ADD symptoms, ADD cannot be said to be the sole or major cause of LD, for many ADD children, even HY ones, learn to read and spell at an age appropriate rate. This observation led us to believe that the major problem for LD children might be in the area of selective attention and for HY children in the area of sustained attention. Moreover, we theorized that the failure of HY children to sustain attention was due to a lack of will to do so (Dykman and Ackerman 1976). Here we moved toward what William James termed *intention.* We further speculated that intention reflects frontal lobe action whereas selective attention, especially as used in reading, reflects temporal lobe involvement.

To test this theory, we modified a paradigm that Karl Pribram (1967) had used to assess frontal and temporal lobe functioning in monkeys (Dykman, Ackerman, and Oglesby 1979; Dykman, Ackerman, and McCray 1980). The

Table I
Summary of Studies Reviewed

	Groups	N	Tests and Measures	Focus
Study I (Dykman et al., 1979; 1980; 1982; Ackerman et al., 1979)	Hyperactive	20	Reaction times and physio-	Selective and
	Reading Disabled	20	logical measures during	sustained
	Hyperactive and		Pribram's visual search	attention;
	Reading Disabled	15	paradigm; Eysenck's	intention; moral
	Normal Controls	20	Junior Personality Inventory; Nowcki-Duke Locus-of-Control Scale; Flavel's 7-Picture Role Taking Test; Selman's moral judgment interview; Davé's structured interview of family situation.	judgment
Study II (Ackerman et al., 1982; 1983; 1984; Dykman et al., 1983)	Hyperactive	27	Reaction times; ERPs and	Nervous system
	Reading Disabled	20	HR to tones ranging from	sensitivity;
	Attention Deficit		55 to 100 db under three	cognitive style;
	Disorder (not HY		reward conditions;	response to
	or RD)	16	Matching Familiar Figures;	reward and
	Mixed HY/RD	11	Children's Embedded Figures; Santostefano's Color Naming and Leveling-Sharpening Tests.	methylphenidate
Study III (Ackerman et al., Ref. notes 1–3; Holcomb et al., in press, Ref. note 4)	Hyperactive	24	Frequency and recency of	Automatic and
	ADD	21	occurrence; speed of	effortful
	Reading Disabled	24	naming and writing; free	information
	Normals	24	and cued recall of acoustic-semantic word pairs; immediate and delayed recall of high and low imagery words; computational efficiency; CPT response, RT, and ERP values; Sternberg Task response, RT, and ERP values.	processing; vigilance; memory scanning

child was asked to scan a visual field, discover the target symbol, learn to stay with the target for five trials, search for a new target, etc. He began with a visual field size of only two symbols, but the field size was increased by steps up to 12 symbols. Symbol presentation was under computer control, and any given symbol could occur in any one of 12 windows on a given trial.

There were two kinds of trials: search trials which involved finding the to-be-rewarded stimulus and after-search reward trials which involved staying with the correct object until it was no longer rewarded (5 trials). The child received one penny for each correct response. Total earnings were continually updated by a computer and displayed on a screen. Failures to choose the target consistently after discovery were not rewarded and were considered after-search lapses. In Pribram's monkeys, after-search lapses were increased by frontal lobe damage and search trials by temporal lobe damage.

Unfortunately for the specifics of the theory, the RD group did not differ from HY children in the number of search trials, after-search lapses, or reaction time (RT). Both clinical groups were, however, inferior to controls. When we later studied mixed HY-RD subjects, they, too, were inferior to controls but not distinguishable from the "pure" clinical groups on Pribram performance measures. If we were to regard Pribram's paradigm as a valid test of selective and sustained attention or brain intactness, we could conclude that both HY and RD children have defective temporal and frontal lobe functioning. This is not to say that the children have lesions but rather could indicate subtle defects in neural connections and/or learned or acquired inattentiveness.

As we pointed out earlier (Dykman and Ackerman 1976), the kinds of behavioral deficiencies produced by injuries of the frontolimbic areas and associated cortex (Milner 1963) are very similar to those seen in ADD children, i.e., hyperactivity, attraction to novelty, task impersistence, impulsivity, perseveration or inability to switch from one motion to another, dissociation of action and verbalization, and disregard for rules and consequences. Half of the HY children told us they had become tired and wanted to quit the Pribram task. The RD children, though tired, did not want to quit, yet they became inattentive as the difficulty of the task increased. The HY boys were more attracted to novelty than the RD children. In the early trials of one procedural condition, where the new symbol added to the visual field was always the one to be chosen for reward, HY children tended to choose the novel stimulus immediately whereas RD children did not (Dykman et al. 1979).

In another sample of ADD, HY, and RD boys, the majority, when unmedicated, exhibited lapses of attention and extraneous responding (key-play) in the intertrial intervals of the Pribram task (Dykman et al. 1980). As with the first sample, the HY boys were far more deviant in extraneous responding than were the RD subjects. Methylphenidate dramatically decreased extraneous responding, particularly in HY subjects, and improved the performance of all clinical groups about equally (Dykman et al. 1980). Interestingly, the drug had a greater effect in decreasing after-search errors than in decreasing search trials, i.e., it improved sustained, more than selective, attention (or memory).

Electrocortical data, obtained from one second before and one second after each display of stimuli, were Fourier transformed and subjected to a principal components analysis. Four components were extracted accounting for 87% of the variance. The first component had strong loadings between 16 and 20 Hz and weaker loadings between 8 and 10 Hz. The RD children had significantly lower scores on this component than the controls, with the HY boys intermediate; however, the mixed HY-RD group, which were expected to be the most impaired, were, in fact, the least impaired of the clinical groups by this measure. We have no good explanation of this finding, but should say that this diagnostic group has been found aberrant in other studies. It may be that the combination HY-RD is compensating in some degree as regards arousal; e.g., RD children try harder (see below) while HY children are more easily aroused than pure RD children. These electrocortical results show that controls exhibited superior task specific arousal (i.e., more beta and alpha activity) to the clinical groups. Previously we had found similar clinical groups to be deficient in physiological arousal, as indexed by heart rate and skin conductance response (Dykman et al. 1971). Lowered task specific arousal has also been reported for animals with frontal lobe dysfunction (see review by Fuster 1980).

Turning to some psychometric data, the above clinical groups did not differ on WISC IQ variables, though all were inferior to controls on the attention-sequential memory triad (Digit Span, Arithmetic, Coding). Unexpectedly, the normal reading HY subjects had higher scores than the RD group on Flavel's 7-picture role-taking task. HY children scored higher on this role-taking task, we believe, not because they are truly inclined to take the perspective of others but because they are more active processors of information, particularly of novelty. Non-hyperactive RD children tend to be passive, compliant, and rule-bound in our laboratory encounters with them. These personality traits could explain the higher scores of RD than HY boys on the Lie (or Defensiveness) Scale of the Eysenck Junior Personality Inventory. RD subjects are not overly defensive; they strive to be, and, in fact, are, good boys. HY and HY/RD children were rated higher on aggressiveness than the pure RD subjects (Conners' parent and teacher ratings). Using a structured interview (Davé 1963), we found that HY children received less home stimulation than either RD or control subjects, perhaps because the HY boys were born to younger mothers (see Ackerman, Elardo, and Dykman 1979 for the above results).

Summary of Pribram Study

RD children did not differ from HY children as predicted on the Pribram task, but the study did yield evidence to suggest that dysfunctioning within certain regions of the frontal and temporal lobes may contribute to difficulties in learning and behavioral control: the assertiveness of HY and the passivity of RD subjects; the excessive key-play of the HY boys and their attraction to novelty; and the inferior search and hold performance of all clinical groups. Also, the sequential and phonetic difficulties of RD subjects implicate the posterior region of the left temporal lobe and associated cortical areas (Galaburda 1983).

Study II

The central focus of this study was again attentional problems. But a new variable related to attention was added, which we have termed sensitivity of the central nervous system (CNS). Russian investigators place this presumably innate response bent along a weak-strong continuum, and Western biologically oriented psychologists such as Buchsbaum (1978), Eysenck (1981), Fowles (1980), Gray (1981), and Zuckerman (1983) believe this response propensity to be an important dimension of personality or cognitive style. Since RD and HY children differ along a dimension of passivity and assertiveness, we hypothesized that these traits might have an underlying physiological basis in CNS sensitivity. According to the Russian literature (Nebylitsin 1972), a person with a strong nervous system responds to louder and louder tones or brighter and brighter lights with an orderly increase in physiological activity and an orderly decrease in reaction times (RTs). By contrast, the sensitive type shows an orderly increase up to a point and then responds less vigorously (i.e., exhibits transmarginal inhibition). Buchsbaum (1978) uses the terms augmentation and reduction to describe such gradients obtained from electrocortical evoked potentials. He reasoned, vis-a-vis the Russian experiments, that strong types augment and weak types reduce.

Following Nebylitsin (1972) we used RT slopes to tones of increasing intensity to characterize ADD and RD subjects as strong and weak (Ackerman, Holcomb, McCray, and Dykman 1982). To classify subjects as augmenters or reducers, we (Dykman, Holcomb, Ackerman, and McCray 1983) used the Buchsbaum measure, the N1–P2 component of the event-related potential (ERP).

We found, as Buchsbaum did, that children diagnosed as HY had more augmenting ERP slopes to tones ranging from soft to loud than did non-hyperactive ADD or RD children (Dykman et al. 1983) but there was considerable overlap (see Figure 1). But we found more HY subjects than those in other groups classified as weak or sensitive on the RT measure (Ackerman et al. 1982). Non-hyperactive ADD children typed strongest on the RT measure. There was little relation, however, between the ERP measure of augmentation and the RT measure of CNS strength. On theoretical grounds, the ERP measure should be a better measure of strength than RT, because it represents CNS activity in the first 200–300 msecs of information processing.

Heart rate (HR) generally decelerates markedly as an individual prepares to respond and then accelerates with the response. While ADD and RD groups exhibited less marked anticipatory HR responses than controls in the sensitivity paradigm, no systematic differences were found among the clinical groups (Ackerman, Holcomb, and Dykman 1984). But, with clinical diagnosis ignored, HR levels were consistently higher in ERP reducers than augmenters, and reducers switched more quickly from HR deceleration to acceleration (see Figure 2).

Figure 3 shows the major relations between experimental variables in the pretreatment session of the sensitivity study and the subsequent clinically titrated methylphenidate doses. Our intent was to determine whether we could predict these carefully titrated dose levels from the pretreatment data. This analysis showed that many of the predictor variables were related at a low level, and that their conjoint effect was highly significant (multiple R = .892, p < .001).

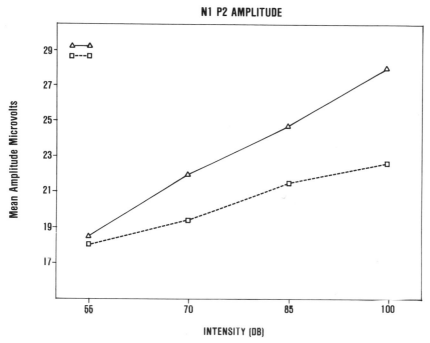

Figure 1.   Mean N1–P2 gradients for two hyperactive (solid line) and two non-hyperactive (broken line) clinical groups.

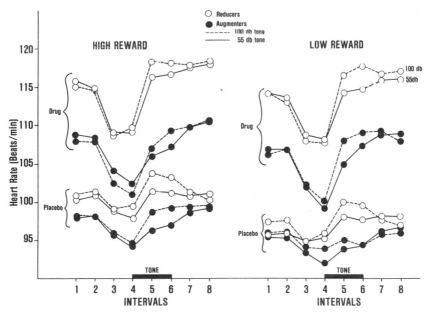

Figure 2.   Mean heart rate levels for 8 contiguous 1-sec. intervals from warning light past tone (imperative stimulus) offset.

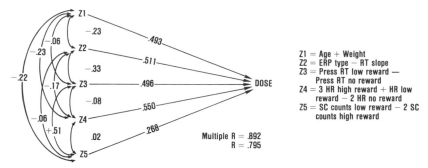

Figure 3. Multiple regression analysis predicting titrated methylphenidate dosage levels from five sets of variables.

In Figure 3, type refers to the RT measure of weak-strong and slope to the ERP measure of augmentation-reduction. In general, we found a highly significant relation between ERP augmentation-reduction and drug-dose and drug-response (Dykman et al. 1983). Relative to reducers, augmenters received smaller doses and had a superior drug response as judged by teacher ratings ($p < .01$).

Turning to cognitive style variables obtained in the sensitivity study (Ackerman, Dykman, Holcomb, and McCray 1982; Ackerman, Dykman, and Oglesby 1983), the clinical groups did not differ on an Embedded Figures Test nor on the Matching Familiar Figures Test. HY children did perform better than RD children on the Leveling-Sharpening test of Santostefano (1970). The solely HY boys were more sensitive to the successive omission of details in an elaborate drawing of a house and its surroundings—evidence, in addition to the Flavel task results, that HY children are more active processors of external change than non-HY RD or ADD children.

Summary of Typology Study

Our most significant findings had to do with the relation of drug titration and response to sensitivity variables as assessed from RT and ERP slopes to tones ranging from soft to very loud. Augmenters were blindly clinically titrated at significantly lower doses of methylphenidate than reducers and they had a much better medication response than reducers. This could mean that ADD reducers need medication other than methylphenidate, no medication at all, or that increasing doses of drug are really not beneficial. Since we have not done a dose-response study, we do not know whether small doses of methylphenidate help reducers as much as or more than large doses. Nearly all children, regardless of diagnostic label, improved in their classroom ratings with the clinically titrated drug dose, and all became more rapid in RT. But, the CNS dimension of sensitivity appears to be a better predictor of drug efficacy than the diagnostic label given a child.

Study III

The third study centered on information processing and consisted of two parts, one contrasting automatic and effortful memory processes and the other vigilance and memory scanning (Ackerman, Holcomb, Dykman, and Anhalt, Reference Note 1; Ackerman, Anhalt, Dykman, and Holcomb, Reference Notes 2 and 3; Holcomb, Ackerman, and Dykman, Reference Note 4). This study utilized four groups of children between the ages of 8 and 12 years: 24 solely HY boys, 24 non-HY but RD boys, 21 boys who were ADD but not HY or RD, and 24 controls. The first part of the study was based on the theory of automatic and effortful processing as outlined by Hasher and Zacks (1979). In order to become proficient in basic school skills, a child must develop highly automatized habits requiring little thinking or effort. Hasher and Zacks point out that some automatic processes appear to be innate, but most are acquired through practice. We theorized that relative to both controls and normal reading ADD subjects, RD children would exhibit certain deficiencies in acquired automatic processing but that HY subjects would differ from controls more in effortful than automatic processing because the former requires sustained attention (or intent to stay with a task).

Several purportedly innate automatic processes were incorporated into the study, e.g., sensitivity to frequency of occurrence of pictures of living creatures and sensitivity to recency of presentation of pictures of common objects. Tasks to measure acquired automatization included speed of picture naming, speed of writing "O's" and one's name, and simple addition and subtraction. Sensitivity to categorical and physical properties of words was also theorized to be automatic in school children with normal language development, and tasks included to assess this type of automatization tapped sensitivity to acoustic and semantic similarities and to words high and low in imagery. Effortful processing was assessed with several memory tasks and by arithmetic problems involving simple borrowing and carrying.

All three groups of clinical children, like controls, gave evidence of intactness of innate processing. That is, they successfully demonstrated in response to probes their sensitivity to the varying number of times they had seen slides of living creatures—from zero to four times for each probe. They were 96% accurate in sorting previously viewed pictures of common objects from pictures they had never seen before from the same categories. And as the literature on levels of processing predicts, all groups showed greater facility at learning and recalling highly imaginable words than words less imaginable, and all groups recalled semantically related words better than acoustically related words. As for acquired automatization of skills, the groups could not be discriminated reliably on speed of naming or speed of writing. All three clinical groups were significantly poorer on all the arithmetic tasks than controls, even with IQ covaried out inasmuch as controls had significantly higher IQs than the clinical groups. But, the clinical groups did not differ from each other in computational efficiency.

Studies that have shown RDs impaired on naming speed (Denckla and Rudel 1976; Garnett and Fleischner 1983) have used a different task (the Boston Rapid Automatized Naming Task, or RAN) than the one we used and have not rigidly controlled for differences in IQ. But, we have not found differences in naming speed on previous studies using a task more like the RAN, i.e., the Santostefano Color Naming Task (Ackerman and Dykman

1982; Ackerman et al. 1983). Perhaps naming speed is more sensitive with subjects younger than 8 years old, and when the task involves recurring alphanumeric stimuli as in the RAN.

The measures which proved most useful in discriminating the RD and ADD groups were from an effortful task, the acoustic-semantic memory task of Weingartner, Rapoport, Buchsbaum, et al. (1980). In brief, the child listened to 20 sets of three words each, having been told to remember as many of the words as possible. For example, the child was asked, "Which word does not belong because of what it means: peas, spinach, house?" Then, "Which word does not belong because of how it sounds: man, can, clock?" Wrong answers were corrected by the examiner. After a distraction task, the child was asked to think back to the sets of words he had heard and to recall as many as possible. This free recall was followed by a cued recall in which the examiner read the child one of the two related words from each set and asked him to name, if he could, the other word of that pair.

We used stepwise discriminant analyses to contrast groups on effortful task variables, removing age and IQ first and second. In the contrast of RD and combined ADD children (both HY and non-hyperactive), the discriminant function yielded 77% correct classifications. This discrimination depended entirely on acoustic-semantic variables, i.e., the discrimination of words that did not rhyme or that were semantically unrelated, the recall of related words in the cued recall task, and the recall of related words in pairs (i.e., clusters) in free recall. Controls could be discriminated from RDs (96% correct) by semantic-acoustic measures, effortful arithmetic, and immediate memory for 12 visually presented first grade level words from three categories. And controls and combined ADDs could be correctly sorted (88% correct) by the effortful arithmetic task, immediate memory for the 12 visually presented words, and delayed memory for low imagery words.

While the contrasts of the clinical groups are of interest, the reality is that many children referred to our service fall between "the cracks" in these arbitrary research cut-offs. Thus, we combined our clinical and control groups in an attempt to arrive at some general conclusions applicable to all children in the age range of the study. In a stepwise regression to predict WRAT reading scores, we forced age and IQ, and then successively removed three variables from the acoustic-semantic task: cued recall of acoustic words, correct detection of unrelated words, and free recall clustering to achieve a multiple R of .59. Adding computational accuracy and delayed recall of low imagery words increased the multiple R to .83, explaining approximately two-thirds of the variance.

Summary of Effortful Processing Results

The finding of impaired phonological sensitivity in the RD group, not only relative to controls but also to children with ADD, corroborates and extends the findings of the Haskins Laboratory group in this country (Liberman, Liberman, Mattingly, and Shankweiler 1980) and Bradley and Bryant (1983) in England. The data from this experiment would also seem to say that ADD impedes automatization of arithmetic computational skills, in that all three clinical groups were poorer than controls. And there is reason to believe that the automatization of arithmetic skills depends on frontal lobe functioning (Fuster 1980). Impaired phonological as well as semantic sensitivity coupled with some long-term memory dysfunction appear to cause reading problems in normally intelligent children. These are temporal lobe functions. Again in this experiment, RD children seemed to be relatively passive encoders and retrievers of more abstract verbal information, which would explain their poor memory for such material, even with cues.

In the second part of this experiment, the same clinical groups and controls as described above were studied on tasks purporting to tap vigilance and memory scanning. Both reaction times (RTs) and event-related potentials (ERPs) were obtained, but only partial results can be reported now. The three tasks used to assess vigilance were an auditory and two visual variants of the much studied Continuous Performance Task (CPT). In the auditory condition, the child was instructed to press a reaction time key as rapidly as possible only when he heard a high pitched tone and at no other time. This target tone occurred on 17% of the 250 trials; a non-target, low pitched tone occurred on 67% of the trials and a non-target burst of white noise on 17% of the trials. The child had practice with the two tones but not the white noise, which was unexpected. In the visual conditions, the stimulus probabilities remained the same. The target was the 3-letter combination *DTM;* the high probability non-target stimulus was the combination *RSC.* For the first visual condition, the novel unexpected stimuli were combinations of three non-alphanumeric symbols (e.g., asterisks, dollar signs, or punctuation marks). For the second visual condition, the novel non-target stimuli were 42 different 3-letter words (e.g., dog, cat, car).

The error data were analyzed with the signal detection measures d' and B, the former being an index of sensitivity or vigilance, the latter an index of risk taking. We also studied mean reaction time to target stimuli and intraindividual RT variability, thought by some to be a better index of attentiveness than mean RT.

In the auditory session, controls had higher d' scores than both RD and HY/ADD children. The groups did not differ in risk taking. Controls had faster RTs than each of the other groups, but only RD children were more variable in RT than controls.

In the two visual CPT sessions, controls were again more sensitive than HY children, particularly in the second session. RD children, however did not differ from controls on d'. In pairwise contrasts, RD children had significantly higher d' scores in the second visual session than the HY subjects. Controls were faster than the RD and ADD children in the visual sessions and had less variable RTs than the two ADD groups.

The analyses of the ERPs to the visual stimuli showed a significant group effect. The group difference was noted in the P3 latencies from the central parietal and occipital leads. Slower P3 latencies are hypothesized to reflect slower evaluation encoding. The RD group had the slowest P3s on the target and non-target stimulus arrays, while the HY group were slowest on the

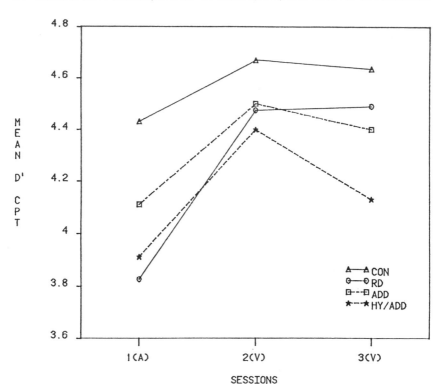

Figure 4.   Continuous Performance Task (CPTs): Mean d' (sensitivity) scores in one auditory (A) and two visual (V) sessions for four groups.

unexpected stimuli, especially the words. Controls had larger amplitude P3s than the ADD and RD children to the expected target and non-target stimuli. To the unexpected novel stimuli, the RD group had considerably lower P3 and slow wave amplitudes to the words than symbols, but controls showed little difference between the two types of novel stimuli. The most intriguing major finding is that young RD subjects had much slower auditory P3 latencies than the young subjects in other clinical groups, but the latencies of the older RD subjects were more in line with the older children in other groups.

A variant of Sternberg's memory scanning task was used to try to shed further light on stages of information processing that might be impaired in the clinical groups. Sternberg manipulated conditions to figure out how long it takes a subject to encode a probe stimulus, scan his memory to determine whether the probe is or is not in a previously presented memory set, make a decision, and execute a response. We used memory sets of 1, 3, and 5 consonant letters. The task was made more effortful in that the size and composition of the memory sets were varied randomly over trials. There were 20 "yes" and 20 "no" trials at each set size.

Overall, controls had higher accuracy scores than each of the clinical groups, but at set sizes 1 and 3, RD subjects were significantly more accurate than the ADD and HY subjects (Figure 5). Thus, RD children appear to perform

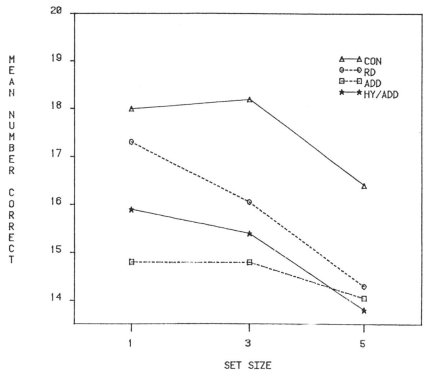

Figure 5.   Sternberg Task: Mean number of correct responses, yes and no, at memory set sizes 1, 3, and 5 letters for four groups.

better than ADD groups until a certain level of complexity is reached. Mean reaction times did not reliably separate the groups, but the two ADD groups had significantly more variable RTs than the controls, with the RD group intermediate.

The event-related potentials of the RDs and controls to the Sternberg stimuli have been analyzed (Holcomb et al. in press). The P3 amplitudes decreased as set size increased, yielding negative slopes, which is what other investigators have reported. At the occipital site, the RD children had significantly more negative slopes than controls, indicating that processing was more difficult for them at larger set sizes. The P3 latency slopes showed controls to have earlier zero intercepts (about 50 msec) than RD children, but this difference was reduced when IQ was partialled out. In this study, the controls' mean IQ was roughly one standard deviation above the mean IQ of RD subjects, and IQ is a significant covariate of P3 latency.

Summary of Information Processing Tasks

The clinical groups had differing patterns of adverse scores in relation to controls but there were only a few significant differences between the clinical groups. The HY group showed a decrease in sensitivity during the second visual CPT session, but the RD group did not and had significantly higher d' scores than HY subjects in this session. Also, the RD group was more accurate than the two ADD groups on the Sternberg with smaller set sizes. On the other hand, the RD group was least sensitive in the auditory version of the CPT, and, whereas two-thirds of controls had faster auditory than visual RTs, 83% of RD subjects had faster visual than auditory RTs (Chi Square = 10.37, p < .01). Thus, RD subjects seem more impaired in auditory than visual vigilance. The opposite is true for HY' subjects. But, Sternberg task results indicate RD children do falter on visual tasks when the information load is heavy, perhaps when they need to employ auditory recoding to keep the information in working memory. Auditory patterns, except for chords, generally require sequential processing, but less complex visual patterns can be processed globally, which seems to be the RD children's preferred mode.

Conclusions

To return to our opening speculations, we are inclined to believe that HY children's inability to sustain attention, their lack of will (effort) to think and remember, their inability to suppress extraneous responses and distracting stimuli, their aggressive or impulsive behavior indicate frontal-limbic dysfunction, most likely subtle defects in the "wiring" of inhibitory connections (Dykman et al. 1979). When information becomes excessive or uninteresting, even normally attentive people exhibit attentional problems similar to those of HY children. The "defect" in these instances would, however, seem to be secondary, or elicited, rather than primary, and we believe that this is the case for most RD children. RD children exhibit attentional problems very similar to those of ADD children but the problems are less noticeable or severe until they are put into effortful information processing situations. When the phonologically handicapped RD child has to discriminate and remember closely related language sounds, his attentional capacity appears overloaded. It is our belief that left hemisphere deficiencies, not necessarily subtle, in the posterior temporal lobe and adjacent regions of the angular gyrus are responsible for the language difficulties of RD children. Moreover, problems in temporal lobe processing (selective attention) can overload frontal lobe processing (sustained attention).

Methylphenidate, like dextroamphetamine, is a nonspecific stimulant that improves performance in a great variety of tasks. These psychostimulants achieve their effect, we believe, by increasing the sensitivity of nonspecific ascending and descending pathways, from and to the reticular system via the limbic system, thalamus, and frontal lobes. We have theorized elsewhere (Dykman et al. 1971) that these drugs have their main effect on the forebrain inhibitory system, which when stimulated suppresses movement. There are other important ascending inhibitory systems that may also be involved (see review by Solanto 1984). Psychostimulants appear to augment selective attention by decreasing (1) the range of stimuli to which a person will respond and (2) competing response tendencies. These drugs also increase the willingness of a person to stay with a task, which is the hallmark of sustained attention. The fact that dextroamphetamine improves the performance of normals (Rapoport, Buchsbaum, Weingartner et al. 1980) does not necessarily mean that the effects of the psychostimulants are identical in normals and clinical cases nor in all clinical cases (see Pelham and Milich 1984).

References Notes

1. Ackerman, P. T., Holcomb, P. J., Dykman, R. A., and Anhalt, J. M. Information processing in educationally troublesome children. Submitted for publication.
2. Ackerman, P. T., Anhalt, J. M., Dykman, R. A., and Holcomb, P. J. Innate and acquired automatization in children with attention and/or reading disorders. Submitted for publication.
3. Ackerman, P. T., Anhalt, J. M., Dykman, R. A., and Holcomb, P. J. In press. Effortful processing deficits in children with reading and/or attention disorders. *Brain and Cognition.*
4. Holcomb, P. J., Ackerman, P. T., and Dykman, R. A. In press. Event-related potentials of RDs during memory scanning. *In* S. J. Ceci (ed.). *Handbook of cognitive, social, and neuropsychological aspects of learning disabilities,* Vol. 2. Lawrence Erlbaum Associates.

References

Ackerman, P. T. and Dykman, R. A. 1982. Automatic and effortful information processing deficits in children with learning and attention disorders. *Topics in Learning and Learning Disabilities* 2:12–22.

Ackerman, P. T., Dykman, R. A., Holcomb, P. J., and McCray, D. S. 1982. Methylphenidate effects on cognitive style and reaction time in four groups of children. *Psychiatry Research* 7:199–213.

Ackerman, P. T., Dykman, R. A., and Oglesby, D. M. 1983. Sex and group differences in reading and attention disordered children, with and without hyperkinesis. *Journal of Learning Disabilities* 16(7):407–415.

Ackerman, P. T., Elardo, P. T., and Dykman, R. A. 1979. A psychosocial study of hyperactive and learning disabled boys. *Journal of Abnormal Child Psychology* 7:91–99.

Ackerman, P. T., Holcomb, P. J., and Dykman, R. A. 1984. Effects of reward and methylphenidate on heart rate response morphology of augmenting and reducing children. *International Journal of Psychophysiology* 1:301–316.

Ackerman, P. T., Holcomb, P. J., McCray, D. S., and Dykman, R. A. 1982. Studies of nervous system sensitivity in children with learning and attention disorders. *Pavlovian Journal of Biological Science* 17:30–41.

Bradley, L. and Bryant, P. E. 1983. Categorizing sounds and learning to read—a causal connection. *Nature* 301:419–421.

Buchsbaum, M. S. 1978. Neurophysiological studies of augmenting and reducing. *In* A. Petrie (ed.). *Individuality in pain and suffering,* Vol. 2. University of Chicago Press.

Chapman, J. J. and Chapman, J. P. 1973. *Disordered Thought in Schizophrenia.* New York: Prentice Hall.

Conners, C. K. 1969. A teacher rating scale for use in drug studies with children. *American Journal of Psychiatry* 126:152–156.

Conners, C. K., Eisenberg, L., and Barcai, A. 1967. Effect of dextroamphetamine on children. *Archives of General Psychiatry* 17:478–485.

Conners, C. K., Rothschild, G., Eisenberg, L., Schwartz, L., and Robinson, E. 1969. Dextroamphetamine sulfate in children with learning disorders: effects on perception, learning and achievement. *Archives of General Psychiatry* 21:182–190.

Davé, R. H. 1963. The identification and measurement of environmental process variables that are related to educational achievement. Unpublished doctoral dissertation, University of Chicago.

Denckla, M. B. and Rudel, R. G. 1976. Naming of object-drawings of dyslexic and other learning disabled children. *Brain and Language* 3:1–15.

Douglas, V. I. 1972. Stop, look and listen: The problem of sustained attention and impulse control in hyperactive and normal children. *Canadian Journal of Behavioral Science* 4:259–281.

Dykman, R. A., and Ackerman, P. T. 1976. The MBD Problem: Attention, intention, and information processing. *In* R. P. Anderson and C. G. Holcomb (eds.). *Learning Disability/ Minimal Brain Dysfunction Syndrome*. Springfield, IL: Charles C Thomas.

Dykman, R. A., Ackerman, P. T., Clements, S. D., and Peters, J. E. 1971. Specific learning disabilities. An attentional deficit syndrome. In H. R. Myklebust (ed.), *Progress in Learning Disabilities*, Vol. II. New York: Grune & Stratton.

Dykman, R. A., Ackerman, P. T., and McCray, D. S. 1980. Effects of methylphenidate on selective and sustained attention in hyperactive, reading-disabled, and presumably attention-disordered boys. *Journal of Nervous and Mental Disease* 168:745–752.

Dykman, R. A., Ackerman, P. T., and Oglesby, D. M. 1979. Selective and sustained attention in hyperactive, learning-disabled, and normal boys. *Journal of Nervous and Mental Disease* 167:288–297.

Dykman, R. A., Holcomb, P. J., Ackerman, P. T., and McCray, D. S. 1983. Auditory ERP augmentation-reduction and methylphenidate dosage needs in attention and reading disordered children. *Psychiatry Research* 9:255–269.

Eysenck, H. J. 1981. General features of the model. *In* H. J. Eysenck (ed.). *A Model for Personality*. New York: Springer-Verlag.

Fowles, D. C. 1980. The three arousal model: Implications of Gray's two factor learning theory for heart rate, electrodermal activity, and psychopathy. *Psychophysiology* 17:87–104.

Fuster, J. M. 1980. *The Prefrontal Cortex: Anatomy, physiology, and neuropsychology of the frontal lobe*. New York: Raven Press.

Galaburda, A. 1983. Developmental dyslexia: Current anatomical research. *Annals of Dyslexia* 33:41–53.

Garnett, K. and Fleischner, J. E. 1983. Automatization and basic fact performance of normal and learning disabled children. *Learning Disability Quarterly* 6:223–230.

Gray, J. A. 1981. A critique of Eysenck's theory of personality. *In* H. J. Eysenck (ed.). *A Model for Personality*. New York: Springer-Verlag.

Hasher, L. and Zacks, R. T. 1979. Automatic and effortful processes in memory. *Journal of Experimental Psychology: General* 108:356–388.

Liberman, I. Y., Liberman, L. M., Mattingly, I., and Shankweiler, D. 1980. Orthography and the beginning reader. *In* J. F. Kavanaugh and R. L. Venezky (eds). *Orthography, Reading, and Dyslexia*. Baltimore: University Park Press.

Milner, B. 1963. Effects of different brain lesions on card sorting. *Archives of Neurology* 9:90–100.

Nebylitsin, V. D. 1972. *Fundamental Properties of the Human Nervous System*. New York: Plenum.

Pelham, W. E. and Milich, R. 1984. Peer relations in children with hyperactivity/attention deficit disorder. *Journal of Learning Disabilities* 17:560–567.

Pribram, K. H. 1967. Memory and the organization of attention. *In* D. B. Lindsley and A. A. Lumsdaine (eds.). *Brain Function and Learning*. Berkeley: University of California Press.

Rapoport, J. L., Buchsbaum, M., Weingartner, H., Zahn, Y. P., Ludlow, C., and Mikkelsen, E. 1980. Dextroamphetamine: Cognitive and behavioral effects in normal and hyperactive boys and normal men. *Archives of General Psychiatry,* 37:933–943.

Santostefano, S. 1970. Cognitive controls versus cognitive styles: An approach to diagnosing and treating cognitive disabilities. *In* S. Chess and A. Thomas (eds.). *Annual Progress in Child Psychiatry and Child Development*. New York: Brunner/Mazel, Inc.

Solanto, M. V. 1984. Neuropharmacological basis of stimulant drug action in attention deficit disorder with hyperactivity: A review and synthesis. *Psychological Bulletin* 95:387–409.

Sprague, R. L., Barnes, K. R., and Werry, J. S. 1970. Methylphenidate and thioridazine: Learning, reaction time, activity, and classroom behavior in disturbed children. *American Journal of Orthopsychiatry* 40:615–627.

Weingartner, H., Rapoport, J. L., Buchsbaum, M. S., Bunney, W. E., Jr., Ebert, M. H., Mikkelsen, E. J., and Caine, E. D. 1980. Cognitive processes in normal and hyperactive children and their response to amphetamine treatment. *Journal of Abnormal Psychology* 89:25–37.

Zuckerman, M. 1983. *Biological Bases of Sensation Seeking, Impulsivity, and Anxiety*. Hillsdale, NJ: Lawrence Erlbaum Associates.

5

Recent Developments in Neuro-Imaging Techniques

Richard Coppola

$\mathcal{W}$e know that human behavior is related to the physiological functioning of the brain. There are very few ways available to study this physiological activity in humans. The variety of neuro-imaging methods currently being developed are providing new windows into the brain. Images of the anatomical or physical structure of the brain are produced by the methods of computerized axial tomography (CAT) and nuclear magnetic resonance (NMR). These images have excellent resolution to show fine detail of structure but they do not give any information about function. (Evolving methods of NMR may lead to images of more interesting chemical structure or function in terms of blood flow but are not presently available.)

It is the techniques of single photon and positron emission tomography (PET) that are able to produce images related to brain activity. Those technologies use radioisotope labeling and detection methods with tracer kinetic models to follow ongoing processes of the brain. Although these tracer and labeling methods can also be used to look at such issues as the distribution of neurotransmitters and receptors, it is blood flow and metabolism that are the aspects of brain function that PET is most used to measure.

Human brain activity can also be measured by the electrical potentials at the scalp, the electroencephalogram (EEG). Although not a direct measure of brain function, as is metabolism, it is well established that the EEG reflects ongoing brain activity meaningfully related to behavior. Current computer and display capabilities enable the production of images of brain activity from multi-lead EEG data, that is, from the electrical activity recorded from many electrodes spaced over the scalp. EEG images, or topographic maps as they are

Richard Coppola, D. Sc.
Senior Staff
Laboratory of Psychology and Psychopathology
National Institute of Mental Health
Bethesda, Maryland 20892

often called, reflect brain activity in quite a different way than blood flow or metabolism and, thus, form a complementary view into brain function.

With all of these neuro-imaging techniques, information can be gained about the brain at rest or during activity, such as performing some cognitive task. Information recorded at rest may be of special interest to determine trait characteristics; however, cognitive activation provides an opportunity to study brain function in relation to specific behaviors. This allows the observation of state characteristics and may be of special interest for the biobehavioral study of normal cognitive processing as well as cognitive dysfunction in a variety of clinical groups. Cognitive activation procedures need to be tailored to particular deficits or abnormalities. The design of appropriate tasks is a challenge to cognitive psychophysiologists to develop paradigms that will work in concert with currently evolving neurophysiological methods.

Each of the neuro-imaging methods provides a different view of brain function. Each has different characteristics in terms of resolution, localization, cost, time, and relation to behavior. The purpose of this chapter is to briefly review these methods and to provide a comparison in terms of what type of information they yield that might be pertinent to the biology of behavior. It is not intended to be a comprehensive review of studies that have been carried out and it will be left to the reader to decide what applications there may be for research on dyslexia.

Methods

Although methods are being developed to utilize X-ray CAT and NMR imaging to get dynamic information about the brain, these techniques are best applied to anatomical studies and thus are of limited use to biobehavioral research. The measures that relate more dynamically to brain function include metabolic activity and blood flow. Three dimensional information relating to these measures can be obtained by positron emission tomography (PET) and single photon emission tomography (SPECT). Regional cerebral blood flow (rCBF) can also be measured in a more planar fashion by equipment less sophisticated than SPECT. The EEG is not a direct measure of activity but it is related dynamically to behavior. It is only these dynamic imaging techniques that will be discussed.

Metabolic Imaging

Glucose is the primary source of energy for neuronal activity. By being able to map the utilization of glucose in the brain, one can infer the distribution of neural activity. Sokoloff and his co-workers (1977) developed the radioactively-labeled 2-deoxy-D-glucose method of autoradiography for mapping metabolic function in serial sections of the brain. The development of PET and the availability of positron emitting radioisotopes allowed the exclusion of this technique for humans.

In PET, the pattern of radioactivity in the brain is imaged in a fashion similar to X-ray CAT (Phelps and Mazziotta 1985; Walker 1984). Certain radioisotopes decay by emitting positrons. The positron travels a very short distance before annihilating by crashing into an electron. This annihilation event gives off two photons traveling 180 degrees apart. Scintillation detectors arranged around the head detect the annihilation event by recording the coincidence of the two photons 180 degrees apart. Thus, the event has been localized to a particular ray path through the head. The amount of radioactivity in each possible ray path is accumulated and a two-dimensional image of the distribution of radioactivity in the slice across the head is reconstructed by the same tomographic methods as used in X-ray CAT. This measure of radioactivity is then related back to the measure of interest by applying the appropriate tracer kinetic model.

The usual PET technique for metabolic mapping is to use the positron emitter fluorine-18 to label fluoro-deoxy-glucose (FDG). FDG is an analog of regular glucose and follows a similar pathway to a certain point where, for practical purposes, it becomes trapped in the cells of the brain. After a bolus injection of FDG, there is a concentration of radioactivity in the blood which eventually decreases to the point where the trapped radioactivity is of sufficiently higher concentration that the actual PET scan can be carried out. Then using the appropriate kinetic model equations, the radioactivity concentration is converted to measure glucose utilization.

The neuronal activity to which this glucose use corresponds is the activity that occurred during the uptake of the FDG. Scanning is usually done about 40 minutes after the bolus injection and the time period of behavior related to uptake thus follows the blood curve during this time. The final glucose image thus reflects an average of about 10 to 20 minutes of neural activity, the period of significant concentration available for uptake as seen in the blood curve.

A stable rest condition must be maintained over this period of time or some behavioral or cognitive activation procedure or sensory stimulation must be carried out by the subject for the same time. The behavioral state of the subject is also influenced by the presence of two I.V. lines (one is required to deliver the FDG, the other to draw samples in order to determine the blood curve).

Multiple slices can be imaged so that glucose utilization throughout the entire brain is obtained. State-of-the-art resolution for PET is about 5 to 7 mm so that neural structures of about one cc can be discerned. One could theoretically detect functional abnormalities in structures about that size. This requires some notion of what the normal values are for the structures of interest. Because the determination of absolute values of glucose utilization is frought with difficulties, relative values must often be used; that is, the ratio of activity in one structure to some other structure or even to the entire slice or hemi-slice activity. This complicates the interpretation of results and has left the field struggling to develop new methods to analyze the complicated distribution patterns that are seen. Qualitative interpretations can be drawn from the image but accurate quantification requires attention to a staggering number of considerations running the gamut from numerous parameters that are needed to characterize the scanner itself in terms of activation, calibration, and correction factors to the possibility of individual differences in parameters of the kinetic model.

The cost of such mapping studies is quite high. Not only is the PET scanner itself very expensive, but a cyclotron and radiochemistry facility are needed to provide the relatively short-lived isotopes that are required.

Blood Flow Studies

Regional cerebral blood flow (rCBF) is another important physiological measure of brain function closely related to neural activity. RCBF is tightly coupled to oxidative metabolism so that increases in neural activity should be reflected by increases in blood flow. Several measuring instruments have been developed harking back to the Kety-Schmidt method (1948).

The most widely used instruments are based on the xenon-133 inhalation method (Risberg 1980). Blood flow is measured by the slope of the clearance curve. Xenon concentration is measured during uptake and then during the washout period. There are several parameters and variations on the kinetic model used to derive blood flow from the clearance curve but the basic method is the same. Xenon-133 is a single photon emitter and its concentration is measured by detecting this radioactivity.

The simpler instruments use 16 or 32 surface mounted detectors that pick up activity from the cortex immediately under the 2 to 3 cm diameter of the detector. The spatial resolution is thus determined by the number and size of the detectors. Localization is limited to the grey matter in the view of the detector. Activity is usually recorded over about a 10-minute period; however, the grey matter flow is mostly determined by the first four minutes. The result is a measure that reflects neural activity over this time period.

Blood flow can be measured by SPECT using the same inhalation method. In one instrument, highly collinated, rapidly-rotating detectors measure radioactivity and tomographic methods are used to reconstruct a slice for each ring of detectors. The concentration values in these slices are then used to construct the clearance curves (Shirahata et al. 1985). SPECT thus gives flow measures for interior structures as well as cortical areas. Spatial resolution for SPECT is currently on the order of $1.7 \times 1.7 \times 2.0$ cm. Other single photon emitters are available besides xenon-133, some of which may offer considerable advantages in terms of sensitivity. Single photon emitters offer a considerable advantage over positron emitters in that they generally have much longer half-lives and can be obtained from remote sources without the need for cyclotron and radiochemistry facilities.

Quantitative measurement of rCBF can also be obtained using PET techniques and short-lived positron emitters, such as oxygen-15 (Huang et al. 1983). PET offers the advantage of a faster and more precise localization of emitted radiation than SPECT. However, the short half-life of oxygen-15 requires that the cyclotron facility needed for its production be immediately adjacent to the scanner. RCBF can be measured using an equilibrium method with continuous inhalation of oxygen-15 labeled carbon dioxide or using a dynamic model with a bolus administration. Dynamic studies may have better temporal resolution than the xenon method with the possibility of following flow changes on the order of one minute. Because of the considerable cost and the complexity of the models involved, this method for flow studies is still evolving.

The bulk of rCBF studies have been carried out using the xenon clearance method with considerable success in the localization of function for different cognitive tasks. As mentioned earlier, the challenge here is to design tasks that tap or unveil both specific cognitive components as well as ones that are neurophysiologically localized.

EEG Imaging

The basic method involves recording EEG from many electrodes placed on the scalp. Such multi-lead data thus leads to localization by inference made from measurements at the different electrode sites. There are several possible measures of the recorded electrical activity, including ones derived from spectrum analysis or event-related potential (ERP) studies. These electro-physiology aspects are discussed elsewhere in this volume. The point of processing such multi-lead data into images is to facilitate the observation of topographic patterns of EEG activity with the view that different patterns reflect different functional organization of the brain.

In order to produce a planar image of EEG or ERP measures, the electrode sites are located on a two-dimensional equal area projection of the three-dimensional scalp. Data values for all the pixels within this scalp outline are obtained by some particular interpolation algorithm. The data itself may consist of instantaneous amplitude values, values for the amount of energy at a particular frequency or within a frequency band, or some measure derived from the ERP, such as a specific component amplitude. Just as with PET and SPECT, there are many issues associated with the image quantification, such as the number and placement of electrodes, reference electrode, projection ge-ometry, signal processing, and analysis (Coppola 1982).

Although it has been clearly demonstrated that EEG is related to behavior in a dynamic fashion the nature of the relation is poorly understood if at all. For event-related potentials, there is just emerging a taxonomy of components each with their particular relation to some aspect of cognitive processing. The utility of the EEG images will be determined by the adequacy of these emerging psychophysiological methods. EEG mapping studies have already been applied specifically to dyslexia (Duffy et al. 1980).

Comparison of Techniques

These neuro-imaging techniques can be compared over several parameters: spatial resolution, localization, temporal resolution, and cost.

EEG imaging is a very indirect measure of brain activity. The scalp recorded EEG results from a convolution and summation of underlying electrical activity from a relatively large area. Even at best, resolution could only be considered to be a few centimeters, regardless of electrode spacing. Additionally confounding is the possibility that the surface activity represents that reflected from a brain region some distance from the recording site. The great advantage of EEG is the ability to reflect changes in brain activity on a millisecond-by-millisecond basis. This allows EEG images to be related to behavior as it is occurring. Indeed it is now possible to display a dynamically changing image and follow its course across behavioral states (Salb and Coppola 1981).

In contrast, PET images have very high resolution, potentially on the order of a few millimeters, and measure in three dimensions activity throughout the brain. Glucose metabolic images, however, have a relatively slow temporal resolution, reflecting the summation of some 10 to 30 minutes of activity. PET derived blood flow images have the same high spatial resolution and a somewhat faster time constant, reflecting activity on the order of one minute. SPECT derived blood flow data still has three-dimensional localization capability but with a somewhat lowered spatial resolution of 1.5 to 2 cm, and a temporal resolution over some few minutes. Surface-only measured blood has only cortical localization with spatial resolution of 2 to 3 cm.

Cost needs to be considered in terms, not only of the dollar amount needed to purchase the instrumentation and provide isotope supplies, but also in terms of the length and number of studies that can be carried out in a single subject. EEG imaging has the lowest cost, after a modest initial investment (less than $100K) there is essentially no incremental cost except for the one hour or so needed to prepare the subject for recording. Because there is no radiation dose involved, any number of repeat slices can be carried out.

Blood flow studies using xenon-133 clearance have a higher investment in instrument cost (several hundred thousand dollars or more), but a low cost per subject since single photon emitters are relatively inexpensive. The radiation dose is low and repeat studies under different activation conditions can be carried out serially over a few hours. The availability of isotope allows greater numbers of subjects to be studied, an important consideration when a considerable degree of individual difference is expected.

PET studies of either metabolism or blood flow are extremely expensive. Initial investment for scanner and cyclotron facility is millions of dollars. Isotope production is also extremely costly with considerable "per subject" cost. FDG studies involve higher radiation doses so that repeat studies can be carried out only in widely spaced time. The logistics of delivery of short-lived isotopes further complicates and increases the cost.

These neuro-imaging techniques hold a vital potential for insight into brain function. They form complementary pictures of what is going on in the brain. Developments in three areas must be pursued in order to realize this potential. Continued technical development will refine the instruments, one hopes with increased resolution and reduced cost. Development of appropriate activation procedures must precede further biobehavioral research. And lastly new statistical and analytical techniques must be developed to deal with the flood of data that neuro-imaging releases.

References

Coppola, R. 1982. Topographic methods of functional cerebral analysis. *In* A. R. Potuin (ed.). *Frontiers of Engineering in Health Care.* New York: IEEE Press.

Duffy, F. H., Denckla, M. B., Bartels, P. H., and Sandini, G. S. 1980. Dyslexia: Regional differences in brain electrical activity by topographic mapping. *Annals of Neurology* 7:412–20.

Huang, S. C., Carson, R. E., Hoffman, E. S., Carson, J., MacDonald, N., Barno, J. R., and Phelps, M. E. 1983. Quantitative measurement of local cerebral blood flow in humans by positron computed tomography and O-15 water. *Journal of Cerebral Blood Flow* 3:141–53.

Kety, S. S. and Schmidt, C. F. 1948. The nitrousoxide method for the quantitative determination of cerebral blood flow in man: Theory, procedure, and normal values. *Journal of Clinical Investigation* 27:476–83.

Phelps, M. E., and Mazziotta, J. C. 1985. Positron emission tomography: Human brain function and biochemistry. *Science* 228:799–809.

Risberg, J. 1980. Regional cerebral blood flow measurements by Xe-133 inhalation: Methodology and applications in neuropsychology and psychiatry. *Brain and Language* 9:9–34.

Salb, J. and Coppola, R. 1982. Dynamic topographic analysis of the EEG in real time. *Proceedings of the 35th Annual Conference on Engineering in Medicine and Biology* New York: IEEE Press.

Shirahata, N., Henriksen, L., Vorstrup, S., Holm, S., Lauritzen, M., Paulson, O. D., and Lassen, N. A. 1985. Regional cerebral blood flow assessed by Xe-133 inhalation and emission tomography: Normal values. *Journal of Computer Assisted Tomography* 9(5):861–66.

Sokoloff, L., Reivich, M., Kennedy, C., DesRosiers, M. H., Patlak, C. S., Pettigrew, K. D., Sakurada, O., and Shinohara, M. 1977. The (C-14) deoxyglucose method for the measurement of local cerebral glucose utilization. *Journal of Neurochemistry* 28:897–916.

Walker, M. D. (ed.). 1984. Research issues in positron emission tomography. *Annals of Neurology* 15(Supplement)

6

Evaluation of Electrophysiological Studies on Dyslexia

John R. Hughes

$\mathcal{A}$ renewed interest can be found in the medical community to establish the neurophysiological correlates of dyslexia. The brain of the dyslexic child must be different in some way from that of the normal and, therefore, there is a neurophysiological basis for dyslexia, if we can only discover it. Electrophysiological techniques have been traditionally used in neurophysiology and they continue to be utilized, especially with the further sophistication of computerized apparatus. This report will briefly summarize the literature up to 1978, then add the more recent studies with emphasis on two related types of investigation in which significant advances have been made.

Electroencephalography (EEG)

General Comments

The general conclusion that the EEG tends to be more abnormal with a greater clinical disturbance remains valid. Thus, children classified as "hyperkinetic" have a higher incidence of EEG disturbance than those considered as only "behavior disorders" (Klingerfuss, Lang, Weinberg, and O'Leary 1965; Anderson 1963; Jasper, Bradley, and Solomon 1938; Knobel, Wolman, and Mason 1959; Stevens, Sachdev, and Milstein 1968) and the "mentally retarded" have a higher incidence than the "learning disabled" (see Hughes 1978). If the deficit is only reading and spelling, then the incidence of an associated EEG abnormality is lower than if the deficit includes other specific cognitive problems (Ingram, Mason, and Blackburn 1970). The 45% incidence of EEG abnormality in dyslexia as an overall mean for 10 studies involving 530 patients is significantly higher than most normal control values (Hughes 1978).

Types of EEG Patterns

The controversial pattern of 6–7 and 14/sec positive spikes had been found in 21% to 55% of dyslexics, but the majority of the EEG community in the United States continues to consider this pattern as a "normal variant" or with great skepticism. However, nearly 100 more papers on this pattern have been published throughout the world during the past two decades (for a review, see Hughes 1983). The findings for Bosaeus and Selldén (1979) are possibly relevant to the present area of concern. These investigators chose 743 children from 1177 subjects, all considered normal on the basis of 13 different criteria. Then 222 were randomly chosen and more carefully examined, especially by a child psychiatrist. One conclusion from this study was that positive spikes was the most common EEG pattern found in children considered normal at first but later found with behavior disorders and also other clinical (neurovegetative) symptoms. The important point here is that these children were initially considered normal with an isolated EEG finding but upon careful investigation were found to have a significant behavior disorder and possibly related EEG pattern. These findings underscore the need to examine carefully patients who initially seem to meet strict criteria for normalcy, but upon further investigation may show significant electro-clinical correlations.

Excessive occipital slow waves have been reported in a number of dyslexics (Hughes 1978) and the location of the primary visual receiving area in the same region provides good neuroanatomical and neurophysiological sense for this possible relationship. However, the data on this pattern are not clear, either with regard to a significantly increased incidence in dyslexia or to the specificity of this EEG pattern in reading disorders. It is well known that excessive occipital slow waves often represent a *nonspecific* EEG pattern in children, found in many different conditions. Also, this *abnormal* pattern is at times difficult to differentiate from the *normal* "occipital slow waves found predominantly in youth" (Aird and Gastaut 1959) and also from the *normal* "rhythmic 2½–4½/sec activity" found on the posterior regions in children under 15 yrs of age, most frequently at 5–7 yrs (Petersén and Eeg-Olofsson 1971).

Diffuse or generalized abnormalities have been reported in some dyslexics, but this finding has not been frequently reported (Hughes and Park 1968). The abnormality may appear in the form of diffuse slow waves (Capute, Niedermeyer, and Richardson 1968) or as an abnormally slow background rhythm in the waking state (Roudinesco, Trélat, and Trélat 1950).

Epileptiform activity occasionally appears, but is an uncommon abnormality among dyslexics (Hughes 1978). Although discharges on the temporal lobe have been emphasized in one study (Torres and Ayers 1968), those on the occipital areas, the visual receiving area, might have been more expected and have been studied by Volterra and Giordani (1966). It remains a mystery and a fascination to electroencephalographers that some children may have such active spike discharges on one or both occipital areas and demonstrate no obvious signs of clinical seizures. However, the possible disturbance within the sphere of reading and/or perception by these discharges has not been fully explored.

Correlations with EEG Abnormalities

An abnormal EEG has been correlated in the previous literature with inadequate visual perception or some type of birth defect (Black 1972), birth complications and an abnormal neurological examination (Gerson, Barnes, Mannino, Fanning, and Burns 1972), brain damage as assessed by birth or developmental history and clinical examination (Ingram et al. 1970), a lower verbal than performance IQ and greater difficulty in perceptual or general academic functions (Burks 1957), and finally a better clinical response to methylphenidate (Satterfield, Lesser, Saul, and Cantwell 1973) or nitrazepam (Fenelon, Holland, and Johnson 1972).

For particular EEG patterns, various correlations have been found for positive spikes, namely the improvement of the verbal and full scale IQ with the use of ethosuximide (Smith, Philippus, and Guard 1968), the greatest difference between the potential and actual achievement in reading, and finally high levels of tension or anxiety and also metabolic rate (Hughes and Park 1968). The absence of any correlations has also been reported (Muehl, Knott, and Benton 1965). For occipital slow waves, correlations have been reported with deafness and decreased photic responses (Hughes 1971), abnormal visuomotor performance (Pavy and Metcalfe 1965) and poor visual duction (Hughes and Park 1968). Diffuse or generalized EEG abnormalities have been correlated with behavior disorders (Stevens et al. 1968), low IQ and visuomotor deficits (Chiofalo, Bravo, Perez, and Villavicencio 1971) and finally retarded speech and motor development (Roudinesco et al. 1950). For epileptiform activity the relationships have been with defects in attention and ideation (Stevens et al. 1968), short attention span (Stores 1973; Green 1961), abnormal stereopsis (Hughes and Park 1968), spatial and verbal communication and writing disorders (Corcelle, Rozier, Dediur, Vincent, and Faure 1968), visual, and also oculomotor disorders, especially if the discharges were occipital in location (Lairy and Harrison 1968).

Frequency Analyses

The past literature has included the results of a frequency analysis of the rhythms recorded from dyslexics compared to normal controls. In dyslexics, Sklar, Hanley and Simmons (1972, 1973) found more 3–7/sec and 16–32/sec activity and less 9–14/sec rhythms at rest, but during reading less of the fast activity than in normals. Coherence function was also assessed and provided the most discriminating feature during reading in that greater coherence was seen within the same hemisphere in dyslexics and between symmetrical regions of both hemispheres in normals. Later (Hanley and Sklar 1976) the left parieto-occipital area was the area of emphasis in that dyslexics showed peaks at 6, 17, 20 and 24/sec without well developed alpha activity especially on that region. Coherence functions again played a role in discriminating the dyslexics as did 3–7/sec activity, and the appearance of 6/sec and disappearance of 18/sec rhythm during reading.

More recent studies have added details to these latter findings. Colon, Notermans, deWeerd, and Kap (1979) compared 44 dyslexics to 49 normal controls, 7–11 years of age with normal IQs. The normal 8-year olds showed more 10–11/sec activity on the central-occipital areas, and the 9-year olds more 11/sec rhythms on the fronto-central areas, similar to mu waves, but the dyslexics in the 10–11 year old group showed an increase in 3–6/sec activity on the temporal areas. This latter increase in theta rhythm in dyslexics was similar to the findings of Sklar et al. (1972, 1973). Even more recently, Fein, Galin, Johnstone, Yingling, Marcus, and Kiersch (1983) compared 31 dyslexics and 32 normals with normal IQs. They found that the absolute power was as reliable as the relative power in the different frequency bands and this reliability of both absolute and relative power in the eyes open and closed condition established a strong empirical basis supporting the use of EEG spectra in assessing the brain function of dyslexics, compared to normals.

All of these studies on EEG have indicated that this routine, uncomplicated test has enough to offer, even without complex spectral analyses, so that the standard EEG should be utilized, at least as a screen, when future studies on dyslexia are planned. Too many significant correlations have been found to disregard this test, although in the wake and sleep EEG we can hope to find significant abnormality in less than one-half of these patients. Frequency analysis offers one more level of sophistication to uncover further differences between the dyslexic and the normal child.

Visual Evoked Potentials (VEP)

Neurophysiologists have found that significant information can be obtained not only from sampling the resting rhythms from the brain, but also from engaging the nervous system in a response to a stimulus. Thus, much can be learned about brain function from the analysis of the visual evoked potential. The past literature includes the report that depressed photic responses on the left side, found during standard EEGs, appeared more often in underachievers than in control groups (Hughes 1971). Conners (1970) reported specifically on poor readers and claimed that the low amplitude of a late wave VI from the left parietal area showed the highest correlation with reading achievement. These studies were criticized on the basis of an inappropriate reference electrode (Kooi 1972), but O'Malley and Conners (1972) later claimed success with the attempt to increase the amplitude of this late wave by alpha feedback training. Later, another study (Preston, Guthrie, and Childs 1974) was published showing a lower amplitude of the VEP not at 600 msec but at 180 msec in the dyslexic group.

More recent studies have served to complicate the VEP picture. On the one hand, Cohen's results (1980) may be considered confirmatory in that he reported a smaller amplitude of the positivity at 200 msec on the occipital area and a longer latency on the temporal area for dyslexics, but he found no evidence for a difference between the dominant (left) and non-dominant (right) hemisphere. He concluded that these studies demonstrated a neurophysiological dysfunction in the processing of visual information in dyslexics.

While the earlier studies placed emphasis on the *late* VEP response, Symman-Louett, Gascon, Matsumiya, and Lombroso (1977) found the major difference between the dyslexics and normals was not in the late but in the *early* components within the first 200 msec. Normals, compared to the dyslexics, showed more early components at all electrode sites, but especially on the left superior and inferior parietal areas where statistical significance was achieved. The dyslexics showed more late components, but none achieved statistical significance. Also, on the central vertex and occipital areas the responses were more similar in the two groups. In the dyslexics with fewer early components, the left and right parietal areas were at times similar, so the authors speculated that these patients may at times have a biparietal abnormality. This finding contributed to the general conclusion that in dyslexia it is likely that there are multiple independent defects and there is no single VEP component from a single location to be determined only by a given task. One other finding was that the dyslexics showed a negativity at 175 msec on the left parietal area, which may or may not have been similar to the negativity in the normals appearing at 120 msec.

Confirmation of the earlier studies was not found in the work of Sobotka and May (1977). These investigators reported a finding opposite to Conners and to Preston et al., viz., that dyslexics, compared to normals, showed a significantly *larger* amplitude on the parietal area of the P_1–N_1 wave and on the occipital area of N_1–P_2 wave. However, the right side did show higher amplitudes than the left, but this finding was true for both the dyslexics and their controls. Normals showed a correlation between the reaction time and the latency of P_2 on both the right parietal and occipital areas, but the dyslexics failed to demonstrate any significant relationship. In addition, no significant correlation was found between these VEP measures and any one of the eight psychometric test scores used. The authors finally concluded that VEP amplitude and asymmetry per se were *not* reliable correlates of dyslexia. Furthermore, they pointed out that amplitude relationships are dependent on whether the measure is peak to trough (theirs) or base to peak (Conners) and also are dependent on whether the stimulus is relevant and attended. Thus, VEP amplitude should be measured both ways, to attended and also ignored stimuli, with behavioral measurements concurrently recorded as a way to evaluate attention as an important factor in dyslexia.

Another group had previously found not a lower, but a higher amplitude of the VEP in a patient group, compared to normal controls. Buchsbaum and Wender (1973) reported an average amplitude of the N_{140}—P_{200} as 17.5 μV in normals, compared to the large 21.4 μV in the child with minimal brain dysfunction. One other finding to increase the complexity of all of these results was that the P_{200} wave generally showed a shorter latency and an increasing latency with the highest intensities in the patients with disabilities, compared to the normals, whose latency decreased with increasing stimulus intensity.

Nearly all permutations and combinations of results have thus been reported in the VEP of the dyslexic. This variability and apparent inconsistency of results might dissuade others from attempting to resolve how the VEP of the dyslexic under different stimulating conditions is different from the normal. However, reading is a visual task and the VEP would seem to be one of the most relevant experimentally controlled tests that can be administered. The literature has now made clear that many variables must be considered in order to properly evaluate the VEP differences between dyslexics and normals. Not only are different stimulating conditions important, but also different recording sites and each of the many wavelets constituting the early and also the late aspect of the total response need to be considered.

Auditory Evoked Potentials (AEP)

Only a few studies have dealt with the auditory sphere in dyslexic patients whose primary problem would seem to be visual. Satterfield et al. (1973) studied children with minimal brain dysfunction in general without indicating a specific dyslexia and reported a lower amplitude and longer latency in the AEP of these patients. More recently, Cohen (1980) reported an average amplitude of 12.8 μV in dyslexics, similar to the 14.2 μV in normals, dealing especially with the wavelets N_{127} and P_{206}. The report of Chuden and Weinmann (1975, 1980) on evoked response audiometry indicated a biphasic summation curve with two negative deflections in some dyslexics. The authors speculated whether this biphasic appearance demonstrated a competition between the right and left hemispheres or whether there was a failure to transmit acoustic information from each ear to the central auditory regions. Thus, the literature on the AEP neither gives hope nor despair that future studies on auditory evoked potentials will be rewarding. However, the logic behind an emphasis on visual, rather than auditory evoked potentials, in a visual disorder is clear. On the other hand, the processing of associative elaboration responses could represent a major problem in dyslexics and then the later components of *any* evoked potential could possibly reveal relevant findings.

Event Related Potentials (ERP)

The ERP refers to very late responses that depend to a great extent upon the informational content of the stimulus or the psychological state of the patient. Perhaps the most carefully studied is the contingent negative variation (CNV), which seems to be related to the psychological variable of expectancy.

CNV

The early literature on CNV includes the studies of Dykman, Ackerman, Clements, and Peters (1971) who reported a reduced response in children with learning disabilities or dyslexia, although these findings were not confirmed two years later by another group (Low and Stoilen 1973). Fenelon earlier (1968) reported a difficulty in obtaining a CNV in a few dyslexics; later, in 1976, Cohen also reported a reduced response in 41 children with learning disorders. More recently Cohen (1980) studied children specifically with dyslexia and reported a significant decrease in amplitude of their CNV at the vertex. The mean amplitude was 13.3 μV for dyslexics, compared to 21.9 μV for the normal controls; none of the 11 dyslexics, as opposed to 8 of 11 normals, showed amplitudes over 20μV. This decrease in CNV in the dyslexics was suggestive of a disorder of attention (Tecce 1972).

Other ERP

Fried, Tanguay, Boder, Doubleday, and Greensite (1981) have studied the ERP in dyslexics and normals to musical stimuli and also to words, finding a larger amplitude: (1) on the temporal-parietal than on frontal areas, (2) on the right than on the left hemisphere and (3) for musical stimuli than for words. Normals showed a larger musical ERP than the dyslexics and also a larger difference in latency between the responses to music and to words. The minority of the dyslexics showed a shorter latency to words than to music, while the majority of the normals demonstrated this difference. Waveform differences to the two stimuli were greater over the left than right hemispheres in normals and also in some dyslexics. However, in some other (dysphonetic) dyslexics there was no word-music waveform difference on the left hemisphere, leading to the speculation that the dominant left side had not fully developed the capacity to process auditory information in a normal manner. Thus, it was as if these individuals essentially had no left cortex, but instead had two right hemispheres.

One further ERP study (Lovrich and Stamm 1983) has been reported on dyslexics. The event related potential to tone pips was investigated in 13 retarded readers and 13 normals. No major group differences were found in the variability of responses, but the poor readers showed on the central-parietal areas less of a difference at 540 msec between responses to attended vs. nonattended signals. Thus, the expected enhancement of the late (positive) components to attended signals did not appear in some of these poor readers. Cortical processing of the stimulus did not differ between the groups until long (540 msec) after stimulus onset. Since the greater negativity to attended vs. nonattended stimuli at 400 msec was similar for the poor and normal readers, the authors concluded that there were no deficiencies in selective attention, as indexed by the ERP to tone pips. Instead, they suggested that the retarded readers processed the task-relevant information in a *different manner* than the normal readers and that this processing was likely less efficient and effective.

These latter studies have emphasized that the dyslexic has more than a problem of attention and that processing of the information hundreds of milliseconds after the simulus is apparently ineffective and inefficient. Further work in this area is clearly justified.

Present Progress in the Neurophysiological Studies on Dyslexia

Two groups have surveyed the literature on the electrophysiological correlates in dyslexia and have proceeded in similar directions to further define the neurophysiological changes in this disorder. They have understood the inadequacy of a few electrodes from a few regions, recording only during a resting state without any stimuli, and looking only for some intermixed patterns of activity that are judged abnormal by commonly used criteria of the clinical electroencephalographer. Instead, these two teams have realized the need to record from all scalp electrodes, with different types of meaningful and meaningless stimuli, but especially analyzed against a computer-based bank of normal values for a given age and for the special set of stimulating conditions.

E.R. John and colleagues—''Neurometrics''

Dr. John and his colleagues (John 1977; Prichep, John, Ahn, and Kaye 1983) have developed a technology—neurometrics—intended to increase the sensitivity and extend the utility of electrophysiological assessment into the domain of sensory, perceptual, and cognitive functions. The authors state that this assessment quantifies features extracted objectively from both the EEG and from multimodal evoked potentials, elicited in different test conditions, and that this technique describes brain dysfunctions in terms of statistically significant deviations from age-related normative values. They utilize a ''Neurometric Test Battery,'' delivered by a microprocessor system that controls the stimulator and sets up 58 different standardized conditions as challenges to a wide variety of brain functions. The data are stored in a digital format with digitally encoded protocols for subsequent automatic retrieval and data analysis. The analysis system involves a logarithmic (or other) transformation to achieve Gaussian distribution and then a Z transformation of each feature extracted from the data, relative to age-appropriate normative values. This statistic provides an objective probability that the observed measure might be obtained from a normally functioning individual of the same age as the patient. The Z-transform is the number of standard deviations by which an individual observation differs from the mean of a reference set.

The features extracted from the EEG include frequency analysis with both absolute and relative power for delta, theta, alpha, and beta frequency bands for each of 8 different bipolar derivations. Also included are percentage of power asymmetry for each frequency band, and finally, coherence, reflecting the degree of wave shape symmetry and synchrony between bilateral derivations for each frequency band.

The measures extracted from the evoked potentials (EPs), elicited by a variety of visual and auditory stimuli, include responses from all electrodes of the 10–20 International System. The variance is computed within each 10 msec latency-interval for 500 msec after stimulus onset. From the raw data quantitative features are extracted: (1) signal strength and signal-to-noise ratios for early, middle, and long latency periods, which may approximate sensory, perceptual, and cognitive processes, respectively; (2) asymmetry of symmetrical electrodes, as seen by the bilateral difference wave; (3) a morphology description, which evaluates the accuracy with which the individual EPs can be reconstructed as a combination of standard factor wave shapes; (4) signal-to-noise ratio of the difference wave between stimulus conditions to assess the significance of differences between EPs elicited from the same electrode by different visual or auditory patterns.

A normative data base has been constructed on 600 normally functioning children, 6–16 years of age. From the criteria similar to Matoušek and Petersén (1973) John and colleagues selected 306 "nonrisk" children, used to calculate age norms for all EEG and EP measures. The computer program also has an automatic artifact rejection, which was tested for validity by comparing the computer selected data to human edited data from 10 records. Consistently high correlations of 0.93 for spectral measures and 0.90 for coherence and power asymmetry established the program as reasonably solid.

The test-retest reliability then compared within session and between session intervals. All test-retest correlations were significant and the average correlation for relative power was 0.83, 0.70, and 0.69 for the short, medium, and long interest intervals, respectively.

These investigators then developed regression equations to describe maturational changes in the EEG. First, they transformed previously published normative tables (Matoušek and Petersén 1973) into regression equations for each measure for each electrode derivation. Fourth degree polynomial functions yielded a satisfactory fit for all measures in this age range. Then, their own group of 306 children was divided into split-half subgroups and an independent set of regression equations was derived. First-order linear equations described these data well. Finally, the data from both groups were compared and it was found that first-order linear equations could describe both groups. Thus, these equations appear to constitute a first approximation to a description of the rules governing the maturation of EEG parameters in the normal healthy human brain.

Generality was established by comparing the data from the United States to those from outside this country, (e.g., Barbados) and no differences were found in 31 of 32 EEG measures.

The next step was to study three different broadly defined groups: (1) patients at risk for neurological disorders such as seizures (474); (2) learning disability (LD) children with generalized disabilities (143); and (3) LD children with specific learning difficulties (163). The significance of difference in the Z values between each of these three groups and the normal children was tested. All three groups showed incidence of deviant values, ranging from 4–44%. In order to avoid false-positives regarding brain dysfunction, the threshold for inferring probable dysfunction was considered twice the number of significant values expected by chance. Using this criterion the incidence of children with "hits" beyond threshold at the p<0.05 level was 54–58% for the three groups and at the <0.01 level was 46–48%. The false positives in the normal children were then only 4% with these criteria.

John and his collegues then studied more specific disabilities, comparing normals (N) to verbal underachievers (VU) (mainly dyslexics), arithmetic underachievers (AU), and a mixed (M) group. The data clearly showed that children with different patterns of underachievement have different neurometric profiles. The VU group had VEP amplitude differences at 200–350 msec, especially on the left parietal and central areas, reminiscent of the data mentioned in the previous section. Unfortunately, the direction of difference was not specified. The AU showed excess theta on the parieto-occipital areas and had VEP amplitude differences at 200–350 msec, predominantly on the right parietal and central areas. The M group showed excessive delta and theta on the posterior regions and had VEP amplitude differences at 100–200 msec on both sides, more on the left central temporal area. The majority of significant differences in these groups appeared in two latency domains, 100–200 msec and 200–300 msec, presumably related to perceptual and cognitive processes, respectively.

The next study involved separating groups based on their neurometric profiles. Five groups were selected: (1) theta excess and LD; (2) delta excess and LD; (3) auditory EP asymmetry and LD; (4) neurometrically normal but LD; (5) neurometrically normal and normally functioning. All children were given five behavioral tasks, including the Wechsler Intelligence Scale for Children, Trail-Making Test, etc. Performance on behavioral tests separated the children along lines correlated with neurometric abnormality. The *theta* excess group showed poor performance on those tasks requiring sustained attention, especially deficits in reaction times and digit span. The *delta* excess group showed deficits in digit span and errors on the Trail-Making Test. The *EP asymmetry* group showed proportionately more errors on the Color-Naming and Trail-Making tests and longer digit span times.

Additional studies especially relevant to dyslexia have been performed by John and his colleagues. One group of children who consistently reversed letters, like b and d, were classified according to (1) lateral errors (b-d), (2) vertical errors (b-p), (3) errors in *verbal* response to *visual* stimulus and (4) errors in *written* response to an *auditory* stimulus. Each group showed some dysfunction on the parieto-occipital area, but distinct differences were also found among the groups. Patterns of abnormalities in the relative power within various frequency bands, presence or absence of asymmetries, and the additional involvement of temporal regions were found to be correlated with specific types of errors in letter reversal. Thus, there were different neurometric EEG profiles correlated with various types of reversal problems, according to these investigators.

Although John and his colleagues have not studied pure dyslexia per se, they have carefully investigated children with learning disabilities, including dyslexia. Most importantly, they have set up a technique called neurometrics as an objective, reliable method for recording and analyzing brain electrical activity; this technique has great promise for investigating disorders like dyslexia. The measures appear to be independent of cultural or ethnic background. Features in the EEG and EP are extracted and quantified and for each feature the probability of deviation from normal is statistically determined. An individual neurometric profile can be constructed for each patient, describing the statistically deviant measures and the regions in which they deviate from normative values. Using these measures, only very few normally functioning children have significant deviations from expected values and there is a high incidence of significant deviations in children with LD. Finally, with respect to differential diagnosis of the heterogenous group called "learning disabled," a variety of specific neurometric profiles seems to be correlated with specific behavioral dysfunctions. Clearly, this technique needs to be applied to many children, specifically those with dyslexia.

F. H. Duffy and Associates—BEAM

Another group has progressed beyond the older, traditional neurophysiological studies on dyslexia, to recording from all electrodes of the 10–20 International System, under many different conditions, and analyzing according to computer-based normal and matched controls. One extra step has been taken by this team in that their data are presented as continuously changing cartoons, representing evolving time after the presentation of the stimulus. Their technique is called brain electrical activity mapping or BEAM.

After recording the electrical activity to any given stimulus or in a resting condition, Duffy and his colleagues transform the data statistically to make visible that which might otherwise remain obscured. Their first transformation is called Significance Probability Mapping (SPM), involving a Z-transform statistic, to delineate regions in which brain electrical activity from an individual subject differs statistically from that of a reference population. These SPMs are primarily used in the delineation of abnormal *regions* during the clinical evaluation of BEAM images. Another manipulation is based upon the student's t-test statistic, used to delineate regional differences between two *groups* of subjects.

In assessing the BEAM images the clinician needs to determine whether a given focal finding indicates regional neuropathology or whether it falls close to or within the normal range of variation. The SPM aids here by showing the degree of deviation, but further judgment may be required as to when statistical abnormality indicates clinical abnormality. The grid sector analysis (GSA) is then used to measure the degree of abnormality. The GSA generates numbers from the numerical matrix underlying the SPM which describe the *degree* of diffuse or focal abnormality.

The first of two companion articles by Duffy, Denckla, Bartels, Sandini, and Kiessling (1980a, 1980b) dealt with eight children 9–11 years old with normal IQs but with dyslexia-pure (Hughes and Denckla 1978), at least with 1.5 years below expected reading levels. Matched normal controls were included in the study. For the EEG, there were 10 different states or conditions, such as speech, music, reading, etc. and for the evoked potentials, VEPs to flash and AEPs to clicks and to different words were recorded.

From the EEG data dyslexics usually showed alpha distributions that were less state dependent and tended to have invariant maxima on the midline or over the left hemisphere. On the medial frontal region, the dyslexics showed activity, different from their controls, only on the left during the conditions of (1) speech, (2) paired associates—instruction, and (3) eyes open. Different activity was seen bilaterally during the conditions of (1) paired associates—testing and (2) reading task—instruction. Also, differences were found on the left mid-temporal area during speech, eyes open and closed, and on the left anterior frontal area during Kimura figures testing. In general, differences between the groups indicated higher mean *alpha* for the dyslexics, suggesting a relative cortical inactivation. For *theta* rhythms between groups, differences were found on the left anterior frontal area for the Kimura figures—instruction. The reading task—instruction showed marked differences on the left mid-temporal area and the left medial and right anterior frontal areas. Also, a difference was noted on the right posterior parietal area during eyes closed. In general, the differences between the groups indicated *higher* mean theta values for the dyslexic children.

The EP also demonstrated differences. For the VEP, a difference was seen at 282 msec with positivity for the dyslexics and negativity for normals; for the AEP, differences appeared at 114, 198, and 342 msec, usually positive for dyslexics and negative for normals. For the AEP to two similar but different words, differences were seen at six latencies from 78 to 186 msec, usually with the dyslexics demonstrating opposite polarity to the normal. The differences were mainly on the left temporal-parietal area.

In summary, this study showed that four different brain regions were distinctive in the dyslexic. These areas were the bilateral medial frontal region (near the supplementary motor area), the left anterior frontal area (near Broca's area) and the left mid-temporal area (the auditory associative area), all determined on the basis of EEG data, and finally the left posterolateral quadrant (Wernicke's area or the parietal and occipital-associative areas), from the EP data. Thus, these studies suggest that the condition of dyslexia-pure may represent a dysfunction within a complex and widely distributed cerebral system rather than involving a discrete lesion.

The next study performed by the Duffy group (Duffy et al. 1980b) followed directly and appropriately from the previous work. The purpose of the next study was to identify diagnostic criteria for dyslexia from BEAM measurements and then to test these criteria on previously unevaluated subjects to establish validity.

First, diagnostic rules were developed on the data gathered from one group of dyslexics and their matched controls from the previous study and then these rules were tested by similar data gathered from an additional group (with only three dyslexics and three normals). Each subject was characterized by measurements from topographic maps of his brain electrical activity under many different conditions and 183 features were obtained during different specific states. The next task was to reduce the number of features from 183 to a significant few. The remaining features were subject to multivariate and classic discriminant analysis. These procedures led to the development of rules for diagnosing subjects as either normal or dyslexic.

The particular results include the 183 measurements, reduced to 55 that were statistically significant, then reduced to 24 best features. The 10 best features were used to represent each subject in multivariate analysis and finally a linear discriminant function analysis demonstrated a significant ($p = 0.0035$) group separation between dyslexics and normals, using these 10 features. Then, with both EEG and EP data, utilized in stepwise linear discriminant function analyses, the combined use of EEG and EP was found to be superior to the separate use of the two, although EP was generally better than the EEG. Finally, nine putative features were developed to diagnose dyslexics, including four from the AEP, one from VEP, three with theta and one with alpha rhythms. The diagnostic success using these criteria to diagnose dyslexia was over 80%. With a clustering program Duffy and his colleagues used only two features, the AEP to different words on the right posterior region and left central-parietal areas and found a diagnostic success rate of about 90% (10/11). These data represent the beginning of real progress in determining the neurophysiological correlates of dyslexia.

Future Direction of Electrophysiological Studies in Dyslexia

The success of John and his colleagues and of Duffy and his colleagues argue strongly for the use of their type of approach in future research efforts. Many different stimulus conditions need to be employed, both resting and evoked activity are important. Computer analysis is needed, especially since the activity from the dyslexic needs to be compared region by region, millisecond to millisecond against computer-based normative values. Very elegant but extremely complex statistical manipulations have been performed by both groups and these maneuvers are justified to determine the most diagnostic features in the electrophysiological correlates of the dyslexic. However, these Bayesian boundaries, stepwise linear discriminant function analyses, Mahalonobis distances, and multivariate analyses must be translated and simplified into the clearest of diagnostic rules to be used by the clinical neurophysiologist in the field. Otherwise, the results are distinctive to one particular study using one set of complex statistical manipulations, never to be replicated or verified by any other investigator or group of researchers.

Particular questions remain, acknowledged by Duffy and his group, who understand that their results do not yet justify full clinical application. Further work is needed to show the relative specificity that would permit dyslexia to be diagnosed as distinct from other kinds of learning disability. Thus, large volumes of data should be gathered from a variety of learning disorders, including dyslexia. A great deal of further work needs to be done on both sensitivity and specificity, especially utilizing many different kinds of stimuli that will help to specify dyslexia as opposed to other kinds of learning disability. These developments should lead to further delineation of the diagnostic rules directed at dyslexia for possible early and objective detection of this disorder. With these rules, subgroups of dyslexia might be found to exist and these data will also help to determine if the condition represents a developmental lag or some special pathophysiological state.

References

Aird, R. B., and Gastaut, Y. 1959. Occipital and posterior electroencephalographic rhythms. *Electroencephalography Clinical Neurophysiology* 11:637–656.

Anderson, W. 1963. The hyperkinetic child: A neurological appraisal. *Neurology* 13:968–973.

Black, F. W. 1972. EEG and birth abnormalities in high and low-perceiving reading retarded children. *Journal of Genetic Psychology* 121:327–32.

Bosaeus, E., and Selldén, U. 1979. Psychiatric assessment of healthy children with various EEG patterns. *Acta Psychiatrica Scandinavicia* 59:180–210.

Buchsbaum, M., and Wender, P. 1973. Average evoked responses in normal and minimally brain dysfunctioned children treated with amphetamine: A preliminary report. *Archives of General Psychiatry* 29:764–770.

Burks, H. F. 1957. The effect on learning of brain pathology. *Exceptional Children* 24:169–174.

Capute, A. J., Niedermeyer, E. F. L., and Richardson, F. 1968. The electroencephalogram in children with minimal cerebral dysfunction. *Pediatrics* 41:1104–1114.

Chiofalo, N., Bravo, L., Perez, M., and Villavicencio, C. 1971. El electroencefalograma en ninos con trastornos del aprendizaje. *Acta Neurologica Latina Americana* 17:164–171.

Chuden, H. G., and Weinmann, H. M. 1975. ERA and dichotic test by Feldmann of dyslexic children. *Archives of Otorhinolaryngology* 209:97–105.

Chuden, H. G., and Weinmann, H. M. 1980. The biphasic response in ERA. *Archives of Otorhinolaryngology* 228:43–50.

Cohen, J. 1976. Learning disabilities and conditional brain activity. *In* R. Karrer (ed.). *Developmental Psychophysiology of Mental Retardation*. Springfield, Ill., Charles C Thomas.

Cohen, J. 1980. Cerebral evoked responses in dyslexic children. *Progress in Brain Research* 54:502–6.

Colon, E. J., Notermans, S. L. H., deWeerd, J. P. C., and Kap, J. 1979. The discriminating role of EEG power spectra in dyslexic children. *Journal of Neurology* 221(4):257–262.

Conners, C. K. 1970. Cortical visual evoked response in children with learning disorders. *Psychophysiology* 7:418–428.

Corcelle, L., Rozier, J., Dediur, E., Vincent, J. D., and Faure, L. 1968. Variations of cortical evoked potentials according to the modality of sensory stimulation in dyslexic children. *Review of Laryngoscopy (Bordeaux)* 89:458–468.

Duffy, F. H., Denckla, M. B., Bartels, P. H., and Sandini, G. 1980a. Dyslexia: Regional differences in the brain electrical activity by topographic mapping. *Annals of Neurology* 7(5):412–420.

Duffy, F. H., Denckla, M. B., Bartels, P. H., Sandini, G., and Kiessling, L. S. 1980. Dyslexia: Automated diagnosis by computerized classification of brain electrical activity. *Annals of Neurology* 7:421–428.

Dykman, R. A., Ackerman, P. T., Clements, S. C., and Peters, J. R. 1971. Specific learning disabilities: An attentional deficit syndrome. *In* H. R. Myklebust (ed.). *Progress in Learning Disabilities* (Vol. II, pp. 56–93). New York: Grune & Stratton.

Dykman, R. A., Holcomb, P. J., Ackerman, P. T., and McCray, D. S. 1983. Auditory ERP augmentation—reduction and methylphenidate dosage needs in attention and reading disorders of children. *Psychiatric Research* 9:255–269.

Fein, G., Galkin, D., Johnstone, J., Yingling, C. D., Marcus, M., and Kiersch, M. E. 1983. EEG power spectra in normal and dyslexic children. I. Reliability during passive conditions. *Electro-encephalography and Clinical Neurophysiology* 55(4):399–405.

Fenelon, B. 1968. Expectancy waves and other complex cerebral events in dyslexic and normal subjects. *Psychonomic Science* 13:253–254.

Fenelon, B., Holland, J. R., and Johnson, C. 1972. Spatial organization of the EEG in children with reading disabilities: A study using nitrazepam. *Cortex* 8:444–464.

Fried, I., Tanguay, P. E., Boder, E., Doubleday, C., and Greensite, M. 1981. Development of dyslexia: Electrophysiological evidence of clinical subgroups. *Brain and Language* 12(1):14–22.

Gerson, I. M., Barnes, T. C., Mannino, A., Fanning, J. M., and Burns, J. J. 1972. EEG of children with various learning problems. I. Outpatient study. *Diseases of the Nervous System* 33:170–177.

Green, J. B. 1961. Association of behavior disorder with an EEG focus in children without seizures. *Neurology* 11:337–344.

Hanley, J., and Sklar, B. 1976. Electroencephalographic correlates of developmental reading dyslexics: Computer analysis of recordings from normal and dyslexic children. *In* G. Leisman (ed.). *Basic Visual Process and Learning Disability.* Springfield, Ill.: Charles C Thomas.

Hughes, J. R. 1971. Electoencephalography and learning disabilities. *In* H. R. Myklebust (ed.). *Progress in Learning Disabilities (Vol. 2).* New York: Grune and Stratton.

Hughes, J. R. 1978. Electroencephalographic and neurophysiological studies in dyslexia. *In* A. L. Benton and D. Pearl (eds.). *Dyslexia: An Appraisal of Current Knowledge.* New York: Oxford University Press.

Hughes, J. R. 1983. Review of the positive spike phenomenon. *In* J. R. Hughes and W. A. Wilson (eds.). *EEG and Evoked Potentials in Psychiatry and Behavioral Neurology.* London and Boston: Butterworths.

Hughes, J. R., and Denckla, M. B. 1978. Outline of a pilot study of electroencephalographic correlates of dyslexia. *In* A. L. Benton and D. Pearl (eds.). *Dyslexia: An Appraisal of Current Knowledge.* New York: Oxford University Press.

Hughes, J. R., and Park, G. E. 1968. The EEG in dyslexia. *In* P. Kellaway and I. Petersen (eds.). *Clinical Electroencephalography of Children.* Stockholm: Almqvist and Wiksell.

Ingram, T. T. S., Mason, A. W., and Blackburn, I. 1970. A retrospective study of 82 children with reading disability *Developmental Medicine and Child Neurology* 12:271–281.

Jasper, H. H., Bradley, C., and Solomon, P. 1938. EEG analysis of behavior problem children. *American Journal of Psychiatry* 95:641–658.

John, E. R. 1977. *Functional Neuroscience: Clinical Application of Quantitative Electrophysiology.* Hillsdale, N. J.: Lawrence Erlbaum Associates.

Klinkerfuss, G. H., Lang, P. H., Weinberg, W. A., and O'Leary, J. L. 1965. EEG abnormalities of children with hyperkinetic behavior. *Neurology* (Minneapolis) 15;883–896.

Knobel, M., Wolman, M. D., and Mason, C. 1959. Hyperkinesia and organicity in children. *Archives of General Psychiatry* 1:310–321.

Kooi, K. A. 1972. Letter to the editor. *Psychophysiology* 9:154.

Lairy, G. C., and Harrison, A. 1968. Functional aspects of EEG foci in children: Clinical data and longitudinal studies. *In* P. Kellaway and I. Petersen (eds). *Clinical Electroencephalography of Children.* Stockholm: Almqvist and Wiksell.

Lovrich, D., and Stamm, J. S. 1983. Event-related potential and behavior correlates of attention in reading retardation. *Journal Clinical Neuropsychology* 5(1):13–37,

Low, M. D., and Stoilen, L. 1973. CNV and EEG in children: Maturational characteristics and findings in the UCS syndrome. *In* W. C. McCallum and J. R. Knott (eds.). *Event Related Slow Potentials and Behavior.* Electroencephalography and Clinical Neurophysiology, Suppl. 33.

Matoušek, M., and Petersén, I. 1973. Frequency analysis of the EEG in normal children and adolescents. *In* P. Kellaway and I. Petersén (eds.). *Automation of Clinical Electroencephalography.* New York: Raven, 1973.

Muehl, S., Knott, J. R., and Benton, A. L. 1965. EEG abnormality and psychological test performance in reading disability. *Cortex* 1:434–440.

O'Malley, J. E., and Conners, C. K. 1972. The effect of unilateral alpha training on visual evoked response in a dyslexic adolescent. *Psychophysiology* 9:467–470.

Pavy, R., and Metcalfe, J. 1965. The abnormal EEG in childhood communication and behavior abnormalities. *Electroencephalography and Clinical Neurophysiology* 19:414.

Petersén, I., and Eeg-Olofsson, O. 1971. The development of the electroencephalogram in normal children from the age of 1 through 15 years—non-paroxysmal activity. *Neuropediatries* 2:247–304.

Preston, M., Guthrie, J. T., and Childs, B. 1974. Visual evoked response in normal and disabled readers. *Psychophysiology* 11:452–457.

Prichep, L., John, E. R., Ahn, H., and Kaye, H. 1983. Neurometrics: Quantitative evaluation of brain dysfunction in children. *In* M. Rutter (ed.) *Developmental Neuropsychiatry.* London: Guilford.

Roudinesco, J., Trélat, J., and Trélat, M. 1950. Étude de quarante cas de dylexie d'évolution. *Enfance* 3:1–32.

Satterfield, J. H., Lesser, L. I., Saul, R. E., and Cantwell, D. P. 1973. EEG aspects in the diagnosis and treatment of minimal brain dysfunction. *In* F. F. de la Cruz, B. H. Fox, and R. H. Robert (eds.) *Annals of the New York Academy of Sciences (Minimal Brain Dysfunction)* 205:274–282.

Sklar, B., Hanley, J., and Simmons, W. W. 1972. An EEG experiment aimed toward identifying dyslexic children. *Nature* (London) 241:414–416.

Sklar, B., Hanley, J., and Simmons, W. W. 1973. A computer analysis of EEG spectral signatures from normal and dyslexic children. *Institute of Electronics and Electrical Engineering Transactions of Biomedical Engineering* 20:20–26.

Smith, W. L., Philippus, M. J., and Guard, H. L. 1968. Psychometric study of children with learning problems and 14–6 positive spike EEG patterns, treated with ethosuximide (Zarontin) and placebo. *Archives of Diseases in Childhood* 43:616–619.

Sobotka, K. R., and May, J. G. 1977. Visual evoked potentials and reaction time in normal and dyslexic children. *Psychophysiology* 14:18–24.

Stevens, J. R., Sachdev, K., and Milstein, V. 1968. Behavior disorders of childhood and the electroencephalogram. *Archives of Neurology* 18:160–177.

Stores, G. 1973. Studies of attention and seizure disorders. *Developmental Medicine and Child Neurology* 15:376–382.

Symann-Louett, N., Gascon, G. G., Matsumiya, Y., and Lombroso, C. T. 1977. Wave form difference in visual evoked responses between normal and reading disabled children. *Neurology* (Minneap.) 27:156–159.

Tecce, J. J. 1972. Contingent negative variation (CNN) and psychological processes in man. *Psychological Bulletin* 77:73–108.

Torres, F., and Ayers, F. W. 1968. Evaluation of the electroencephalogram of dyslexic children. *Electroencephalography and Clinical Neurophysiology* 24:281–294.

Volterra, V., and Giordani, L. 1966. Considerazioni electrocliniche su 193 soggetti con EEG caratterizzato da punte e punte-onda in regione occipitale. *Geornali Di Psichiatria and Di Neuropatologia* 94:337–373.

7

Electrophysiological Studies of Reading-Disabled Children: In Search of Subtypes

David Wm. Shucard, Katharine R. Cummins,
Elizabeth Gay, Judy Lairsmith, and Phillip Welanko

$\mathcal{G}$n this chapter we will describe some of our findings that have been obtained from electrophysiological studies of cerebral functional specialization in reading-disabled and normal readers. This work represents a component of the Colorado Reading Project (see DeFries, Olson, and Decker and Vandenberg chapters in this volume).

Cerebral Specialization of Function and Reading Disability

The notion that the two cerebral hemispheres of the human brain are specialized for qualitatively different types of information processing has been fairly well substantiated from anatomical, clinical, behavioral, and neuro-physiological evidence. Areas of the left hemisphere, in most right-handed individuals, are believed to play a significant role in language comprehension and production and in analytical information processing. Areas of the right hemisphere appear to be more specialized for tasks that require spatial and holistic processing. (See Broca 1865; Wernicke 1874; Geschwind and Levitsky 1968; Geschwind 1976; Wada, Clark, and Hamm 1975; and Sperry 1973 for clinical and anatomical evidence: see Kimura 1973; Kimura, and Durnford 1974; Kinsbourne 1972; and Galin and Ornstein 1974 for behavioral evidence: see Morrell and Salamy 1971; Molfese, Freeman, and Palermo 1975; Doyle, Ornstein, and Galin 1974; Galin and Ellis 1975; Friedman, Simson, Ritter, and Rapin 1975; Shucard, Shucard, and Thomas 1977; and Galin 1979 for electro-

This work was supported in part by NICHD Grant HD11681.

We are grateful to John Hill and Deborah Minarick for their technical assistance with data collection and Dr. David G. Thomas and Janet Shucard for their valuable comments.

physiological evidence: see Galin 1974; and Nebes 1974 for more general reviews.)

A number of different deficits and models that emphasize brain dysfunction have been proposed to account for the symptomatology of dyslexia. For example, Duane (1979) in a review of the literature, cited the following: malformed or malfunctioning angular gyrus, impaired cerebral dominance, delayed cerebral maturation, cerebral biochemical imbalance, impaired sensorimotor integration, environmental toxins, nutritional deficiency, and pre, peri, or postnatal cerebral insult. In addition, a critical evaluation of the literature pertaining to major etiological explanations of dyslexia led Vellutino (1977) to conclude that dyslexia is caused by specific deficits in aspects of linguistic functioning and/or verbal processing.

Findings pertaining to the functional organization of the human brain and in particular, cerebral specialization of function, suggest that at least some poor readers may be distinguished from normal readers by the degree to which functions are lateralized, by peculiarities in their pattern of lateralization (e.g., bilateral language representation), by some dysfunction within a cerebral hemisphere, or by a disturbance in normal interhemispheric transfer of information (e.g., Orton 1928). Literature reviews of behavioral and electrophysiological studies of cerebral specialization and cerebral functioning that compare normal and reading-disabled children have concluded that there does seem to be a consistent tendency for deviant cerebral organization and poor reading to appear together (see Benton 1975; Rourke 1978; Hughes 1978; Denckla 1978; Conners 1978).

Models of Dyslexia that Focus on Cerebral Specialization. A number of models of dyslexia have as their focus cerebral specialization of function. For example, Satz and Sparrow (1970) proposed that the failure "to acquire normal reading proficiency despite conventional instruction, sociocultural opportunity, average intelligence and freedom from gross sensory, emotional, or neurological handicap" (p. 17) is due to a delay in the development of left-hemispheric specialization. Masland (1975) emphasized left hemisphere dysfunction and argued that "the specific task of analysis of symbolic visually presented material is at some time transferred from the right to the left hemisphere" (p. 4). In other words, reading is an interhemispheric process. He suggested however, that the connections *within* hemispheres are more easily affected than connections *between* hemispheres and that overdevelopment of the right hemisphere impedes the functional development of the left hemisphere. Both of these models emphasize some abnormality of the left hemisphere.

Witelson's (1977a; 1977b) interference model is similar to that of Masland's in that both point to right hemisphere functions as being responsible for abnormal left hemisphere functioning. Witelson proposed that dyslexia may be associated with bihemispheric representation of spatial functions as opposed to right hemisphere specialization of spatial functions in normal children. Therefore, if the left hemisphere was more involved in spatial processing in dyslexics than in normal individuals, there would be *interference* with left hemisphere linguistic processes. This type of cerebral organization may contribute to a spatial holistic reading strategy that may be inefficient in learning to read phonetically coded languages like English.

Recently Bakker (1983) proposed two types of dyslexics, i.e., L-type and P-type. L-type readers may be sensitive to the linguistic aspects of text, whereas P-type readers may be more attuned to the perceptual features. This typology relies on the purported functional differences between the two cerebral hemispheres and a two-stage process when learning to read. According to Bakker, "the L-type dyslexic may rely on left-hemispheric strategies at too early a stage," whereas the P-type dyslexic "may fail to adapt such a strategy in time" (p. 504).

Other more functionally oriented models of reading disability, such as that of Boder (1973), have derived subgroups of reading disabilities (e.g., dysphonetic versus dyseidetic) that could conceivably correspond to individuals with different patterns of cerebral specialization. Further, the behavioral symptomatology present in at least some individuals who have difficulty with reading, coupled with the deficits seen in individuals with specific brain lesions suggests that at least a subset of the reading-disabled population may have a neurological disturbance related to a deficit or deficits in the functional organization of the brain. In support of this conjecture are the striking behavioral similarities observed between adults who acquire alexias and dyslexias through trauma or surgery and children who have a reading disability (see Hynd and Hynd 1984a; Bogen 1969; and Geschwind 1976).

In a recent review of neuroanatomical and neurolinguistic perspectives of dyslexia, Hynd and Hynd (1984a) presented a neurolinguistic model adapted and modified from Sevush (1983). This model describes major cortical regions thought to be involved in normal reading and identifies three different types of dyslexias (i.e., deep dyslexia, phonological dyslexia and surface dyslexia) each with a deficit in a specific part of the cortical reading pathway. Thus, this model relates the purported functional asymmetries of areas in the left and right cerebral hemispheres to the reading system, and deficits in specific cortical areas may result in subtypes of dyslexia.

As conceptualized by Luria (1966) and reviewed by Hynd and Hynd (1984b), a functional system of reading must exist in which visual stimuli are registered in the occipital cortex, associations are made cross-modally through the angular gyrus with information in the temporal region, and sharing occurs with Broca's area via the arcuate fasciculus. Therefore, a deficit within any of these regions could affect the individual's ability to read. The model proposed by Sevush (1983) above, is similar to this one in its conceptualization of reading difficulties. The processes involved in the functional system of reading correspond with those capacities for information processing believed to reside differentially in areas of the two cerebral hemispheres.

Behavioral Studies of Reading Disability and Cerebral Specialization. Behavioral studies of the relationship between cerebral specialization and reading disability have not led to clear conclusions. It is not certain whether tasks and measures used to date, such as dichotic listening (Bryden 1970), dichotomous haptic presentation of shapes (Witelson 1977a), and visual half-field presentations of various stimuli (Marcel, Katz, and Smith 1974; Yeni-Komshian, Isenberg, and Goldberg 1975), are even reliable indicators of cerebral specialization, let alone sensitive enough to be able to distinguish among *degrees* of cerebral specialization (Shankweiler and Studdert-Kennedy 1975; also see Schwartz and Kirsner 1984 for a critique of laterality indices). Rourke (1978) concluded that "the relationship between ear advantage, cerebral asymmetry, and disabilities in reading must, at least for the present, remain something of a mystery" (p. 159).

Although three studies that used visual half-field presentations (Witelson 1977a; Yeni-Komshian et al. 1975; Marcel and Rajan 1975) all indicated that there *are* differences in cerebral specialization between good and poor readers, the degree and type of differences reported are not consistent among the studies. In fact, studies that have used visual half-field presentations have come under strong criticism due to lack of control of the way subjects approached the task, failure to control the subjects' central fixation, failure to demonstrate that the same types of stimuli were recognized by normal and poor readers, failure to take into account strategy differences between normal and poor readers, and failure to compare groups of normal and poor readers matched on reading ability (Young and Ellis 1981).

Previous behavioral studies, in general, relating cerebral specialization to reading disabilities have not taken into account a number of subject and task variables that are known to influence measures of cerebral specialization. These variables include: (1) whether subjects write with the hand ipsilateral or contralateral to the hemisphere specialized for language and verbal processing (see Milner, Branch, and Rasmussen 1966; Hughes 1978, for example), (2) the sex and age of the subjects (see Witelson 1977a; 1977b for a discussion of develomental sex differences in cerebral specialization), and (3) the demand the task places on the subject. This latter point is related to the level of activation, or loading, the task imposes on each cerebral hemisphere (see Kinsbourne 1970; Kinsbourne 1973; Hillige and Cox 1976; Friedman and Polson, 1981), and to the level and type of processing required by a given task (see Moscovitch, Scullion and Christie 1976; Morrison, Giordiani and Nagy 1977).

Electrophysiological Studies of Reading Disability and Cerebral Specialization. Earlier studies using electrophysiological measures to detect possible differences in brain functioning between reading-disabled and normal individuals have relied on two methods: the standard clinical electroencephalogram (EEG), and the event-related potential (ERP) to simple discrete stimuli such as tones and flashes. Hughes (1978) in a review of EEG and neurophysiological studies in reading disability, cited evidence for relationships that were obtained between various EEG patterns (e.g., positive spikes) and reading disability. In addition, based on studies by Sklar, Hanley, and Simmons (1972 and 1973) and the degree of synchronization of various EEG frequencies (alpha, beta, theta) within and between the cerebral hemispheres may be different in those individuals with reading disabilities. Many other relationships between EEG variables and poor reading have also been reported. For example, more occipital slow waves, diffuse abnormalities, and epileptiform activity have been seen in disabled readers as compared to normals (Hughes 1978).

In a critical review of the EEG literature related to reading disabilities, Conners (1978) pointed out a number of difficulties and methodological flaws with these studies, including non-blind readings of EEGs, improper or lack of matching of experimental and control samples, and the lack of consistent findings across studies with respect to either the locus or type of EEG abnormality associated with reading disability. Conners (1978) argued that there was little reliable evidence to support a conclusion that there is a greater incidence of EEG abnormalities among reading-disabled as compared to normals. More recently, Pirozzolo and Hansch (1982) suggested that EEG studies should be conducted under conditions of complex task involvement. This procedure would represent a step forward in the assessment of neuro-electric correlates of brain dysfunction in reading-disabled individuals. Hughes, in this volume, reviews the more recent findings from the EEG literature.

Event-related potential methods offer another means of directly measuring brain electrical events and thus another way of studying brain-behavior relationships in the reading-disabled. A number of event-related potential (ERP) studies showed differences between disabled readers and normals. For example, Conners (1971) reported visual event-related potential (VERP) amplitude attenuation in the left parietal area of reading-disabled individuals. In a study which examined left-right hemisphere responses, Preston, Guthrie, Kirsch, Gertman, and Childs (1977) reported larger VERP differences between words and flashes from the left parietal electrode (referenced to linked mastoids) for normals as compared to reading-disabled adults. Sobotka and May (1977) found an overall hemispheric VERP amplitude asymmetry to dim flashes in both occipital and parietal leads referenced to the vertex for both experimental and control subjects. However, the reading-disabled children, in contrast to the control sample, exhibited an *increased* amplitude to unattended stimuli and slower reaction time to attended stimuli.

In a study (Symann-Louett, Gascon, Matsumiya, and Lombrosco 1977) using visually presented discrete word stimuli, VERP wave form differences were obtained between disabled and normal readers. Although these differences were not statistically significant, normal readers were reported to exhibit more waves in the early components (<200 msec) recorded over the left superior and inferior parietal areas. Reading-disabled subjects appeared to show two peaks between 200 and 350 msec instead of the single one exhibited by the controls.

In reviewing this earlier ERP work, the following points are clear: (1) The findings have been inconsistent (see Preston et al. 1977; Weber and Omenn 1977; and Sobotka and May 1977); and (2) none of these studies has attempted to examine brain activity during the *ongoing* processing of complex information, such as verbal passages; they generally used simple stimuli such as light flashes, auditory tones, or discrete word stimuli to elicit the response.

With respect to the latter point, it has been strongly suggested by Conners (1978) and others, as well as Pirozzolo and Hansch (1982) for EEG studies, that the brain be actively challenged during recording. If the brain is actively challenged with stimuli, such as verbal input, that require higher level processing rather than simple clicks or flashes, for example, effects are more likely to show clearer localization of function, particularly over the angular gyrus (Conners 1978). Support for this approach comes from a report by Morrison, Giordiani, and Nagy (1977) whose results suggested that reading-disabled children showed no perceptual deficits for visual stimuli as compared to controls when the task involved only immediate, low level processing. However, the data did suggest that reading disability involves some problem in the processing of information in stages following the initial perception, perhaps with encoding, organizational, or retrieval skills. In addition, these investigators found that difficulties with higher level functioning are not limited to verbal material, since poor readers also performed poorly on tasks involving geometric and abstract forms. Thus, from these findings, it appears that *some* poor readers may also be deficient in other forms of perceptual, and perhaps memorial, processing. Lack of or improper integration of stimuli from different modalities (e.g., visual and auditory) may also be a factor in some poor readers (Rourke 1978).

In keeping with this notion of different etiological mechanisms in reading disability, Mattis, French, and Rapin (1975) proposed the presence of multiple independent deficits in higher cortical functioning as opposed to a single causal deficit for reading disability. This proposal was based on neuropsychological observations but, according to Symann-Louett et al. (1977), could be based on neurophysiological observations as well. Symann-Louett et al. (1977) proposed studying many aspects of the visual ERP, not just VERP components derived from a single recording site. In addition, they emphasized the importance of studying VERPs under different tasks in order to differentiate between normal versus disabled readers and within disabled readers themselves. Following these suggestions, Duffy, Denckla, Bartels, and Sandini (1980) and Duffy, Denckla, Bartels, Sandini, and Kiessling (1980) have described differences in topographic maps of the brain's electrical activity (EEG and ERP) between dyslexics and normals during both resting and non-resting conditions. Their findings indicated four distinct regions of difference between normal and dyslexic subjects: the medial frontal lobe, the left lateral frontal lobe, the left mid-temporal lobe, and the left posterior quadrant (including Wernicke's area, left posterior lobe, and left posterior parietal lobe). Consistent differences for auditory ERP measures were seen in the left posterior temporoparietal region. Because of their sample size they were unable to evaluate the possibility of subtypes in their population.

Most recently Johnstone, Galin, Fein, Yingling, Herron, and Marcus (1984) taking a multi-method approach that included a comprehensive battery of both electrophysiological and behavioral measures, reported findings obtained in a group of 34 control and 32 dyslexic 10-to-12 year old, right-handed boys. The data reported focused on VERPs obtained while subjects performed silent and oral reading at two levels of difficulty. Using a visual probe technique, Johnstone et al. (1984) obtained a number of interesting findings, including different patterns of VERP asymmetry during silent versus oral reading between the two groups. The difference in VERP asymmetry between normal and disabled readers was seen at the mid-temporal recording sites. With the probe procedure used in this study, *task-irrelevant* visual stimuli (pattern flashes) elicited the VERPs while subjects were performing the ongoing tasks. In this chapter we will describe results obtained with an auditory probe procedure used in our laboratory.

Summary

Although the behavioral and electrophysiological findings are somewhat inconsistent they are also encouraging. The inconsistency may be due to differences in methods as well as to heterogeneity within the reading-disabled population itself. It is obvious that further studies are needed that follow the recommendations of Conners (1978) and Pirozzolo and Hansch (1982) and that use large enough sample sizes to permit an individual-differences approach that takes into account (1) the possibility that the reading-disabled population is composed of subgroups with different etiologies, (2) task factors such as the type and amount of processing required by a given task and, (3) subject variables such as age, sex, and the relationship between handedness and the cerebral hemisphere predominantly specialized for verbal processing.

Further, it is important that cerebral specialization related to reading disability be studied during tasks requiring the *ongoing processing* of different types of information (both linguistic and non-linguistic) designed to engage differentially one or the other hemisphere. Measures used should be: (1) demonstrably reliable indicators of cerebral specialization and/or functional organization, (2) sensitive to individual differences, and (3) quantifiable. Finally, a multi-method approach, such as one that uses electrophysiological, behavioral, and genetic techniques to study the same population, may allow us to identify and characterize etiologically distinct subtypes of reading disability.

Findings Obtained in Our Laboratory

Over the past several years we have developed an electrophysiological technique to measure cerebral functional organization and have applied it to the study of a number of different populations. For example, we have used this procedure to study cerebral specialization of function in normal adults (see Shucard, Shucard, and Thomas 1977; Shucard, Cummins, Thomas, and Shucard 1981), in patients with brain damage (Selinger, Shucard, and Prescott 1980) as well as in infants (Shucard, Shucard, Cummins, and Campos 1981). A number of other investigators have employed similar methods in their studies of brain organization (see Papanicolaou and Johnstone 1984, for review). The event-related potential (ERP) probe procedure lends itself, in contrast to more classical ERP methods, to the study of electrophysiological events associated with *ongoing* information processing. Thus, the probe technique is less restrictive in the types of stimuli and paradigms that could be used in ERP studies.

In discussing our findings, we will focus on data obtained from a subset of the population studied as part of the Colorado Reading Project. A total of 282 children (141 reading-disabled and 141 Controls) were studied, ranging in age from 7 years, 11 months to 16 years, 11 months with a mean age of 12 years, 10 months. Further information about the population is provided in this volume by DeFries and in previously published reports (see Shucard, Cummins, and McGee 1984, for example).

The data discussed in this chapter will pertain to electrophysiological findings associated with two experimental conditions: Letter Sounds and Letter Shapes. Although during these two conditions subjects do not actually read text, they do perform mental operations that are involved in more complex reading tasks. In later studies, a Reading Condition was incorporated into the experimental procedures.

During the *Letter Sounds Condition,* three separate 15 × 24 inch visual displays were presented to each subject while seated in a comfortable chair in a sound-attenuated-electrically-shielded room. Each visual display contained a 22 × 34 array of all of the lower-case letters of the alphabet and was projected on a screen 55 inches (±2 inches) from the subject using a slide projector. Interspersed at different locations within each array were target letters. There were nine target letters in each array. The targets were letters that had a long "e" sound (viz., b, c, d, e, g, p, t, v, z). Subjects were told to scan each line in each array from left to right and to press two microswitches simultaneously with both index fingers when they found a letter with a long "e" sound. It was hypothesized that this task required visual-phonemic transfer of information similar to that which is presumed to occur during the reading process.

During the *Letter Shapes Condition,* subjects were presented with the same visual arrays as used in the Letter Sounds Condition except here subjects had to identify letters having either closed circular shapes (viz., a, b, d, g, o, p, q) or only straight lines (viz., k, l, t, v, w, y, x, z). As in the Letter Sounds Task, subjects had to indicate their recognition of the targets by pressing the microswitches. Also, as in the Letter Sounds Task, there were nine target letters in each array. It was hypothesized that this task required only recognition of the shape of the letter (visual information processing) rather than visual-phonemic processing as in the Letter Sounds Condition.

While subjects performed these tasks, pairs of *task-irrelevant* auditory tone pips (100 msec, 600 HZ, 65 ± 1 db SPL) were presented to them binurally over headphones. Tone pips had an intrapair interval of 2 sec and a variable interpair interval (no less than 6 sec). The tones served as probe stimuli. A discussion of the rationale for this method is presented in Shucard et al. (1977). Event-related potentials (ERPs) were recorded from scalp leads to these probe stimuli while the subject's state was monitored by means of a video system, by observation of the ongoing EEG and by recording the subject's response to the target stimuli. Eye movements were also monitored in order to determine visual search strategies, to track each subject's place in a given array and to control the presentation of tone stimuli during the performance of each task so that eye movement artifact would have minimal effect on the ERPs.

Summary of Findings Related to Left-Right Asymmetries

Comparisons between a Homogeneous Group of Reading-Disabled and Normal Readers. The most consistent and significant difference found to date between normal and disabled readers was in the pattern of auditory event-related potential (AERP) amplitude asymmetry between 30 normal and 30 disabled readers who were closely matched on age (X = 14 yrs, 8 mo; SD = 1 yr, 3 mo), sex (all males) and handedness (all strongly right handed) and who reported similar task performance strategies (see Shucard et al 1984).

In this phase of the analysis we attempted to control for variables that were not well controlled in previous electrophysiological studies, such as handedness and sex in order to examine electrophysiological data for a more homogeneous subset of reading-disabled and normal readers and obtain measures that could be used in further analyses of more heterogeneous subsets.

Figure 1 is a computer printout illustrating the morphology of an AERP waveform obtained from a reading-disabled subject. Four peaks were identified for each subject's AERPs derived from left and right mid-temporal electrodes referred to the vertex (T3-Cz, T4-Cz, respectively). The mean latencies and standard deviations in milliseconds for these peaks across conditions for all subjects were: P1 latency = 62.9 msec (SD = 14.6); N1 latency = 107.0 msec (SD = 8.6); P2 latency = 171.2 (SD = 13.4); and N3 latency = 247.2 (SD = 33.8).

As can be seen from Figures 2 and 3, in the Letter Sounds Condition, for example the reading-disabled group showed relatively higher amplitude left-hemisphere, Tone 2 response than right ($p < .01$), whereas the normal readers showed relatively higher amplitude right-hemisphere responses than left ($p < .05$). Also, during the Letter Sounds Condition, disabled readers showed a higher left-hemisphere, Tone 2 response than normal readers ($p < .05$). Further, chi-square analyses indicated that during both conditions of the experiment a majority of normal readers showed a higher amplitude right-than left-hemisphere AERP Tone 2 response, whereas the reverse was true for the majority of disabled readers.

In brief, the pattern of hemispheric AERP amplitude asymmetry found for the disabled readers was opposite that found for the normal readers, suggesting that the same reading-related, visual-phonemic tasks may have involved different cerebral processes in the two groups studied. These findings were obtained for AERP Peaks 2 (N1-P2) and 3 (P2-N3) (see Figure 1) and were most prominent for the Letter Sounds Condition. In addition, there were significant between-group differences in speed and accuracy measures obtained while subjects performed the experimental tasks. As might be expected, reading-disabled children were less accurate than normal readers. They were also slower on the Letter Sounds Task. These findings are discussed in more detail in Shucard et al. (1984).

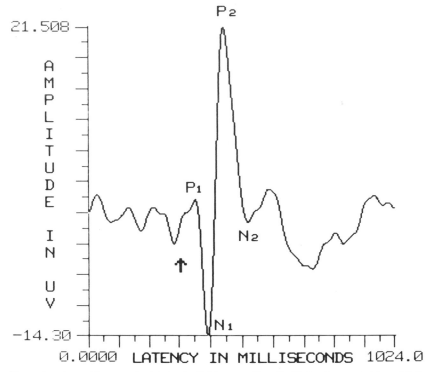

Figure 1.   An auditory event-related potential for a reading-disabled male recorded from T4-Pz
            during the Letter Shapes Condition. The vertical arrow indicates stimulus onset.
            Peaks 1, 2, and 3 refer, respectively, to the negative-going peak from P1 to N1, the
            positive-going peak from N1 to P2, and the negative-going from P2 to N2. Positivity at
            Pz with respect to T4 is up.

*Comparisons Between Reading-Disabled and Normal Readers Across a
Larger Subset of Subjects.*   Based on the robustness of the findings obtained
for the homogeneous subset of 30 reading-disabled and 30 normal subjects, we
wished to determine whether a similar relationship between EEG variables and
groups existed for a larger subset of the sample. In this analysis, data from 180
male subjects (90 reading-disabled and 90 normals[1]) were examined. The
findings proved to be similar to those obtained for the 30 pairs, in that
reading-disabled and normal subjects had different patterns of AERP amplitude
asymmetries. As can be seen from Figure 4, these asymmetries were in the
same direction, albeit not as robust as those obtained for the 30 pairs described
above. This effect was most potent for AERP Peak 3 Tone 2 during the Letter
Sounds Condition. Also, contrary to that for the 30 pairs, in this subset both age
and handedness varied.

*Comparisons Between Reading-Disabled and Normal Readers Matched
on Performance IQ.*   Since there was considerable variation between the

---

[1]Complete data for Peak 3 across both Conditions were available for 66 of the 90 subject pairs
examined. If one subject of a pair had any missing data, both members of the pair were excluded
from the data analysis.

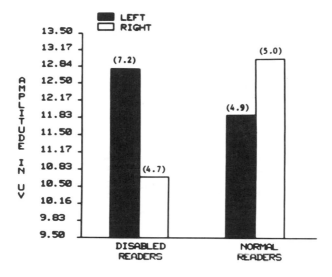

LETTER SOUNDS TASK

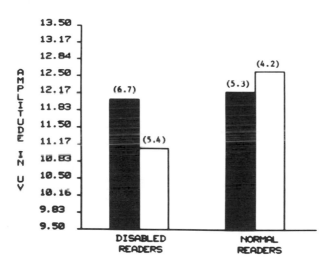

LETTER SHAPES TASK

Figure 2. Left-and right-hemisphere bipolar AERP amplitude responses for normals (N = 30) and disabled readers (N = 30) during the Letter Sounds and Letter Shapes Conditions. Data are for Peak 3 AERP amplitudes for Tone 2. Standard deviations (in parentheses) are shown at the end of each bar (Shucard, Cummins, and McGee 1984).

reading-disabled and normal subjects on Full Scale, Performance and Verbal IQ, we were interested in determining what relationships would be obtained between these two groups if they were matched as closely as possible on Performance IQ. Matching on Performance IQ is a common procedure, since reading deficits may produce a depression on Verbal IQ. Subject pairs were selected who were matched according to our original selection criteria (see

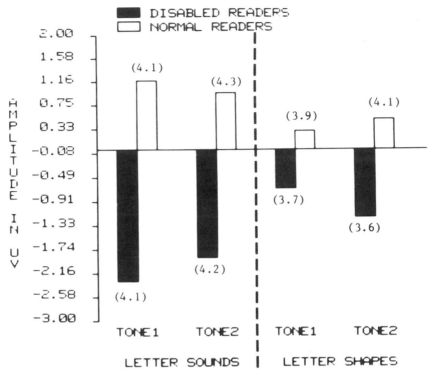

Figure 3.   Mean amplitude difference scores for AERP Peak 3 Tone 2 obtained during the Letter
           Sounds and Letter Shapes Conditions for 30 normal and 30 disabled readers. A
           positive value indicates that the mean right-hemisphere AERP amplitude was greater
           than the left, whereas a negative value indicates that the mean left-hemisphere AERP
           amplitude was greater than the right. Standard deviations (in parentheses) are shown at
           the end of each bar (Shucard, Cummins, and McGee 1984).

Shucard et al. 1984). In addition, each member of the pair had to be within 9
points of the other on Performance IQ. Thirty-five subject pairs met these
criteria.

Table I presents a summary of the means and standard deviations of a
number of behavioral variables that were of interest to us in this subset. It can be
seen from Table I that reading-disabled subjects were lower than normals on
Full Scale IQ, Verbal IQ and reading recognition.

The same AERP amplitude measure found to best differentiate between
reading-disabled and normal readers in the 30 pairs reported above was
examined in these data. The results showed a similar, but less pronounced,
pattern of amplitude asymmetry differences between reading-disabled and
normal subjects as that obtained for the 30 pairs. The group means for the R-L
Peak 3 AERP amplitude difference measure are represented graphically in
Figure 5 below.[2]

---

[2]Complete data for Peak 3 across both Conditions were available for 24 of the 35 subject pairs
examined. If one subject of a pair had any missing data, both members of the pair were excluded
from the data analysis.

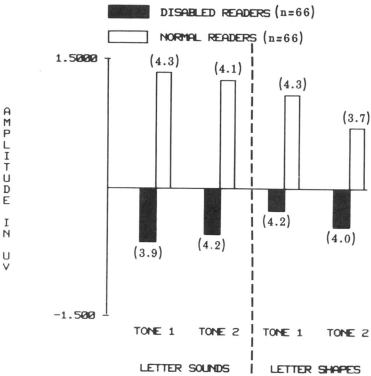

Figure 4. Mean amplitude difference scores for AERP Peak 3 Tone 2 obtained during the Letter Sounds and Letter Shapes Conditions for normal (N = 66) and disabled readers (N = 66). A positive value indicates that the mean right-hemisphere AERP amplitude was greater than the left, whereas a negative value indicates that the mean left-hemisphere AERP amplitude was greater than the right. Standard deviations (in parentheses) are shown at the end of each bar.

As can be seen in Figures 3–5, showing the mean R-L difference scores for each subset, the means for the reading-disabled subjects from the 30 pairs showed the greatest R-L differences reflecting higher amplitude left hemisphere responses, followed by the 66 pairs and then the 24 pairs. These data indicate that there was a range in the degree of R-L AERP amplitude asymmetries within the reading-disabled population. For example, the mean R-L Peak 3 Tone 2 AERP difference scores across the 30 pairs, 66 pairs, and 24 pairs for the normals were + 1.0 μv, + 1.3 μv and + 1.6 μv, respectively. For the reading-disabled subjects these R-L amplitude differences were − 2.0 μv, − .54 μv and − .34 μv, respectively.

The relationship between the magnitude of R-L amplitude asymmetry and other variables may provide further information leading to the delineation of subtypes within the reading-disabled population. That is, it may be that subjects with the greatest R-L amplitude asymmetries are those who do poorly on certain types of information processing that affect their reading skills. These relationships are being studied further. In the next section the potential of this approach is illustrated.

Table I

Summary of Behavioral Variables that Characterized Reading-Disabled and Normal Subjects
Matched on Performance IQ

Variable	Reading-Disabled		Normal	
	Mean	S.D.	Mean	S.D.
PIAT Reading Recognition				
Grade Equivalent	5.3	2.5	8.9	2.6
Verbal IQ	101.1	14.3	112.4	9.4
Performance IQ	105.2	7.5	105.6	7.0
Full Scale IQ	103.2	10.6	110.2	8.3
Age in years	12.9	2.5	12.8	2.5
Handedness	11.5	6.7	9.1	8.7

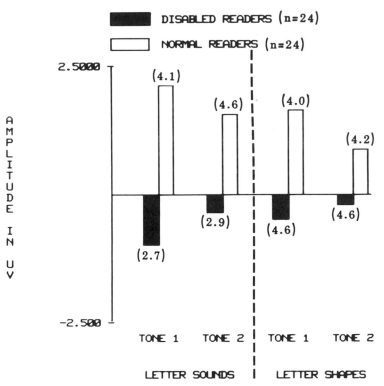

Figure 5.   Mean amplitude scores for AERP Peak 3 Tone 2 obtained during the Letter Sounds and
Letter Shapes Conditions for normal (N = 24) and disabled readers (N = 24). A
positive value indicates that the mean right-hemisphere AERP amplitude was greater
than the left, whereas a negative value indicates that the mean left-hemisphere AERP
amplitude was greater than the right. Standard deviations (in parentheses) are shown at
the end of each bar.

Examination of Cross Component Relationships. Our approach to uncovering possible interrelationships between behavioral and electrophysiological variables has consisted of both macroscopic and microscopic analyses. For example, factor analytic procedures have been and are being used to reduce the number of variables and create more reliable measures for use in analyses across the different components of the Colorado Reading Project (see DeFries, this volume). In addition, we have been examining the data through tests of specific hypotheses of theoretical interest that relate to the reading disabilities literature. In this section, we will present one such approach and associated findings.

First, as was described in the previous sections, an AERP amplitude asymmetry measure was obtained that yielded significant differences between reading-disabled and normal subjects. Using this measure, we attempted to determine whether it related to individual differences across reading-disabled and normal individuals on several composite scores derived from the WISC-R. In this section we will focus on the Bannatyne (1974) recategorization of nine of the WISC-R subtests into three composite ability dimensions thought to measure Conceptual (C), Spatial (Sp) and Sequential (Sq) performance. Using these composite scores, Bannatyne (1971) proposed the existence of a "genetic dyslexic" form of reading disability based on an ordered profile of scores (Spatial > Conceptual > Sequential). The Spatial score was composed of a composite of Picture Completion + Block Design + Object Assembly. The Conceptual score was composed of Comprehension + Similarities + Vocabulary and the Sequential Score was composed of Digit Span + Arithmetic + Coding. Bannatyne (1971) emphasized that the Sp > C > Sq pattern was specific to only 30% of those children who had been diagnosed as reading-disabled and that there were reading problems among their relatives; thus, the notion of a genetic subtype of reading disability. Attempts to validate this Sp > C > Sq profile as a diagnostic tool using group data have lent some support to the idea that this pattern occurs among disabled readers (Rugel 1974). However, in a recent report that came out of the Colorado Reading Project, Decker and Corley (1984) failed to find significant differences between the Sp > C > Sq subtype of disabled readers and a non-specific group of disabled readers on any other cognitive or academic achievement tests. They concluded that the Bannatyne distinction showed no efficacy that could be related to educational manifestations of the disorder as measured by the PIAT subtests. They also questioned the notion of the Sp > C > Sq profile characterizing a genetic subtype.

We attempted to explore possible relationships between the Bannatyne profile and our electrophysiological measures. In addition to the more classical composite scores, a Spatial minus Sequential (Sp − Sq) variable was also derived. We reasoned that the difference between these measures would provide interval level data that would describe the range of the discrepancy between Sp and Sq scores across reading-disabled subjects. Pearson Product-Moment correlations were then performed between Sp-Sq, Sp, Sq, and C scores and the R-L Peak 3 Tone 2 AERP amplitude difference score for both the 30 pairs and the 66 pairs of reading-disabled and normal subjects. The correlations for the normals and reading-disabled were done both separately and combined. A major finding of interest was a significant correlation of − .42 (p <.01) between Sp-Sq and R-L Peak 3 Tone 2 AERP amplitude for the 30, strongly right handed, 12–16 year old reading-disabled males. There were no noteworthy correlations between the Sp-Sq variable and the electrophysiological measures for the normals or other reading-disabled subjects. In addition, it is important to note that neither the Sq score nor the Sp score by themselves correlated with the AERP amplitude measures.

From these findings it was predicted that when the reading-disabled group was divided into those subjects above and below the mean of their group's Sp-Sq score, those subjects who fell below the mean would show the greatest R-L asymmetry with greater left hemisphere amplitude. Further, it would be these subjects who would account for the difference in the pattern of AERP amplitude asymmetry previously reported between normal and reading-disabled subjects (Shucard et al. 1984). It can be seen from Figure 6, that the

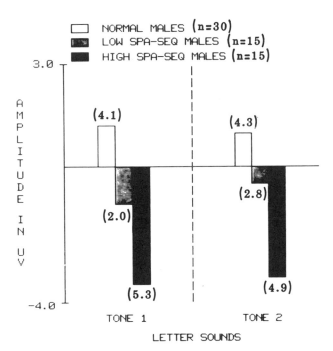

Figure 6.   Mean amplitude difference scores for 2 AERP Peak 3 Tone 1 and Tone 2 during the Letter Sounds Condition for normal male readers (N = 30), low Spatial-Sequential reading-disabled males (N = 15), and high Spatial-Sequential reading-disabled males (N = 15). A positive value indicates that the mean right-hemisphere AERP amplitude was greater than the left, whereas a negative value indicates that the mean left-hemisphere AERP amplitude was greater than the right. Standard deviations (in parentheses) are shown at the end of each bar.

results were as predicted. The mean R-L Tone 2 μv difference was approximately $+1.0$ μv for the normals, the reading-disabled subjects with a Sp-Sq difference below their group mean (closer to that of the normal readers) was $-.49$ μv, whereas those subjects with a Sp-Sq difference greater than the group mean had a mean R-L amplitude asymmetry of -3.26 μv. The degree of Sp-Sq difference for the three groups was as follows: normal readers: $\bar{X} = 4.7$ (S.D. $= 7.6$, N $= 30$), reading-disabled subjects with a Sp-Sq score below the reading-disabled mean: $\bar{X} = 6.6$ (S.D. $= 4.7$, N $= 15$), reading-disabled subjects with a Sp-Sq discrepancy above the reading-disabled mean: $\bar{X} = 15.8$ (SD $= 3.6$, N $= 15$). The mean PIAT reading recognition grade equivalent for both reading-disabled subgroups was 5.8. The normals had a mean reading recognition score of 10.7.

These findings suggest that subjects showing a greater degree of R-L AERP amplitude asymmetry with higher amplitude left-hemisphere responses also tend to have the greater discrepancy between their Sp and Sq abilities with sequential being lower than spatial. Further analyses are being conducted that include variables such as reading style obtained by Dr. Olson (see Olson, this volume).

Summary and Conclusions Based on Findings Discussed

The results of the findings to date indicate that (1) electrophysiological measures may provide important data relevant to the search for individual differences within the reading-disabled population; (2) the relationships obtained between electrophysiological and behavioral variables are complex and most likely interact with variables such as age, sex and handedness, thus it is important to take these variables into account in studies of reading-disability; (3) measures of R-L peak AERP amplitude asymmetries are significantly different between certain subjects of the reading-disabled population we have studied and their matched controls; (4) these measures are also related to differences within the reading-disabled population on such behavioral variables as the degree of discrepancy between spatial and sequential abilities. This relationship may be indicative of differences in the functional organization of the brain among subsets of reading-disabled individuals. However, the precise nature of the disturbance is unclear at this point. In any event, it is fair to conclude, based on our findings, that when sex, age, and handedness were controlled, reading-disabled subjects showed a different electrophysiological pattern than normals. In addition, certain disabled readers show a different pattern of electrophysiological activity than others as defined by their performance on particular abilities tests. Further clarification of these findings and related theoretical issues is needed and can be obtained through studies that take a multidisciplinary approach. Such studies should provide a clearer understanding of brain-behavior relationships among individuals in the reading-disabled population.

References

Bakker, D. J. 1983. Hemispheric specialization and specific reading retardation. *In* M. Rutter (ed.). *Developmental Neuropsychiatry*. New York: The Guilford Press.

Bannatyne, A. 1971. *Language, Reading & Learning Disabilities*. Springfield, Ill.: Charles C Thomas.

Bannatyne, A. 1974. Diagnosis: A note on recategorization of the WISC scaled scores. *Journal of Learning Disabilities* 7:13–14.

Benton, A. L. 1975. Developmental dyslexia: Neurological aspects. *In* W. J. Friendlander (ed.). *Advances in Neurology*. New York: Raven.

Boder, E. 1973. Developmental dyslexia: A diagnostic approach based on three atypical reading-spelling patterns. *Developmental Medicine and Child Neurology* 15:663–687.

Bogen, J. E. 1969. The other side of the brain. I. Dysgraphia and Dyscopia following cerebral commissurotomy. *Bulletin of Los Angeles Neurological Society* 34:73–105.

Broca, P. 1865. Du siege de la faculte du langage article. *Bulletin of the Society for Anthropology* 6:377–393.

Bryden, M. P. 1970. Laterality effects in dichotic listening. Relations with handedness and reading ability in children. *Neuropsychologia* 8:433–450.

Conners, C. K. 1971. Cortical visual evoked response in children with learning disorders. *Psychophysiology* 7:418–428.

Conners, C. K. 1978. Critical review of "Electroencephalographic and neurophysiological studies in dyslexia." *In* A. L. Benton and D. Pearl (eds.). *Dyslexia: An Appraisal of Current Knowledge*. New York: Oxford University Press.

Decker, S. N., and Corley, R. P. 1984. Bannatyne's "Genetic Dyslexia" subtype: A validation study. *Psychology in the Schools* 21:300–304.

Denckla, M. B. 1978. Critical review of "Electroencephalographic and neurophysiological studies in dyslexia." *In* A. L. Benton and D. Pearl (eds.). *Dyslexia: An Appraisal of Current Knowledge*. New York: Oxford University Press.

Doyle, J. C., Orstein, R., and Galin, D. 1974. Lateral specialization of cognitive mode: II. EEG frequency analysis. *Psychophysiology* 11:567–578.

Duane, D. D. 1979. Theories about the causes of dyslexia and their implications. *Pediatric Annals* 8:632–640.

Duffy, F. H., Denckla, M. B., Bartels, P. H., and Sandini, G. 1980a. Dyslexia: Regional differences in brain electrical activity by topographic mapping. *Annals of Neurology* 7:412–420.

Duffy, F. H., Denckla, M. B., Bartels, P. H., Sandini, G., and Kiessling, L. S. 1980b. Dyslexia: Automated diagnosis by computerization classification of brain electrical activity. *Annals of Neurology* 7:421–428.

Friedman, A., and Polson, M. C. 1981. Hemispheres as independent resource systems: Limited-capacity processing and cerebral specialization. *Journal of Experimental Psychology: Human Perception and Performance* 7:1031–1058.

Friedman, D., Simson, R., Ritter, W., and Rapin, I. 1975. Cortical evoked potentials elicited by real speech words and human sounds. *Electroencephalography & Clinical Neurophysiology* 38:13–19.

Galin, D. 1974. Implications for psychiatry of left and right cerebral specialization. *Archives of General Psychiatry* 31:572–583.

Galin, D. 1979. EEG studies of lateralization of verbal processes. *In* C. L. Ludlow and M. F. Doran-Quire (eds.) *The Neurological Basis of Language Disorders in Children: Methods and Directions for Research*. Washington, D.C.: U.S. Department of Health, Education and Welfare, NIH Publication No. 79–440.

Galin, D., and Ellis, R. R. 1975. Asymmetry in evoked potentials as an index of lateralized cognitive processes: Relation to EEG alpha asymmetry. *Neuropsychologia* 13:45–50.

Galin, D., and Ornstein, R. 1974. Individual differences in cognitive style. I. Reflective eye movements. *Neuropsychologia* 12:367–376.

Geschwind, N. 1976. Language and the brain. *In Readings from Scientific American, Progress in Psychobiology*. San Francisco: W. H. Freeman and Co.

Geschwind, N., and Levitsky, W. 1968. Human brain: Left-right asymmetries in temporal speech region. *Science* 161:186–187.

Hillige, J. B., and Cox, P. J. 1976. Effects of concurrent verbal memory on recognition of stimuli from the left and right visual fields. *Journal of Experimental Psychology: Human Perception and Performance* 2:210–221.

Hughes, J. R. 1978. Electroencephalographic and neurophysiological studies in dyslexia. *In* A. L. Benton and D. Pearl (eds.). *Dyslexia: An Appraisal of Current Knowledge*. New York: Oxford University Press.

Hynd, G. W., and Hynd, C. R. 1984a. Dyslexia: Neuroanatomical/neurolinguistic perspectives. *Reading Research Quarterly* 19:482–498.

Hynd, G. W., and Hynd, C. R. 1984b. Dyslexia: Two priorities for the 1980s. *International Journal of Neuroscience* 23:223–230.

Johnstone, J., Galin, D., Fein, G., Yingling, C., Herron, J., and Marcus, M. 1984. Regional brain activity in dyslexic and control children during reading tasks: Visual probe event-related potentials. *Brain and Language* 20:233–254.

Kimura, D. 1973. The asymmetry of the human brain. *Scientific American* March:360–368.

Kimura, D., and Durnford, M. 1974. Normal studies on the function of the right hemisphere in vision. *In* S. J. Dimond and J. G. Beaumont (eds.). *Hemisphere Function in the Human Brain*. New York: Halstead Press.

Kinsbourne, M. 1970. The cerebral basis of lateral asymmetries in attention. *Acta Psychologia* 33:193–201.

Kinsbourne, M. 1972. Eye and head turning indicates cerebral lateralization. *Science* 176: 539–541.

Kinsbourne, M. 1973. The control of attention by interaction between the cerebral hemispheres. *In* S. Kornblum (ed.). *Attention and Performance IV*. New York: Academic Press.

Luria, A. R. 1966. *Higher Cortical Functions in Man*. New York: Basic Books.

Marcel, T., Katz, L., and Smith, M. 1974. Laterality and reading proficiency. *Neuropsychologia* 12:131–139.

Marcel, T., and Rajan, P. 1975. Lateral specialization for recognition of words and faces in good and poor readers. *Neuropsychologia* 13:489–497.

Masland, R. L. 1975. Neurological bases and correlates of language disabilities: Diagnostic implications. *Acta Symbolica* 6:1–34.

Mattis, S., French, J. H., and Rapin, I. 1975. Dyslexia in children and young adults: Three independent neuropsychological syndromes. *Developmental Medicine and Child Neurology* 17:150–163.

Milner, B., Branch, C., and Rasmussen, T. 1966. Evidence for bilateral speech representation in some non-right-handers. *Transactions of the American Neurological Association* 91:306–308.

Molfese, D., Freeman, R., and Palermo, D. 1975. The ontogeny of brain lateralization for speech and nonspeech stimuli. *Brain and Language* 2:356–368.

Morrell, L., and Salamy, J. 1971. Hemispheric asymmetry of electrocortical responses to speech stimuli. *Science* 174:164–166.

Morrison, F. J., Giordiani, B., and Nagy, J. 1977. Reading disability: An information processing analysis. *Science* 196:77–79.

Moscovitch, M., Scullion, D., and Christie, D. 1976. Early versus later stages of processing and their relation to functional hemispheric asymmetries in face recognition. *Journal of Experimental Psychology: Human Perception and Performance* 2:401–416.

Nebes, R. D. 1974. Hemispheric specialization in commissurotomized man. *Psychological Bulletin* 81:1–14.

Orton, S. T. 1928. Specific reading disability—strephosymbolia. *Journal of the American Medical Association* 90:1095–1099.

Papanicolaou, A. C., and Johnstone, J. 1984. Probe evoked potentials: Theory, method and applications. *International Journal of Neuroscience* 24(2):107–132.

Pirozzolo, F. J., and Hansch, E. C. 1982. The neurobiology of developmental reading disorders. *In* R. M. Malatesha and P. G. Aaron (eds.). *Reading Disorders: Varieties and Treatments*. New York: Academic Press.

Preston, M. S., Guthrie, J. T., Kirsch, I., Gertman, D., and Childs, B. 1977. VERs in normal and disabled adult readers. *Psychophysiology* 14:8–14.

Rourke, B. P. 1978. Neuropsychological research in reading retardation: A review. *In* A. L. Benton and D. Pearl (eds.). *Dyslexia: An Appraisal of Current Knowledge*. New York: Oxford University Press.

Rugel, R. P. 1974. WISC subtest scores of disabled readers: A review with respect to Bannatyne's recategorization. *Journal of Learning Disabilities* 7:48–55.

Satz, P., and Sparrow, S. S. 1970. Specific developmental dyslexia: A theoretical formulation. *In* D. J. Bakker and P. Satz (eds.). *Specific Reading Disability: Advances in Theory and Method*. Rotterdam: Rotterdam University Press.

Schwartz, S., and Kirsner, K. 1984. Can group differences in hemispheric asymmetry be inferred from behavioral lateral indices? *Brain and Cognition* 3:57–70.

Selinger, M., Shucard, D. W., and Prescott, T. 1980. Relationships between behavioral and electrophysiological measures of auditory comprehension. *In* R. H. Brookshire (ed.). *Clinical Aphasiology Conference Proceedings*. Minneapolis, Minnesota: BRK Publishers.

Sevush, S. 1983. The neurolinguistics of reading: Anatomic & neurological correlates. Paper presented at the Annual Conference of the International Neuropsychological Society, Mexico City.

Shankweiler, D., and Studdert-Kennedy, M. 1975. A continuum of lateralization for speech perception? *Brain and Language* 2:212–225.

Shucard, D. W., Cummins, K. R., and McGee, M. G. 1984. Event-related brain potentials differentiate normal and disabled readers. *Brain and Language* 21:318–334.

Shucard, D. W., Cummins, K. R., Thomas, D. G., and Shucard, J. L. 1981. Auditory evoked potentials as probes of hemispheric functioning—A replication and extension. *Electroencephalography and Clinical Neurophysiology* 52:389–393.

Shucard, D. W., Shucard, J. L., and Thomas, D. G. 1977. Auditory evoked potentials as probes of hemispheric differences in cognitive processing. *Science* 197:1295–1298.

Shucard, J. L., Shucard, D. W., Cummins, K. R., and Campos, J. J. 1981. Auditory evoked potentials and sex related differences in brain development. *Brain and Language* 13:91–102.

Sklar, B., Hanley, J., and Simmons, W. W. 1972. An EEG experiment toward identifying dyslexic children. *Nature* 240:414–416.

Sklar, B., Hanley, J., and Simmons, W. W. 1973. A computer analysis of EEG spectral signature from normal and dyslexic children. *IEEE Transactions of Biomedical Engineering* 20:20–26.

Sobotka, K. R., and May, J. G. 1977. Visual evoked potentials and reaction time in normal and dyslexic children. *Psychophysiology* 14:18–24.

Sperry, R. W. 1973. Lateral specialization of cerebral function in the surgically separated hemispheres. *In* F. J. McGuigan and R. A. Schoonover (eds.). *The Psychophysiology of Thinking*. New York: Academic Press.

Symann-Louett, N., Gascon, G. G., Matsumiya, Y., and Lombrosco, C. T. 1977. Wave form differences in visual evoked responses between normal and reading disabled children. *Neurology* 27:156–159.

Vellutino, F. R. 1977. Toward an understanding of dyslexia: Psychological factors in specific reading disability. *In* A. L. Benton and D. Pearl (eds.). *Dyslexia: An Appraisal of Current Knowledge*. New York: Oxford University Press.

Wada, J., Clark, R., and Hamm, A. 1975. Cerebral hemispheric asymmetry in humans. *Archives of Neurology* 32:239–246.

Weber, B. A., and Omenn, G. S. 1977. Auditory and visual evoked responses in children with familial reading disabilities. *Journal of Learning Disabilities* 10:153–158.

Wernicke, C. 1874. *Der Aphasische Symptomcomplex*. Breslau: Max Cohn and Weigert.

Witelson, S. F. 1977a. Developmental dyslexia: Two right hemispheres and none left. *Science* 195:309–311.

Witelson, S. F. 1977b. Early hemispheric specialization and interhemispheric plasticity: An empirical and theoretical review. *In* S. J. Segalowitz and F. A. Gruber (eds.). *Language Development and Neurological Theory*. New York: Academic Press.

Yeni-Komshian, G., Isenberg, D., and Goldberg, H. 1975. Cerebral dominance and reading disability: Left visual field deficit in poor readers. *Neuropsychologia* 13:83–94.

Young, A. W., and Ellis, A. W. 1981. Asymmetry of cerebral hemisphere function in normal and poor readers. *Psychological Bulletin* 89:183–190.

8

Colorado Reading Project

J. C. DeFries

S ince 1979, research at the University of Colorado concerning the etiology
of reading disability has been supported in part by a program project grant
from the National Institute of Child Health and Human Development. The
long-range objectives of this project are the identification, characterization,
and validation of etiologically distinct subtypes of reading disability. To
accomplish these objectives, a newly developed test battery that includes
measures of cognitive abilities, reading and language processes, and patterns of
electrophysiological activity is being administered to a sample of identical and
fraternal twin pairs in which at least one twin is reading disabled, to identical
and fraternal twin pairs of normal reading ability, to nontwin reading-disabled
and control children who were previously tested in our project, and to the
parents and siblings of these children. Resulting twin and family data are being
used to validate alternative typologies and to conduct genetic, longitudinal, and
risk analyses.

For administrative and logistical convenience, the program project includes four components: Psychometric Assessment/Family Study; Twin Study;
Reading and Language Processes; and Patterns of Electrophysiological Activity. The primary objectives of the present report are to review the background of this project and to summarize results of several recent analyses
conducted within the Psychometric Assessment/Family Study component.
Results obtained in the other components of the project are described elsewhere
in this volume by S. N. Decker and S. G. Vandenberg, R. K. Olson, and D. W.
Shucard, K. R. Cummins, E. Day, J. Lairsmith, and P. Welanko.

This work was supported in part by grants from the Spencer Foundation and NICHD (HD-11681) to
J. C. DeFries.

    I wish to acknowledge the invaluable contributions of staff members of the many school
districts in Colorado who referred subjects to us and of the families who participated in the study. I
also thank Michele C. LaBuda and George P. Vogler for performing the data analyses and Rebecca
G. Miles for expert editorial assistance.

Colorado Family Reading Study

Our first attempt to study the etiology of reading disability was the Colorado Family Reading Study (FRS), supported initially by a small grant from the Spencer Foundation. The primary objectives of that study were as follows: (1) to construct a battery of tests that differentiates children with reading problems (probands) from matched controls; (2) to assess possible cognitive and reading deficits in parents and siblings of probands; and (3) to study the transmission of reading disability in families of probands.

Probands and matched control children were ascertained by referral from local school districts in Colorado. The referral criteria employed for probands included an IQ score of 90 or above as measured by a standardized intelligence test; a reading achievement level of one-half grade level expectancy or lower as measured by a standardized reading test (e.g., a child in the fourth grade who is reading at or below second-grade level); chronological age between 7.5 and 12 years; residence with both biological parents; no known emotional or neurological impairment; and no uncorrected deficits in auditory or visual acuity. A control child whose reading level was equal to or greater than current grade placement was matched to each proband on the basis of age (within 6 months), sex, grade, school, and home neighborhood. Before a proband or control child was scheduled for testing, school records were reviewed by our staff to ensure that the referral criteria were being met.

Siblings (7.5–18 years of age) and parents of probands and control children were also tested. Thus, in addition to the obvious comparison between probands and controls, the very simple design of the FRS (see Figure 1) facilitated comparisons between siblings of probands and siblings of controls and between parents of probands and parents of controls. If reading disability or its correlates are heritable to any extent, then relatives of probands should manifest at least some deficits on reading-related tests.

During the initial 15 months of that study, members of 58 matched pairs of proband and control families were individually administered a 3-hour battery of psychometric tests by trained examiners. Based upon analyses of those data, a 2-hour battery that retained the most discriminating and reliable tests was developed for subsequent testing during the remainder of the study.

Between October 1, 1973, and July 30, 1976, 125 probands (96 boys and 29 girls), their parents and siblings, and members of 125 matched control families (total $N = 1,044$) were tested. Test descriptions and sample statistics for individual tests were reported by Foch, DeFries, McClearn, and Singer (1977) and DeFries, Singer, Foch, and Lewitter (1978). In the present chapter, composite scores based upon seven tests (Peabody Individual Achievement Test: Reading Recognition, Reading Comprehension, and Spelling [Dunn and Markwardt 1970]; Nonverbal Culture Fair Intelligence Test [Institute for Personality and Ability Testing 1973]; Primary Mental Abilities [PMA] Spatial Relations Test [Thurstone 1963]; Wechsler Intelligence Scale for Children [WISC] Coding, Form B [Wechsler 1949]; and the Colorado Perceptual Speed

PROBAND FAMILY   **CONTROL FAMILY**

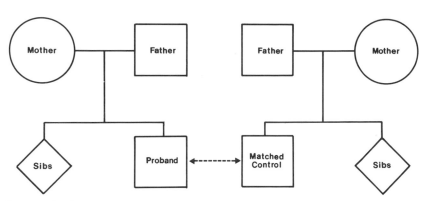

Figure 1.   Design of the Colorado Family Reading Study. (From DeFries and Decker 1982.)

Test: Rotatable Letters and Numbers) administered to all FRS subjects are reported.

Because the test battery was administered to subjects across a wide age range, individual test scores were adjusted for age differences. First, the sample was divided into three age groups: children under ten years of age; children ten and older; and adults. Each score was then expressed as a deviation from expectation based upon a linear and quadratic regression equation estimated from control data. Resulting deviation scores were transformed to T-scores (mean of 50 and a standard deviation of 10 for each variable in each control group) and then intercorrelated in the combined sample.

Principal component analysis with Varimax rotation of the resulting correlation matrix yielded evidence for three readily interpretable ability dimensions: reading, symbol-processing speed, and spatial/reasoning. As shown in Table I, the reading component correlates highest with Reading Recognition, Reading Comprehension, and Spelling; symbol-processing speed

Table I
Varimax Rotated Principal Component Loadings

Test	Reading	Symbol-Processing Speed	Spatial/Reasoning
Reading Recognition	0.89	0.19	0.17
Reading Comprehension	0.83	0.13	0.30
Spelling	0.85	0.31	0.01
Nonverbal Intelligence	0.40	0.12	0.76
PMA Spatial Relations	0.02	0.20	0.89
WISC Coding	0.13	0.88	0.19
Colorado Perceptual Speed	0.37	0.79	0.15
Percent Common Variance	45	28	27

has highest loadings on WISC Coding and Colorado Perceptual Speed; and spatial/reasoning has highest loadings on Nonverbal Intelligence and PMA Spatial Relations. Principal component analysis of various subsets of the total data set (e.g., families of probands, families of controls, probands only, control children only) yielded highly congruent results.

In previous analyses (e.g., Decker and DeFries 1980, 1981), principal component scores were computed for each subject by summing the products of standardized test scores and factor score coefficients across tests. However, for the present analyses, composite scores were obtained for reading, symbol-processing speed, and spatial/reasoning by calculating unweighted means of age-adjusted T-scores from the measures with the highest principal component loadings. Thus, for example, a composite reading measure was obtained for each individual by calculating the mean of that individual's Reading Recognition, Reading Comprehension, and Spelling T-scores. This method was employed, for the present report, to yield scores which characterize the three dimensions, but which retain covariation among them for the multivariate path analysis described later in this chapter.

Group Means

Average reading, symbol-processing speed, and spatial/reasoning scores of probands, matched controls, siblings, and parents are presented in Table II. Multivariate analyses of variance yield evidence for significant group and gender differences for each of the three comparison samples (probands versus controls; siblings of probands versus siblings of controls; and parents of probands versus parents of controls). As expected, the largest univariate group difference is that between probands and controls for the reading composite, over 2 standard deviations on the average. Probands also score more than 0.7 of a standard deviation lower than controls on both symbol-processing speed and spatial/reasoning. With regard to gender differences, girls obtain somewhat higher scores on symbol-processing speed (about 0.5 of a standard deviation), whereas boys obtain higher scores on spatial/reasoning (about 0.4 standard deviations). The absence of significant multivariate and univariate interactions between group and gender in the proband data suggests that reading-disabled girls on the average are no more or less impaired than reading-disabled boys. Thus, despite the marked difference in prevalance rate for boys and girls in this study (about 3.3:1), there is little or no evidence for gender bias in diagnosis.

With regard to sibling data, the difference in reading performance between brothers of probands and brothers of controls (about 1 standard deviation) is larger than that between sisters of probands and sisters of controls (about 0.4 standard deviations), resulting in a significant univariate interaction for this measure. This result suggests that brothers of probands are at higher risk for reading disability than are sisters of probands. Significant differences between siblings of probands and those of controls are also evident for symbol-processing speed and spatial/reasoning, as is a gender difference in favor of girls for symbol-processing speed.

Table II

Multivariate Analysis of Variance of Composite Reading, Symbol-Processing Speed, and Spatial/Reasoning Scores

| | Mean Scores | | | | F Values | | | |
| | Males | | Females | | | | | |
	Reading Disabled	Control	Reading Disabled	Control	Group	Gender	Group × Gender	df
Probands								
Reading	29.77	50.33	28.44	52.12	480.93*	0.04	1.85	1,245
Symbol processing	41.56	48.68	45.72	54.07	58.83*	17.43*	0.29	1,245
Spatial	43.37	52.16	41.28	47.06	60.30*	8.53*	1.50	1,245
Multivariate					162.58*	11.72*	1.55	3,243
N	96	95	29	29				
Siblings								
Reading	39.49	49.49	45.67	49.17	36.62*	7.58*	7.99*	1,286
Symbol processing	42.41	46.39	50.79	54.50	11.60*	61.35*	0.02	1,286
Spatial	46.19	49.38	47.07	48.43	5.35*	0.00	0.80	1,286
Multivariate					12.34*	24.17*	3.21	3,284
N	81	76	73	60				
Parents								
Reading	41.38	49.69	45.09	50.50	52.65*	5.75*	2.35	1,492
Symbol processing	42.87	48.66	46.98	51.35	35.93*	16.11*	0.70	1,492
Spatial	49.36	52.96	46.15	47.19	8.97*	33.72*	2.74	1,492
Multivariate					20.48*	35.55*	1.22	3,490
N	123	123	125	125				

*$p < 0.05$.

Parents of probands obtain lower scores than do parents of control children for each of the three measures. In accord with the sibling data, differences are somewhat greater for fathers (about 0.8 standard deviations) than for mothers (about 0.5 standard deviations) for the reading measure; however, the differential effect is not sufficiently large to result in a significant group-by-gender interaction for the parental data. With regard to gender differences, mothers obtain higher average scores than fathers for reading and symbol-processing speed, but lower scores for spatial/reasoning.

Genetic Analyses

Results of the multivariate analyses of variance outlined above conclusively demonstrate the familial nature of reading disability. But what about the genetics of reading disability? Familial resemblance may be necessary, but it is not sufficient evidence for genetic influence. In order to test for possible genetic influence, the FRS data have been subjected to various genetic analyses (DeFries and Decker 1982). For example, as predicted by the sex-influenced polygenic threshold model (Carter 1973), relatives of reading-disabled girls are at higher risk for reading disability than are relatives of reading-disabled boys. However, other models (e.g., sex-influenced major-gene or environmental threshold models) could also account for this pattern of results.

Tests of hypotheses of major-gene influence were also undertaken, but with mixed results. For example, variances of reading scores for relatives of probands are significantly greater than those for relatives of controls, in accordance with expectation based upon the major-gene model. However, little or no evidence for sex linkage was obtained, and complex segregation analyses of the total data set provided no evidence for autosomal major-gene influence (Lewitter, DeFries, and Elston 1980). On the other hand, when data from only the families of female probands were analyzed, the hypothesis of single-gene, recessive inheritance could not be rejected. Thus, results of segregation analysis of FRS data provide some evidence for autosomal recessive inheritance in families of reading-disabled girls. (For a recent review of the genetics of reading disability, see DeFries, Vogler, and LaBuda in press.)

Heterogeneity

Perhaps, in retrospect, mixed results from genetic analyses of the total FRS data set should not have been unexpected. If there are several etiologically distinct forms of reading disability, some may be heritable whereas others may be due to environmental influences. Of the heritable forms, one or more may be due to autosomal recessive inheritance, others may be dominantly inherited, etc. In an initial attempt to explore this heterogeneity issue, principal component scores representing each of the three ability dimensions were plotted for each proband and the resulting profiles were categorized into subtypes (Decker and DeFries 1981). The validity of this tentative typology was then assessed by applying the same classification system to profiles of affected relatives and cross-tabulating them as a function of the proband's subtype. Our rationale was similar to that used to test for heterogeneity in the psychoses (DeFries and

Plomin 1978): If a given subtype has biological validity, then affected relatives of probands of a given subtype should be more likely to be of the same subtype than expected on the basis of chance alone. Although some evidence was obtained for profile similarity between probands and their affected siblings, subtype resemblance was not apparent between probands and their parents. Thus, we reluctantly concluded that this particular typology did not meet our validity criterion. Nevertheless, results of this study illustrate how family data may be used to test the validity of alternative typologies, and it would be interesting to see how other typologies would fare when subjected to the same validity test. (For recent reviews of the subtype literature, see McKinney 1984, and Vogler, Baker, Decker, DeFries, and Huizinga in press.)

The validity test employing family data should be particularly powerful when data are available for twin pairs in which both members are affected. Moreover, a comparison of subtype similarity in identical and fraternal twins would provide evidence concerning the heritable nature of different subtypes. For example, assume that a particular typology hypothesizes the existence of four subtypes. The frequencies of these subtypes in co-twins could be cross-tabulated as a function of proband subtype in a 4×4 contingency table. To the extent that the frequencies tend to cluster along the main diagonal, twin resemblance for subtypes would be indicated. If this tendency were greater for identical twins than for fraternals, genetic factors would be implicated. Such analyses will be undertaken with the twin data currently being collected in the Colorado Reading Project.

Colorado Reading Project

Although our initial attempt at differential diagnosis using family data was encouraging, it was almost certainly circumscribed by the relatively narrow range of behavioral assessments employed. In order to obtain data for a broader array of measures, a program project application (Differential Diagnosis in Reading Disability, abbreviated DDRD) was submitted and eventually was funded in 1979. During the initial 3-year project period, a test battery that includes measures of cognitive abilities, reading and language processes, and electrophysiological activity was developed and administered to a core sample of 140 reading-disabled and 140 matched control children. In addition, a number of analyses of these data were undertaken.

Our goal during the current 3-year project period is to administer our test battery to 30 identical and 30 fraternal twin pairs in which at least one twin is reading disabled, to the same numbers of control twins, to 50 nontwin reading-disabled and 50 nontwin control children who were tested during the initial project period, and to as many parents and siblings of these children as time and resources permit. Preliminary analyses of the twin data are described in the chapter by Dr. Decker and analyses of data collected in the Reading and Language Processes and Patterns of Electrophysiological Activity components are discussed in the chapters by Drs. Olson and Shucard.

The component of the program project for which I am chiefly responsible is the Psychometric Assessment/Family Study. A number of analyses of data collected by this component have recently been undertaken, but only four will be outlined below: (1) a multivariate analysis of variance of reading and IQ data; (2) an analysis of longitudinal data; (3) a risk analysis; and (4) a multivariate path analysis of family data.

Reading and IQ Data

Means and standard deviations for WISC-R IQ (Wechsler 1974) and PIAT Reading Recognition (grade equivalent) scores of subjects tested during the initial program project period are presented in Table III. In order to assess the significance of group differences in IQ, a two-way multivariate Roy-Bargman stepdown analysis of variance comparing the effects of group (proband versus control), gender, and their interaction was performed using the WISC-R Verbal, Performance, and Full-Scale IQ scores as dependent measures. As expected, given the correlation between verbal and reading abilities, the two groups differ significantly in Verbal IQ. However, they do not differ significantly with respect to Performance or Full-Scale IQ when differences in Verbal IQ are partialed out.

As may be seen in Table III, group differences in PIAT Reading Recognition are highly significant, even after covariance adjustment for differences in Verbal IQ. Thus, the group difference in reading performance is not due to the IQ difference. In fact, given that the F value for the Reading Recognition group comparison after covariance adjustment exceeds that for Verbal IQ, it seems more likely that the IQ difference is due to the group difference in reading performance. It may also be seen from this table that probands on the average read at approximately one-half the grade level of the control group. Moreover, the lack of a significant group-by-gender interaction suggests that the unequal sex ratio of reading-disabled males to females (3.8:1 in this sample) is not due to a gender ascertainment bias. Thus, we may conclude that the proband and control groups differ substantially in reading performance (about 2 standard deviations on the average), but that they are well matched for Performance IQ when the data are adjusted for differences in Verbal IQ.

Longitudinal Analysis

Of the 280 children for whom valid psychometric test data were collected during the initial program project period, 69 matched pairs had also been tested as part of the FRS 5 years earlier. Several analyses of these longitudinal data have recently been reported (Baker, Decker, and DeFries 1984; DeFries and Baker 1983a, 1983b). For example, when principal component reading and symbol-processing speed scores were computed for each subject at both ages (mean ages of 9.4 and 14.8 years at the time of initial and follow-up testing, respectively) and subjected to a mixed-model multivariate analysis of variance, significant effects due to group (proband versus control), time (initial versus follow-up test sessions), and their interaction were found (DeFries and Baker 1983a). As may be seen in Figure 2, the rate of improvement across the 5-year

Table III
Means $\pm$ SD for WISC-R and Reading Recognition Scores of Reading-Disabled and Control Children Tested in the Colorado Reading Project

	Group				F Values		
	Reading Disabled		Control				
	Males	Females	Males	Females	Group	Gender	Group × Gender
WISC-R[a]							
Verbal IQ	100.18 ± 11.34	97.14 ± 11.07	114.56 ± 11.62	111.62 ± 12.85	107.94*	3.43	0.04
Performance IQ	104.46 ± 10.11	101.86 ± 10.42	112.65 ± 12.83	111.31 ± 13.01	2.35	0.15	0.19
Full-Scale IQ	102.16 ± 9.89	99.10 ± 9.86	115.13 ± 11.78	112.52 ± 12.83	2.23	0.68	0.18
PIAT Reading Recognition[b]	5.09 ± 2.27	4.69 ± 1.87	9.45 ± 2.63	9.30 ± 2.69	124.72*	0.12	0.15
N	111	29	111	29			

[a] F values for the WISC-R were obtained using the multivariate Roy-Bargman stepdown F test.
[b] Grade equivalent scores. The F value for the PIAT was obtained using a univariate F test after covariance adjustment for Verbal IQ.
*$p < 0.001$.

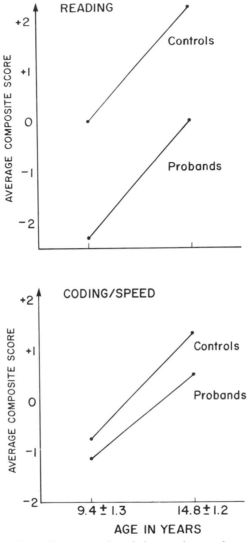

Figure 2.   Mean reading performance and symbol-processing speed component scores of 69
matched pairs of reading-disabled and control children tested at two different ages.
(From DeFries and Baker 1983a.)

test-retest interval for symbol-processing speed is significantly lower for
probands than for controls. However, with regard to the reading measure, the
rate of change is highly similar for the two groups, i.e., reading-disabled and
control children differ substantially on the average at both ages, but by a
constant amount. Thus, results of this longitudinal study clearly demonstrate
the persistent nature of reading disability.

    In contrast to the similarity in rate of improvement in average reading
performance of probands and controls across the 5-year interval, the stability
correlation is significantly lower for the reading-disabled children ($r = 0.2$ and

0.5 for probands and controls, respectively). Therefore, initial test scores may be less informative for predicting subsequent reading performance of probands than of controls. Because of the familial nature of reading disability, we hypothesized that the accuracy of predicting reading performance of reading-disabled children over the 5-year test-retest interval could be significantly improved by incorporating parental data into a prediction equation. Age-adjusted scores of probands who participated in both phases of the study were subjected to a hierarchial multiple regression analysis in which a child's score at retest was predicted from the initial test score and from the parents' test scores. As hypothesized, there is a significant increase in the squared multiple correlation for reading performance of probands when parental data are added to the prediction equation (DeFries and Baker 1983a). However, no significant increase occurs when parental data are added to the prediction equation for reading performance of control children or to the regression equation used to predict later symbol-processing speed scores of either group. These results suggest that the accuracy of long-term prognoses for reading disability may be significantly improved by including parental data in clinical case studies.

Risk Analysis

Identification of children at risk for reading disability prior to the onset of serious academic problems could facilitate preventive intervention and early remediation. Parental data, of course, may be used for such risk analysis. Employing the principles of Bayesian inverse probability analysis, we recently estimated the probability that a child will become reading disabled from parental self-report data.

During the initial program project period, no psychometric test data were obtained from parents of reading-disabled or control children. However, each parent completed a questionnaire regarding reading habits and abilities. One question asked was whether or not the parent encountered any serious difficulty learning to read. From these data, the probability that a parent will self-report a difficulty learning to read given that his or her child is either reading disabled or not can be computed directly. However, the prediction is more informative if it is made the other way around, i.e., the probability that a child will become reading disabled given that a parent self-reports a problem learning to read.

In order to estimate the probability that a child will become reading disabled as a function of parental self-reported reading status, self-report data obtained from parents of 174 probands and 182 control children who participated in either the FRS or the DDRD program project were analyzed (Vogler, DeFries, and Decker 1985). Separate risk estimates were obtained for boys and girls assuming a sex ratio of 3.5:1 and various population prevalence rates. For a prevalence rate of 5%, estimated posterior probabilities indicate that sons of fathers who report a problem learning to read have about a 40% risk of developing a reading disability. This risk estimate is approximately 7 times greater than that for sons of fathers who report no such problems. Sons of mothers who report a difficulty learning to read have a risk of about 35%, or about 5 times greater than that for sons of mothers who report no reading problems. For daughters of parents with a positive history, the absolute risk is lower (17%–18%) than that for sons; however, the relative risk is 10 to 12 times higher than that for daughers of parents with no history of reading problems.

Results of this analysis clearly indicate that parental self-reported history of reading disability is a powerful risk factor. Parental self-reports are easily obtained, and we have recently established that they have considerable validity (Decker, Vogler, and DeFries in press). Thus, such data should be routinely employed to aid in the early identification of children at risk for reading disability.

Multivariate Path Analysis

In order to study the etiology of covariation between composite measures of reading performance and symbol-processing speed, FRS data were recently subjected to bivariate path analysis (Vogler and DeFries 1985). A path model that incorporates measures of phenotypic assortative mating and cross-assortative mating was formulated and applied to the joint transmission of the two characters in families of probands and in those of controls. Using this method, phenotypic variances for the two characters and their covariance were partitioned into components due to familial (genetic and/or environmental) influences and specific, nontransmissible environmental influences. In brief, resulting parameter estimates obtained from data on families of probands and those of controls are highly similar and indicate that familial sources of variation are important for both reading performance and symbol-processing speed; moreover, more than half of the observed phenotypic correlation between the two measures is due to transmissible influences.

Bivariate path models are useful for analyzing the etiologies of variation and covariation in multivariate systems; however, because the diagrams are complex, error-free expectations are difficult to derive. When the next level of complexity is examined, i.e., trivariate path analysis, these difficulties are compounded. Thus, application of path analysis to complex multivariate data sets is seriously limited using this approach. However, a significant advance in multivariate behavioral genetic analysis was recently made in our laboratory. A graduate student, Mr. George P. Vogler, extended path analysis to the general multivariate case (Vogler 1985; Vogler and DeFries 1984). Latent and observed variables of the traditional path model are replaced by column vectors of standardized deviations from the mean; correlations indicated by double-headed arrows are replaced by matrices of correlations; and path coefficients are replaced by matrices of path coefficients. By observing the standard rules for path analysis, as well as a few simple additional rules for multivariate path analysis, multivariate expectations can be readily derived. The beauty of this approach is that matrices of expectations can be derived from a path diagram that is no more complex than that used for the univariate case.

In theory, any number of variables can be analyzed using multivariate path models. In practice, however, there are limitations that depend upon the size and speed of the computer, the efficiency of the optimization program, the complexity of the model, and the fit of the model to the observed data. We have recently undertaken a trivariate analysis of FRS reading, symbol-processing speed, and spatial/reasoning composite scores and encountered no serious difficulty in obtaining a solution (LaBuda, Vogler, DeFries, and Fulker in press). Expected correlations among family members were derived using the multivariate path diagram depicted in Figure 3 (symbols are defined in Table IV). In order to fit the model, a maximum-likelihood estimation procedure was employed that simultaneously equates observed and expected covariance matrices of different size (Fulker and DeFries 1983). Resulting parameter estimates were then used to partition the observed phenotypic correlation matrix into components due to familial and specific environmental influences. As may be seen in Table V, the pattern of results is highly similar for families of probands and those of controls. In both groups, familial influences account for 30% to 50% of the observed variance in the three measures. Of even greater interest, however, is the finding that approximately two-thirds of each of the three phenotypic correlations between the characters is due to these transmissible influences. This result suggests that individual differences in reading performance, symbol-processing speed, and spatial/reasoning are due to many of the same genetic and/or family-environmental factors.

Concluding Remarks

Results of family studies, as well as those of the twin study described by Dr. Decker in this volume, strongly suggest that reading disability is highly

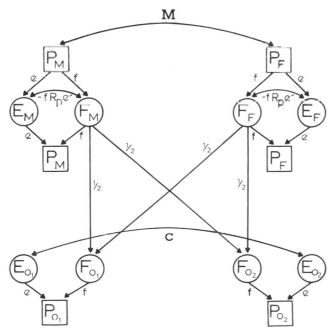

Figure 3.   Multivariate path diagram of familial resemblance (symbols defined in Table IV). (From LaBuda, Vogler, DeFries, and Fulker in press.)

Table IV
Variables, Path Coefficients, and Correlations Used in the Multivariate Path Model

Symbol	Description
P_M, P_F, P_{O_1}, P_{O_2}	A column vector of phenotypes for reading ability, symbol-processing speed, and spatial/reasoning in mother (M), father (F), and two offspring (O_1 and O_2)
F_M, F_F, F_{O_1}, F_{O_2}	A column vector of familial factors for all three composites in mother, father, and two offspring
f	A diagonal matrix of the influences of familial factors on the phenotype for all composites
e	A diagonal matrix of the influences of nontransmissible environmental factors on the phenotype for all composites
R_F	A symmetric matrix of the familial correlations among all composites
R_E	A symmetric matrix of the nontransmissible environmental correlations among all composites
M	A non-symmetric matrix of spouse phenotypic correlations among all composites
c	A non-symmetric matrix of sibling nontransmissible environmental correlations among all composites

Note. From LaBuda, Vogler, DeFries, and Fulker (in press).

heritable. Establishing the mode or modes of inheritance for this condition would be of considerable theoretical and practical significance; however, results of carefully designed family studies can also provide other important information. For example, results of our program project already demonstrate the importance of family data for risk analysis, for predicting the long-term consequences of reading disability, for studies of subtype validity, and for analyses of the etiology of covariation among reading-related measures. (For a more detailed discussion of the importance of studying the genetics of reading disability, see Finucci 1978.)

Table V
Partitioning of Phenotypic Correlation Matrices into Parts Due to Familial and Environmental Influences[a]

Families of Probands

$$
R_P = fR_Ff' + eR_Ee'
$$

$$
\begin{bmatrix} 1 & .46 & .46 \\ & 1 & .48 \\ & & 1 \end{bmatrix} = \begin{bmatrix} .41 & .23 & .35 \\ & .33 & .32 \\ & & .54 \end{bmatrix} + \begin{bmatrix} .59 & .23 & .11 \\ & .67 & .16 \\ & & .46 \end{bmatrix}
$$

Families of Controls

$$
R_P = fR_Ff' + eR_Ee'
$$

$$
\begin{bmatrix} 1 & .38 & .29 \\ & 1 & .35 \\ & & 1 \end{bmatrix} = \begin{bmatrix} .34 & .27 & .24 \\ & .34 & .26 \\ & & .51 \end{bmatrix} + \begin{bmatrix} .66 & .11 & .05 \\ & .66 & .09 \\ & & .49 \end{bmatrix}
$$

Note. From LaBuda, Vogler, DeFries, and Fulker (in press).
[a]Variables defined in Table IV.

Reading disability is an important public health problem because of its relatively high prevalence among school-age children and young adults. Recent evidence suggests that it may be a heterogeneous disorder with different subtypes displaying different patterns of performance. In order to achieve rational remediation and preventive measures, these different subtypes must be identified and characterized. The Colorado Reading Project is a systematic effort by researchers at the University of Colorado to accomplish the differential diagnosis of etiologically distinct subtypes of reading disability and to increase our understanding of its genetic and environmental bases.

References

Baker, L. A., Decker, S. N., and DeFries, J. C. 1984. Cognitive abilities in reading-disabled children: A longitudinal study. *The Journal of Child Psychology and Psychiatry and Allied Disciplines* 25:111–117.

Carter, C. O. 1973. Multifactorial genetic disease. *In* V. A. McKusick and R. Clairborne (eds.). *Medical Genetics.* New York: HP Publishing Company.

Decker, S. N., and DeFries, J. C. 1980. Cognitive abilities in families with reading disabled children. *Journal of Learning Disabilities* 13:517–522.

Decker, S. N., and DeFries, J. C. 1981. Cognitive ability profiles in families of reading-disabled children. *Developmental Medicine and Child Neurology* 23:217–227.

Decker, S. N., Vogler, G. P., and DeFries, J. C. in press. Validity of self-reported reading disability by parents of reading-disabled children. *Acta Paedologica.*

DeFries, J. C., and Baker, L. A. 1983a. Colorado Family Reading Study: Longitudinal analyses. *Annals of Dyslexia* 33:153–162.

DeFries, J. C., and Baker, L. A. 1983b. Parental contributions to longitudinal stability of cognitive measures in the Colorado Family Reading Study. *Child Development* 54:388–395.

DeFries, J. C., and Decker, S. N. 1982. Genetic aspects of reading disability: A family study. *In* R. N. Malatesha and P. G. Aaron (eds.). *Reading Disorders: Varieties and Treatments.* New York: Academic Press.

DeFries, J. C., and Plomin, R. 1978. Behavioral genetics. *Annual Review of Psychology* 29:473–515.

DeFries, J. C., Singer, S. M., Foch, T. T., and Lewitter, F. I. 1978. Familial nature of reading disability. *British Journal of Psychiatry* 132:361–367.

DeFries, J. C., Vogler, G. P., and LaBuda, M. C. in press. Colorado Family Reading Study: An overview. *In* J. L. Fuller and E. C. Simmel (eds.). *Behavior Genetics: Principles and Applications,* Vol. II. Hillsdale, NJ: Lawrence Erlbaum Associates.

Dunn, L. M., and Markwardt, F. C. 1970. *Examiner's Manual: Peabody Individual Achievement Test.* Circle Pines, MN: American Guidance Service.

Finucci, J. M. 1978. Genetic considerations in dyslexia. *In* H. R. Myklebust (ed.). *Progress in Learning Disabilities,* Vol. IV. New York: Grune and Stratton.

Foch, T. T., DeFries, J. C., McClearn, G. E., and Singer, S. M. 1977. Familial patterns of impairment in reading disability. *Journal of Educational Psychology* 69:316–329.

Fulker, D. W., and DeFries, J. C. 1983. Genetic and environmental transmission in the Colorado Adoption Project: Path analysis. *British Journal of Mathematical and Statistical Psychology* 36:175–188.

Institute for Personality and Ability Testing. 1973. *Measuring Intelligence with Culture Fair Tests: Manual for Scales 2 and 3.* Champaign, IL: Author.

LaBuda, M. C., Vogler, G. P., DeFries, J. C., and Fulker, D. W. in press. Multivariate familial analysis of cognitive measures in the Colorado Family Reading Study. *Multivariate Behavioral Research.*

Lewitter, F. I., DeFries, J. C., and Elston, R. C. 1980. Genetic models of reading disability. *Behavior Genetics* 10:9–30.

McKinney, J. D. 1984. The search for subtypes of specific learning disability. *Journal of Learning Disabilities* 17:43–50.

Thurstone, T. G. 1963. *Examiner's Manual: Primary Mental Abilities*. Chicago: Science Research Associates.

Vogler, G. P. 1985. Multivariate path analysis of familial resemblance. *Genetic Epidemiology* 2:35–53.

Vogler, G. P., and DeFries, J. C. 1984. Application of multivariate path analysis to data from the Colorado Family Reading Study. *Behavior Genetics* 14:618.

Vogler, G. P., and DeFries, J. C. 1985. Bivariate path analysis of familial resemblance for reading ability and symbol processing speed. *Behavior Genetics* 15:111–121.

Vogler, G. P., DeFries, J. C., and Decker, S. N. 1985. Family history as an indicator of risk for reading disability. *Journal of Learning Disabilities* 18:419–421.

Vogler, G. P., Baker, L. A., Decker, S. N., DeFries, J. C., and Huizinga, D. H. in press. Cluster analytic classification of reading disability subtypes. *British Journal of Educational Psychology*.

Wechsler, D. I. 1949. *Examiner's Manual: Wechsler Intelligence Scale for Children*. New York: Psychological Corporation.

Wechsler, D. I. 1974. *Examiner's Manual: Wechsler Intelligence Scale for Children. Revised*. New York: Psychological Corporation.

9

Colorado Twin Study of Reading Disability

Sadie N. Decker and Steven G. Vandenberg

*F*rom the earliest reports at the turn of the century to the more recent systematic family studies, convincing evidence for the presence of important genetic factors in the etiology of reading disability has been accumulating (Decker and DeFries 1980; Finucci 1978). However, attempts to fit single-gene genetic models of inheritance to the data have yielded contradictory results. These apparent inconsistencies suggest that reading disability is a heterogeneous disorder, with multiple subtypes, some which have a genetic origin and some which do not. It is also becoming clear that more than one genetic form of the disorder exists. For example, it is now recognized that the 47XXY sex chromosome anomaly frequently results in a specific form of reading disability (see Decker and Bender in press). However, because the 47XXY karyotype occurs in only 1 out of 800 live male births, and because it is not passed from one generation to the next, it can not account for a significant proportion of the reading disability cases, nor can it explain a familial pattern of reading disorders. Nevertheless, it does confirm that genetic abnormalities can cause a reading disability, and that more than one genetic form of reading disability seems likely.

It is also possible that multiple genetic systems may interact to produce a wide range of phenotypic expression, or that environmental factors may increase the variability of the observed symptoms. Therefore, lacking any clear-cut biological marker for the diagnosis of a hereditary form of reading disability, the most effective strategy for studying the relative contributions made by specific genetic and environmental factors is the twin study.

This work was supported by a grant from NICHD (HD-11681) to Sadie N. Decker and Steven G. Vandenberg.

The authors wish to acknowledge the invaluable assistance of the 20 school districts that participated in this study and of the twins and their families for making this project possible. We also thank Rebecca G. Miles for her expert editorial assistance.

The Twin Study Method

Vandenberg (1976) has described the twin study method as a naturally existing experiment which allows investigators to study the etiology of a disorder by partitioning genetic and environmental variation into more clearly defined dimensions. Although the twin method can be derived from general quantitative genetic theory (Vandenberg 1965), it may also be viewed as an epidemiological technique for validating causal models for the differential diagnosis of reading disability.

In the United States, twin births typically occur at a rate of approximately 1 in 83 live births. Of these, about 28% are identical, or monozygotic (MZ), twins, 36% are same-sex fraternal, or dizygotic (DZ), twins, and 36% are opposite-sex fraternal twins. Because MZ twins have identical genotypes, any dissimilarity between the twins must be attributed to environmental factors either prenatally or postnatally. However, same-sex DZ twins share on the average only 50% of their genes, just as do non-twin sibling pairs. Thus, if the two types of twins show the same degree of similarity for a trait such as reading disability, we know that the greater genetic similarity of the MZ twins has not made a difference, and we can conclude that genetic factors are not the primary determinants of the traits. However, if the degree of similarity between MZ twins is greater than that for DZ twins, we can conclude that genetic factors are indeed playing an important etiological role. Furthermore, if home and school environments are of significantly greater importance than genetic factors, there should be little or no difference between the incidences of the trait in MZ and same-sex DZ twins.

A necessary assumption of the twin study design is that the degree of environmental similarity is approximately the same for the two types of twins. This is typically referred to as the "equal environments assumption." If this assumption is not correct (e.g., if identical twins experience greater similarity in their home or school environment than do fraternal twins), then observations of greater phenotypic similarity between identical twin pairs might be due in part to greater environmental similarity (not greater genetic similarity). Several studies have addressed this question, and the data generally support the validity of the equal environments assumption (Vandenberg 1976, 1984).

The Colorado Twin Study Design

The major objective of this twin study is to delineate how environmental and genetic factors may contribute to individual differences in the expression of reading disability. In order to accomplish this goal, 60 pairs of twins (30 MZ and 30 DZ), in which at least one twin of each pair has been diagnosed as having a reading disability (index cases), are currently being tested by each project domain of the Colorado Reading Study. These 60 twin pairs constitute the reading-disabled sample. In addition, control twin pairs are being selected and matched to the reading-disabled twin pairs on the basis of age (within 6 months), sex, and zygosity. Figure 1 illustrates the design of the study.

Colorado Twin Study of Reading Disability

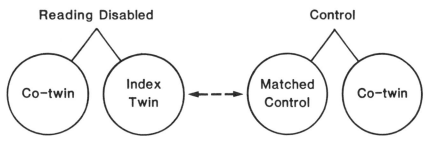

Figure 1.   Design of the Colorado Twin Study of Reading Disability.

When the first phase of the study is completed in 1985, there will be 30 matched pairs of reading-disabled and control MZ twins and 30 matched pairs of reading-disabled and control DZ twins for a total sample of 240 individuals.

Selection Criteria

Subjects for the study are being chosen using school records obtained from the major school disticts within a 100-mile radius of Denver. The criteria for selection of the reading-disabled index cases are as follows: (1) chronological age between 8.5 and 18 years; (2) a reading level at or below the 41st percentile as measured by the Reading Recognition subtest from the Peabody Individual Achievement Test (PIAT, Dunn and Markwardt 1970);[1] (3) no known neurological, emotional, or behavioral disorders; (4) an IQ of at least 90 as measured by either the Verbal or Performance scale of the WISC-R (Wechsler 1974) or the WAIS-R (Wechsler 1981), (5) no uncorrected visual or auditory acuity deficits; and (6) no unusual educational circumstances that could account for their poor reading ability. The matched control twins met all of the same criteria, except that they were reading at or above the 50th percentile.

The analyses for this first report of these data are based upon 20 pairs of MZ twins, in which at least one twin was diagnosed as having a reading disability, and 20 pairs of similarly ascertained DZ twins. In order to insure the comparability of the two types of twins, the MZ and DZ twins were matched for sex (9 female pairs and 11 male pairs), age (within 6 months), and the absence of any history of seizures among the index cases. This additional exclusionary criterion was added because we have found an unexpectedly high frequency of self-reported seizures among a subset of our reading-disabled sample. Thus, all index cases who reported a history of seizures were excluded from these analyses.

By utilizing both inclusionary and exclusionary selection criteria, it was

---

[1]The 41st percentile was found to be the point which best separated the two distributions of Reading Recognition scores for normal vs. disabled readers in the Colorado Family Reading Study. Percentiles are based on age, not grade placement, an important consideration in view of the fact that reading-disabled children occasionally repeat a grade.

possible to select a non-clinical, representative sample of disabled readers whose unexpected reading problems could not be attributed to other neurological disorders, poor teaching, environmental deprivation, or low intellectual capability. Typically, the families are middle to upper-middle class Caucasians, and English is always the language spoken in the home.

Zygosity Determination

Zygosity of the twins is being determined by an updated version of the Nichols and Bilbro (1966) zygosity questionnaire which has a reported accuracy of 95% (copies are available from Dr. Decker). For twin pairs for which zygosity is uncertain, blood samples are taken from each twin and 16 blood markers are compared by the Minneapolis War Memorial Blood Bank. These markers include six blood type systems, eight serum proteins and RBC enzymes, and Gm and Inv$_1$ typing. Therefore, the determination of the zygosity of the twins is done with a high degree of certainty.

Psychometric Assessment

Because reading disability is a psychometrically defined disorder, the process of establishing baseline markers for differential diagnosis depends upon standardized psychometric assessment. Our "benchmark" indices are standardized tests for which substantial amounts of normative data are available and they meet several important requirements of a study in which large numbers of individuals are tested over a wide age range. These basic requirements include the following: (1) the test must be suitable for use over a wide educational and developmental period; (2) it must measure the same basic constructs in both children and adults; (3) it must be highly reliable since analyses of twin similarity may be underestimated if test reliabilities are low; and (4) it must be designed so that it may be efficiently and accurately administered within a typical educational or psychological testing situation.

A 2.5-hour battery of psychometric tests is being individually administered to each subject by a trained examiner. A 15-minute break for rest and refreshment separates the testing session into two approximately equal segments.

The test battery is divided into two parts: a standardized portion and an experimental portion (see Table I). The standardized measures were selected in order to maintain consistency with the data being collected in a family study and with previously existing longitudinal data. The experimental portion consists of three newly developed neurolinguistic tests which were designed to assess expressive verbal fluency, rapid automatic naming, and perceptual speed. These measures were developed as part of the Colorado Adult Reading Project which was completed in 1982. The tests and detailed psychometric data are available from the first author—also see Decker and Bender (in press). Since testing on the experimental measures is not yet complete, only the standardized reading and IQ measures were used for the analyses reported here.

Table I
Psychometric Test Battery

Tests	Reliability	Source
Standardized Tests		
Peabody Individual Achievement		Dunn and Markwardt (1970)
Test (PIAT)		
Reading Comprehension	0.64	
Reading Recognition	0.89	
Mathematics	0.74	
Spelling	0.65	
Primary Mental Abilities Test		Science Research Associates (1965)
Spatial Relations	0.78	
Wechsler Adult Intelligence Scale-	*	Wechsler (1981)
Revised (WAIS-R)		
Wechsler Intelligence Scale for	*	Wechsler (1974)
Children-Revised (WISC-R)		
Detroit Tests of Learning Aptitude		Baker and Leland (1959)
Auditory Attention Span for	**	
Unrelated Words		
Auditory Attention Span for	**	
Related Syllables		
Educational Testing Service		French, Ekstrom, and Price (1963)
Identical Pictures Test	0.82	
Experimental Tests		Decker and Bender (in press)
Expressive Verbal Fluency		
Letters	0.59	
Categories	0.69	
Rapid Automatic Naming		
Pictures	0.80	
Colors	0.82	
Numbers	0.86	
Letters	0.86	
Colorado Perceptual Speed Test-		
Revised		
Phonetically Similar	0.80	
Phonetically Dissimilar	0.91	
Pronounceable Non-Words	0.92	

*Subtest reliabilities range from 0.65 to 0.97.
**To be determined.

Results

Descriptive Data

As a preliminary analysis to check for sex effects which might create an ascertainment bias, a one-way ANOVA was calculated to test for mean differences between male vs. female index twins on the PIAT Reading Recognition measure. Results of this analysis indicated that there were no significant differences ($F = 0.35, p > 0.05$); thus, the data for males and females could be combined.

Because members of twin pairs covary perfectly for age, it is important that all test scores be age-corrected in order to eliminate the effect of covariance due to age on twin correlations. For the Reading Recognition scores, the linear and quadratic effects of age were removed by expressing each subject's score as a deviation from a quadratic regression line derived from control data provided by the family study (see Decker and DeFries 1980). For the standard scores and percentiles, the age corrections were provided by the conversion tables from the respective test manuals.

Means and standard errors for the 20 matched pairs of MZ and DZ twins are presented in Table II. As anticipated, both the MZ and DZ index twins are reading at approximately one-half the expected level for comparable normal readers. The means for the Verbal and Performance IQ scales indicate that the reading-disabled twins tend to have a lower Verbal IQ than Performance IQ. It is important to note that one of the ascertainment criteria was that *either* the Verbal or Performance IQ score had to be equal to at least 90. Thus, the lower Verbal IQ scores *do not* reflect an ascertainment bias; rather, they reflect the typical pattern of lower verbal scores that is characteristic of disabled readers (Vellutino 1979).

It is also the case that the MZ co-twins do not differ significantly from the MZ index cases on any of these measures. However, the scores of the DZ co-twins do differ significantly from those of the DZ index twins for Reading Recognition ($F = 22.05, p < 0.01$) and verbal IQ ($F = 5.00, p < 0.05$), a result which warrants further analyses.

Concordance Rates

Twin similarities can be expressed by concordance rates when a dichotomous diagnostic categorization is of interest. Concordance rates may be calculated two different ways: probandwise or pairwise. Probandwise cal-

Table II
Means ± SE for Reading-Disabled Twin Sample

Measure	Identical (MZ) Twins		Same-Sex Fraternal (DZ) Twins	
	Index Twins ($N = 20$)	Co-Twins ($N = 20$)	Index Twins ($N = 20$)	Co-Twins ($N = 20$)
Reading Recognition[a]	24 ± 1.14	26 ± 1.15	21 ± 1.09	38 ± 1.21
Verbal IQ	95.4 ± 1.68	97.3 ± 1.90	90.9 ± 1.93	98.6 ± 2.83
Performance IQ	99.6 ± 2.36	101.7 ± 2.01	102.9 ± 2.44	103.3 ± 3.09
Age	13.4 ± 0.55		13.3 ± 0.57	

[a]Percentile.

Table III
Concordance Rates for Reading Disability

	MZ Twins (N = 20 Pairs)	DZ Twins (N = 20 Pairs)	X² (Corrected)
Reading Level ≤ 41st Percentile	0.80	0.45	3.84*
Discriminant Function Composite	0.85	0.55	4.98*

*$p \leq 0.05$.

culations are appropriate when each affected twin is selected independently and when comparisons are to be made with population incidence rates. However, for small studies in which twins are ascertained through the selection of one affected member of the twin pair (the index case), pairwise concordance rates are appropriate.

Pairwise concordance rates are calculated by counting each pair of twins only once, and the concordance rate is simply the proportion of pairs in which both members of the pair are similarly affected (Gottesman and Shields 1972). Of the few small twin studies of reading disability that have been published, the typical pairwise concordance rates range from 84% to 100% for MZ pairs and from 29% to 30% for DZ pairs (for a review, see Finucci 1978).

As a first step in estimating concordance rates for our twins, the selection criterion for the Reading Recognition test (i.e., reading level at or below the 41st percentile) was confirmed for all the index cases (20 MZ and 20 DZ). When the co-twins were similarly classified, the concordance rate for DZ twins was significantly lower than that for the MZ twins (see Table III). Because spurious discordance may occur when the difference is only a matter of degree, it is important to analyze the reading scores for both concordant and discordant twins.

Table IV presents the means and standard errors for the normal and reading-disabled MZ and DZ co-twins. The reading scores indicate that the DZ co-twins who were classified as "normal" are indeed well within the typical range for average or above readers. However, the large standard error term for the MZ co-twins who are classified as "normal" readers indicates that there is considerable variability in their scores. Inspection of the distribution of their reading scores indicates that two of the so-called "normal" readers have percentile scores of 43 and 44 respectively. Thus, concordance rates may fluctuate as a function of the arbitrary cut-off point on any continuous measures.

Table IV
Means ± SE for Reading-Disabled and Normal-Reading Co-Twins

	MZ Co-Twins		DZ Co-Twins	
Measure	Disabled (N = 16)	Normal (N = 4)	Disabled (N = 9)	Normal (N = 11)
Reading Recognition[a]	24 ± 1.17	50 ± 5.48	28 ± 0.87	55 ± 2.89
Verbal IQ	96.3 ± 2.33	100.3 ± 3.52	93.1 ± 3.23	102.8 ± 4.06
Performance IQ	101.4 ± 2.17	100.3 ± 5.87	107.1 ± 5.24	100.1 ± 3.57

[a]Percentile.

It is also interesting to note that the "normal" co-twins Verbal IQ scores are higher, but that their Performance IQ scores do not differ markedly from the scores of the other co-twins who were classified as "reading-disabled." Thus, Verbal IQ and reading disability may have a common etiological relationship.

Because the reliable diagnosis of reading disability involves considerations other than an arbitrary cut-off point on a single reading test, other diagnostic criteria must be considered as well. In order to provide a more complete, empirically derived, diagnostic index, a separate and independent sample of reading-disabled and control subjects was selected from the family study and matched to the index twins and their matched controls on the basis of age (within 6 months) and sex. Thus, 80 non-twin subjects (40 reading disabled vs. 40 controls) were used to calculate a multivariate composite which could then be applied to the twin sample for concordance calculations. The PIAT Reading Recognition, Reading Comprehension, and Spelling subtests, along with the Verbal and Performance IQ scales and the mother's report of whether or not the child had difficulty learning to read, were entered into a direct discriminant function analysis (Hull and Nie 1981). The resulting composite was able to correctly classify 93% of the reading-disabled and 97% of the control subjects into their previously determined correct group. Thus, the composite index has considerable diagnostic validity. When the same composite was used to classify the twins, all 40 index twins were classified as being reading disabled, while the concordance rates for the co-twins were approximately 5% higher than for the selection criteria alone (see Table III). However, it must be acknowledged that potentially important individual differences may be masked by the use of multivariate composites.

These concordance analyses confirm the consistency of the selection criteria across samples, which in turn lends credence to the prediction and diagnosis of reading disability among the co-twins of this study. Accuracy in calculating concordance rates is an essential first step toward differential diagnosis and the delineation of etiologically distinct subtypes. Only by knowing precisely which twins are affected are we able to study potential genetic and environmental influences on the disorder. However, the reliability of any classification system will influence concordance calculations.

Environmental Factors

Before examining potential hereditary causes of reading disability, the similarity of the twins' environments becomes a question of crucial importance. For example, if the MZ twins experience more similar educational environments than do the DZ twins, any method of estimating the hereditary contribution to the disorder will be spuriously inflated with the environmental variance. Unfortunately, the fact is that we know very little about differences in the educational correlations of MZ and DZ twins. Furthermore, if such differences exist, we do not know how large they might be.

It is also possible that various methods for teaching reading may influence twin similarities and differences. For example, Vandenberg (1976) reported a study by Naeslund in which 10 pairs of identical twins were separated during school hours for the first three school semesters from 1953 to 1955. The members of each pair were placed at random in two different classes—one class used the phonics approach to reading instruction, and the other used the whole word method. At the end of a year and a half, the twins were tested for speed and accuracy of reading and for reading comprehension. It was found that the whole word method was superior for teaching children of lower intellectual ability; for the more intelligent children, there was no difference between the two methods.

A series of educational questions were developed for the twin study in order to assess the twins' attitudes toward school and the degree to which twins have the same teachers and classes. Likewise, home environment questions were developed to assess parental treatment of the two types of twins and the degree of similarity in their general life experiences.

Table V presents an analysis of the school and home environment questionnaire measures. When the twins were asked how they liked school and whether or not they found various subjects to be difficult, 63% of the MZ twins and 65% of the DZ twins were found to have a positive attitude toward school. Hence, differences in reading scores between MZ and DZ twins do not appear to be related to attitudes toward school.

When the mothers were asked to rate how often their twins had similar teachers and whether or not they were currently in the same classrooms, the mothers replied that only 20% of the MZ twins and 25% of the DZ twins were placed with the same teachers and in the same classes. In fact, discussions with school personnel indicate that both parents and teachers make an effort to separate twins so that they may be treated as individuals.

A slightly different pattern of results emerged from the family environment questionnaire data. When the mothers were asked questions concerning the degree to which they treated their twins in a similar way with respect to such things as punishment, rewards, dressing alike, and so on, approximately 70% of the mothers of MZ twins indicated that they treated their twins in similar manner as compared to 50% of the DZ twins. A similar pattern of results was obtained for the life experience measures, which looked at such things as extended separations of the twins, major illnesses, or any other types of important experiences which were not common to both twins. Although these

Table V

Proportion of Twins Who Respond Similarly to Family and School Questionnaire Items

Measure	MZ Twins ($N = 20$ Pairs)	DZ Twins ($N = 20$ Pairs)	X^2 (Corrected)
Educational			
Positive Attitude Toward School	0.63	0.65	0.30
Similar Teachers and Classes	0.20	0.25	0.56
Family Environment			
Similar Parental Treatment	0.70	0.50	0.94
Similar Life Experiences	0.70	0.55	0.43

differences failed to reach statistical significance, it is important to acknowledge the possibility that MZ twins may share a more common home environment than DZ twins. However, as a general rule, it seems only sensible to focus
more attention on the educational environment, given a school system which
systematically devotes a substantial part of every school day to the teaching of
reading.

Hereditary Factors

Results from studies of normal-reading twins, which span almost 40
years, consistently show a substantial hereditary contribution to reading ability.
More specifically, Matheny and Dolan (1974) found that intraclass correlations
based upon reading subtest scores from the California Achievement Test
ranged from a low of 0.84 to a high of 0.89 for MZ twins, whereas the range for
DZ pairs was 0.52 to 0.61. Tests for the significance of the difference between
the MZ and DZ correlations were all significant ($p < 0.05$). There are,
however, conflicting views about the degree of differential genetic influence.

Ho, Foch, and Plomin (1980) have developed another approach for
analyzing twin differences on continuous measures. Their hierarchical multiple
regression model is particularly well suited for analyzing small data sets and for
providing tests of significance for the difference between MZ vs. DZ twins
using measures of index and co-twin similarity. For both types of twins, the
index twin's score on a psychometric test may be used to predict the co-twin's
score, zygosity, and an interaction term consisting of the index twin's score and
zygosity. The model is

$$\hat{Y} = B_1X_1 + B_2X_2 + B_3X_1X_2 + A \text{ (constant)},$$
$$\quad\;\; \text{step 1} \qquad\quad \text{step 2}$$

in which $\hat{Y}$ is the predicted score of the co-twin, X_1 is the index twin's score,
and X_2 is the categorical variable representing zygosity. The product X_1X_2 is
indicative of a conditional relationship between the co-twin's predicted score
and the index twin's score and zygosity. B_1 is the partial regression of $\hat{Y}$ on X_1
(a measure of twin resemblance); B_2 is the partial regression of $\hat{Y}$ on X_2 (a
measure of the influence of zygosity); and B_3 is the partial regression of $\hat{Y}$ on
the two-way interaction X_1X_2. A significant B_3 would indicate a conditional
relationship between the predicted score of the co-twin and the index twin's
score and zygosity. Thus, the partial regression coefficient for the two-way
interaction (B_3) measures the extent to which the mixture of genetic and
environmental influences differs as a function of zygosity.

Results for the hierarchical multiple regression analyses using the Reading
Recognition, Verbal and Performance IQ scores, and height are presented in
Table VI. As recommended by Ho et al. (1980), height was included as a
"benchmark" variable. The partial regression coefficients (B_3) for the two-
way interaction between the index twin's score and zygosity were statistically
significant for the reading measure and for height, but not for Verbal or
Performance IQ. Thus, these comparisons do provide evidence for a heritable
component of reading ability. Moreover, these results are consistent with the

Table VI

Partial Regression Coefficients and F-Values for Two-Way Interaction Between Index Twin's Score and Zygosity

Measure	Partial Regression Coefficient	F-Value
Reading Recognition	−0.432	8.29**
Verbal IQ	−0.042	0.30
Performance IQ	0.035	0.04
Height	−0.269	2.82*

*$p < 0.10$.
**$p < 0.01$.

findings obtained by Matheny and Dolan (1974) for twins not selected for reading disability. It is also interesting to note that the regression model was able to account for 51% of the total variance for the reading measure, with 11% of that variance being uniquely explained by the two-way interaction.

If, in fact, reading disability does have a more specific differential hereditary component than does Verbal or Performance IQ, then the relative MZ twin similarities should be greater for the reading measure than for other cognitive variables. It may also be the case that the presence of a reading disability may unduly influence the relative mixture of environmental and genetic effects on IQ scales. These questions concerning the differential genetic and environmental effects will be more completely explored when all of the twins have been tested and comparison data from our control twins are available.

Discussion

These preliminary analyses from the Colorado Twin Study of Reading Disability indicate that reading ability in general appears to have a substantial hereditary component. Whether or not these genetic influences can be related to a specific form of reading disability is not clear. For example, it may well be that certain reading-disabled individuals represent only the lower end of a normal distribution of reading scores. For others, a specific genetic form of the disorder may be present. Data from the electrophysiological domain of the project will provide important diagnostic information concerning the specificity of these genetic effects on neurological functioning. To the extent that reading disability may be caused by a specific genetic factor, it seems reasonable to expect that observable neurological deficits should also be present.

With respect to environmental influences on the expression of the disorder, the discordance of some MZ co-twins confirms that environmental factors are contributing to the expression of the disorder. To what extent these effects are artifacts of measurement error or correlated variables will be more clearly understood when the data on the control twins become available. However, results of analyses of the school questionnaire data were somewhat surprising in that both parents and educators appear to make a concerted effort to provide a separate educational environment for each twin. Thus, differences between MZ and DZ twin similarities in reading cannot be attributed to more common educational experiences among MZ twins.

Finally, it is important to mention that twins may be more susceptible to cognitive and neurological dysfunction than are singletons. Results of the Collaborative Perinatal Project conducted by the National Institute of Neurological and Communicative Disorders and Stroke have led to the conclusion that poor prenatal environmental conditions may be partly responsible for the higher incidence of congenital malformations in twins, especially those of the central nervous system (Myrianthopoulos, Nichols, and Broman 1976). This susceptibility is particularly relevant to our study given that we have encountered an unexpectedly high incidence of self-reported (or parent-reported) seizures among reading-disabled twins. Therefore, it is imperative that the co-existence of reading disability with other neurological disorders be carefully documented.

Upon the completion of this phase of the study in 1985, data on the new neurolinguistic measures, as well as data from the other domains of the project, will provide new insights into the genetic and environmental bases of reading disability which, in turn, will provide valuable information concerning differential diagnosis.

References

Baker, H. J., and Leland, B. 1959. *Detroit Tests of Learning Aptitude*. Indianapolis: Test Division of Bobbs-Merrill.

Decker, S. N., and Bender, B. (in press). Converging evidence for multiple genetic factors in reading disability. *In* H. A. Whitaker and A. Caramazza (eds.). *Studies in Neuropsychology*. Hillsdale, NJ: Lawrence Erlbaum Associates.

Decker, S. N., and DeFries, J. C. 1980. Cognitive abilities in families with reading disabled children. *Journal of Learning Disabilities* 13:517–522.

Dunn, L. M., and Markwardt, F. C. 1970. *Examiner's Manual: Peabody Individual Achievement Test*. Circle Pines, MN: American Guidance Service.

Finucci, J. M. 1978. Genetic considerations in dyslexia. *In* H. R. Myklebust (ed.). *Progress in Learning Disabilities*, Vol. IV. New York: Grune and Stratton.

French, J. W., Ekstrom, R. G., and Price, L. A. 1963. *Manual for a Kit of Referenced Tests for Cognitive Factors*. Princeton, NJ: Educational Testing Service.

Gottesman, I. I., and Shields, J. 1972. *Schizophrenia and Genetics: A Twin Study Vantage Point*. New York: Academic Press.

Ho, H-Z., Foch, T. T., and Plomin, R. 1980. Developmental stability of the relative influence of genes and environment on specific cognitive abilities during childhood. *Developmental Psychology* 16:340–346.

Hull, C. H., and Nie, N. H. 1981. *SPSS UPDATE 7–9*. New York: McGraw-Hill.

Matheny, A. P., and Dolan, A. B. 1974. A twin study of genetic influence in reading achievement. *Journal of Learning Disabilities* 7:99–102.

Myrianthopoulos, N. C., Nichols, P. L., and Broman, S. H. 1976. Intellectual development of twins—Comparison with singletons. *Acta Geneticae Medicae et Gemellologiae* 25:376–380.

Nichols, R. C., and Bilbro, W. C. 1966. The diagnosis of twin zygosity. *Acta Geneticae Medicae et Gemellologiae* 16:265–275.

Science Research Associates, Inc. 1965. *Primary Mental Abilities: Technical Report*. Chicago: Author.

Vandenberg, S. G. 1965. Multivariate analysis of twin differences. *In* S. G. Vandenberg (ed.). *Methods and Goals in Human Behavior Genetics*. New York: Academic Press.

Vandenberg, S. G. 1976. Twin studies. *In* A. R. Kaplan (ed.). *Human Behavior Genetics*. Springfield, IL: Charles C Thomas.

Vandenberg, S. G. 1984. Does a special twin situation contribute to similarity for abilities in MZ and DZ twins? *Acta Geneticae Medicae et Gemellologiae* 33:219–222.

Vellutino, F. 1979. *Dyslexia: Theory and Research*. Cambridge, MA: MIT Press.

Wechsler, D. I. 1974. *Examiner's Manual: Wechsler Intelligence Scale for Children-Revised*. New York: Psychological Corporation.

Wechsler, D. I. 1981. *Examiner's Manual: Wechsler Adult Intelligence Scale-Revised*. New York: Psychological Corporation.

10

Approaches to Subtype Validation Using Family Data

Joan M. Finucci

Introduction

*T*he idea that there are subtypes among developmental dyslexics had its genesis in observations of differences among dyslexics in clinical settings. For instance, Ingram and his colleagues described the difficulties of 82 dyslexic patients as being predominantly audio-phonic, predominantly visuo spatial, or as having a combination of difficulties of both types (Ingram, Mason, and Blackburn 1970; Ingram 1971). Johnson and Myklebust (1967) described two main types of dyslexia and appropriate treatments for each, based on their clinical observations. Visual dyslexics have a primary disturbance in learning through the visual modality; auditory dyslexics have primary difficulties in auditory processing. Myklebust (1978) extended the subtype description to include two additional types. Intermodal dyslexics have visual and auditory processing intact but have difficulty in transferring information processed in one modality to another modality (e.g., visual to auditory). Inner language dyslexics are described by Myklebust as individuals with an integrative-neurosensory deficit; they are able to perceive graphemes and transduce them into their auditory equivalents (word-calling), but they cannot code the names to meaning. This "subtype" is similar to the hyperlexics described by Huttenlocher and Huttenlocher (1973) and Healy (1982) and perhaps dyslexic is not an apt description of such individuals.

An additional reason for suggesting that there are subtypes of dyslexia is to explain the heterogeneity in the data of research studies with dyslexics. For example, family studies of dyslexia have shown the condition to cluster in families, yet there are subjects with one or both parents affected, only sibs affected, or no affected relatives (Finucci, Guthrie, Childs, Abbey, and Childs

The work was supported by funds from The John F. Kennedy Institute and NIH Grant HD 00486.

137

1976). Such heterogeneity across families may reflect genetically distinct subtypes of developmental dyslexia.

Springing from such observations have been experimental studies whose purpose has been to characterize in a systematic fashion subtypes of dyslexia. Most of these studies have been described in reviews by Satz and Morris (1981), Lyon (1983), and Malatesha and Dougan (1982). Subtyping studies may be differentiated on the basis of the variables or the techniques used to determine subtypes or, in the case of a few more recent studies, on the basis of the means of validating subtypes. For instance, with respect to the variables used, the studies of Doehring (Doehring and Hoshko 1977 and Doehring, Trites, Patel, and Fiedorowicz, 1981), of Boder (1971, 1973), and of Lovett (1984a,b) based the classifications on measures of reading and spelling skill or components of those skills (e.g., speed of letter naming). In contrast, studies of Mattis (Mattis, French, and Rapin 1975; Mattis, 1978) and of Rourke (Petrauskas and Rourke 1979; Fisk and Rourke 1979) used as classifying variables a number of cognitive and neuropsychological variables other than reading and spelling skill, such as scores from Raven's Progressive Matrices, the Benton Test of Visual Retention, Peabody Picture Vocabulary Test, WISC or WISC-R subtests, or tests of tactile skills.

With respect to methods used in subtyping, the main distinction is between the use of clinical observations and the use of statistical classification techniques. The clinical approach is typified by the study of Mattis et al. (1975) in which 29 developmental dyslexics, 53 brain-damaged dyslexics, and 31 brain-damaged readers were administered a battery of neuropsychological tests. The battery included tests of naming, language comprehension, imitative speech, fine motor coordination, and visuo-spatial analysis. The investigators' clinical judgment was that the dyslexics presented with one of three patterns of disorder: a disorder in language development, a motor-speech difficulty often associated with grapho-motor dyscoordination or a visuo-spatial perceptual disorder. Based on these clinical observations, three syndromes were defined quantitatively. That is, ". . . to assure the exclusion of deficiencies irrelevant to dyslexia, criteria were established for each syndrome such that no false positives would be detected in the brain-damaged readers group." (p. 154).

Illustrative of multivariate statistical approaches to classification are the studies of Doehring and Hoshko (1977), Fisk and Rourke (1979), and Lyon and Watson (1981). In the study of Fisk and Rourke, 100 nine- and ten-year olds, 100 eleven- and twelve-year olds, and 64 thirteen- and fourteen-year olds were given a battery of tests which yielded 44 measures. Raw scores from these were converted to T scores based on normative data and a correlational analysis of the pooled samples was carried out. Twenty-one of the measures from each of six skill areas (auditory-verbal, sequencing, visual-spatial, tactile, motor, and abstract-conceptual) were selected for Q factor analyses within each age sample. Those subjects whose factor loadings were $\geq .50$ on a single factor were used to define a subtype which was characterized by those subjects' average pattern of performance on the 21 measures. Six subtypes emerged in each age group and 80% of the subjects could be classified into a subtype. Two subtypes were replicated across all three age groups and a third across the two younger age groups. The investigators suggested that the third subtype might be a variation of one of the first two. Both the first and second subtypes were characterized by relatively poor auditory-verbal processing and psycholinguistic skills and average or better visual-perceptual and visual-spatial abilities. However, the first showed marked impairment in tactile finger localization whereas the second showed relatively intact tactile-kinesthetic and kinesthetic-perceptual abilities. The subjects in this second subtype showed the largest WISC VIQ-PIQ discrepancy; on average, Performance IQ was approximately 21 points higher than Verbal IQ.

Validation of Subtypes

The number of subtyping studies is now relatively large. Malatesha and Dougan (1982) reviewed 29 studies in which two or more subtypes emerged. The more consistent the subtypes among the various studies the more likely that they have clinical and statistical validity. But, in fact, there is a lack of consistency, owing partly to the variance in measures that are used and partly to the variance in techniques. In recent years, some studies designed to determine subtypes have also included a validation component; other studies have selected subjects based on the characteristics of subtypes defined by other investigators and have had as their purpose the validation of those subtypes. The chief method of attempting to show that a classification has validity has been to show that subtypes defined by one set of variables can be differentiated using a second set of variables or that they are predictive of or predicted by a second variable or set of variables.

Among such studies are those which have attempted to show that dyslexics subtyped by the Boder method (1971, 1973) differ on other variables. For example, studies by Aaron, Grantham, and Campbell (1982), Rosenthal, Boder, and Calloway (1982) and van den Bos (1984) explored the relationship of the Boder subtypes to different sets of variables. Van den Bos conducted two experiments with 22 "dysphonetic" children, 9 "dyseidetic" children and 17 "mixed" children, defined by the decision criteria of a Dutch version of the Boder Reading-Spelling Pattern Test (Boder and Jarrico 1982). In the first experiment, he tested the prediction that auditorily presented letter sets should be processed better by dyseidetic than by dysphonetic readers. In the second experiment he tested predictions that there would be differential performance by dyseidetic and dysphonetic readers in a task requiring subjects to make rapid determinations about whether two letters of a pair (e.g., ee, EM, EF, dD, Dm, Dp) shared the same name. Neither prediction was confirmed. Acknowledging that the experiments focused on letter processing only and allowing that there may be processes that differentiate between dysphonetic and dyseidetic subjects, van den Bos concluded that all three dyslexic groups showed similar difficulty in accessing phonetic representations in the speeded test situations used.

Rosenthal et al. (1982) studied a sample of adult dyslexics, 12 of whom were classified as dysphonetic, 11 as dyseidetic, and 10 as mixed using the Camp and Dolcourt (1977) modification of the Boder test. The purpose of the study was to determine if there are electrophysiological correlates of the three types. Specifically they measured visual and auditory event-related potentials from left and right parietal leads using attentive and passive conditions. Because certain amplitude measures in the 250–450 msec latency band produced significant differences between dyseidetic and dysphonetic subjects the investigators concluded that their results lent support to the construct validity of the Boder subtypes. Their data suggest, however, that fewer than half of the subjects in each group account for the differences between groups.

The study by Aaron et al. 1982 examined whether dysphonetic and dyseidetic dyslexic subjects show a differential response to remediation efforts. In two separate experiments, one lasting four weeks and one lasting an academic year, a total of 8 dyseidetic subjects and 9 dysphonetic subjects were trained using either a phonetic-sequential method or a whole-word method. Small sample sizes prohibited valid statistical analysis, but the investigators concluded that the dyseidetics did better under the phonetic-sequential method and the dysphonetics under the whole-word method. Their conclusions, however, were based on visual inspection of gain scores, and there was no adjustment made for different lengths of training between groups.

Other investigators have also raised the question of whether subtypes show differing responses to remediation. For example, Lyon (1983) reported a study in progress in which he examined the responses of subjects in each of six different subgroups to one hour of extra reading instruction per week for 26 weeks. The teaching approach was a synthetic phonics program that was well-sequenced, offered systematic drill, and introduced phonics concepts. Five subjects were in each of the six groups, and they were equated for reading level, age, sex, and IQ. There were significant differences in reading recognition gain scores among the samples at the end of the intervention period. The two groups that made the most gain were those in which subjects manifested no severe deficits in auditory discrimination, auditory memory, and sound blending, that is, in skills important for phonics development, whereas the two groups which made no improvement had significant deficits in auditory memory, auditory comprehension, and sound-blending. The investigators caution, however, that their results should be regarded as tenuous because, although the subgroups were matched on preintervention reading recognition level, they did not compute preintervention regression between aptitude and achievement which might have differed among subgroups.

Finally, Doehring (1984) discussed the complexity of designs that are necessary for evaluating whether the effectiveness of remediation varies as a function of subtype. For example, he suggested that to determine if there is a "best" method to use with just one subtype, each of the subjects of that type might be assigned to one of five treatment groups with training in each group focusing on a) deficient reading skills, b) underlying nonreading deficits, c) compensatory skills and strategies, d) deficits and compensatory skills, or e) on no training at all (a control group). To expand this design to determine if "best" methods exist for two subtypes, which may also serve to differentiate and validate the subtypes, ten training groups would be necessary. Thus, research on subtype-treatment interactions has involved compromises to such designs and no such research with dyslexics has produced definitive results.

Validity Testing with Family Data

Another approach to the validation of subtypes of dyslexia is to show within-family homogeneity and between-family heterogeneity with respect to characteristics that define the subtype. Much of the remainder of this chapter will describe the approach, review some studies where the method has been used and discuss some considerations that need to be made in future studies.

The approach is based on some observations and assumptions that are listed in Table I.

The first observation is that a significant number of cases of developmental dyslexia are familial. In 1905, two reports of multiple cases in the same family were reported and the authors of both suggested that the condition had a tendency to run in families (Fisher 1905, Thomas 1905). Since then several studies have been carried out which have shown that reading and spelling level among relatives of dyslexics is poorer than that of relatives of controls (Owen, Adams, Forrest, Stolz, and Fisher 1971; DeFries, Singer, Foch, and Lewitter 1978) and that the frequency of dyslexia among relatives of dyslexics is higher than would be expected if there were a random distribution of cases in the general population (Hallgren 1950; Walker and Cole 1965; Finucci et al. 1976). Because these non-random distributions occur in families in which a disadvantaged environment, lack of motivation, and lack of schooling have been ruled out as possible explanations for the occurrence of dyslexia and because in many families there is evidence from parental emotional and financial investment in the children's education, that reading ability is valued, we state our first assumption: that there is a biological basis for the multiple cases of dyslexia within families. This assumption was given further support from the studies of Smith, Kimberling, Pennington, and Lubs (1983). They conducted a genetic linkage analysis among 12 kindreds comprising 105 individuals in which there

Table I
Observations (O) and Assumptions (A) Underlying the Familial Approach to Subtyping

O: Familial nature of dyslexia

A: Common biologically-based explanation of dyslexia within families.

A: Error in development of neurological mechanism subserving reading.

O: Different dissociations in cognitive processing skills among different forms of acquired dyslexia.

A.: Subtypes within families of developmental dyslexia can be defined by dissociations of cognitive processing skills.

was evidence of developmental dyslexia in three generations, consistent with an autosomal dominant pattern of inheritance. Their purpose was to determine if dyslexia could be shown to be linked with a known genetic marker. The results of those initial studies suggested that in most of these families, developmental dyslexia is linked to a marker on the short arm of chromosome 15, implicating the same genetic etiology of dyslexia within the families. It should be noted, however, that upon collection of additional data (Kimberling, et al. 1985) the investigators were unable to replicate their earlier results. Thus, there may have been greater genetic heterogeneity among their second group of families than among the first (the first group might be more representative of a specific genetic subtype) or their initial results may have been spurious.

Our next assumption is that, given that developmental dyslexia is a cognitive deficit, the biological basis for dyslexia is rooted in one or more errors in the development of neurological mechanisms that subserve the cognitive processing components of reading. The logic of this assumption is supported by observations of disruptions in reading and spelling as a result of acquired neurological impairments among adults. In particular, the study of acquired dyslexia among adults has led to the observation of dissociations in components of reading and spelling abilities that reflect impairment to different cognitive processing functions (Marshall and Newcombe 1966; Coltheart, Patterson and Marshall 1980; Patterson 1981). Finally, we make the assumption that similarly, the reading and spelling patterns of developmental dyslexics within the same family will reflect impairment of the same cognitive processing components and that the differences in reading behavior between families will reflect the fact that different neurological mechanisms are impaired in different families.

Studies of Within-Family Likeness

The geneticist's interest in the subtyping issue is motivated by the need to have homogeneous subgroups in which to test hypotheses about genetic transmission. Boder was attuned to the significance of within-family homogeneity. She noted in her early paper (Boder 1971) that ''there is evidence that a genetic factor may exist in each of the three reading-spelling patterns; all but two of the sets of dyslexic siblings in our sample—a total of 39 siblings from 16 families—fall into the same reading-spelling pattern group'' (p. 313). The studies that have examined within-family likeness to date have looked at rather broad cognitive or electrophysiological measures.

In our family studies in Baltimore (Finucci and Childs 1983; Childs and Finucci 1983) we have looked at within-family data for spelling error type. Our classification of spelling errors is dichotomous—either a subject's misspelling could be produced by the use of rules for phonology-to-orthography correspondence or it is not a phonologically equivalent rendering of the target word. In Boder's terms the error is phonetic or it is dysphonetic. The scheme differs from Boder's though, in that no judgment is made with respect to the visual similarity of the error to the target word. In Figure 1 are shown the distributions of the proportions of subjects' errors that are dysphonetic for two groups of dyslexic children, 69 from Baltimore who, with one exception, were in grades 3 to 8 and 88 from the Gow School near Buffalo who were in grades 7 to 12. It can be seen that even dyslexics made more phonologically appropriate errors than dysphonetic errors, but these distributions are skewed farther to the right than those for normal readers, Groups II and III in the figure, and within these distributions are represented dyslexics of equal severity—some whose errors are primarily phonetic and others whose errors are primarily dysphonetic (Finucci, Isaacs, Whitehouse, and Childs 1983).

Among adults we have also shown that there is a high correlation between the tendency to make dysphonetic spelling errors and difficulty in reading

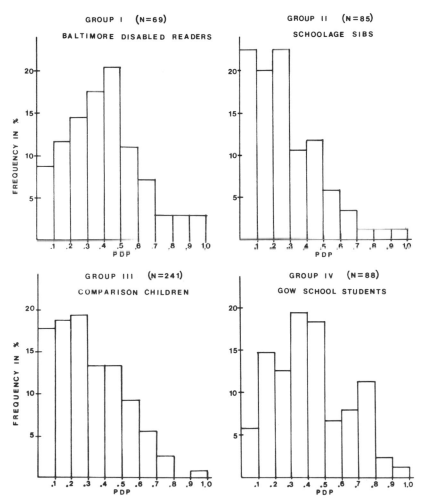

Figure 1.   Distribution of proportion dysphonetic errors in four groups of subjects (From Finucci, Isaacs, Whitehouse, and Childs, 1983). Reprinted from *Brain and Language* by permission of Academic Press.

Table II
Relationship between Proportion Dysphonetic Spelling Errors (PDP)
and Errors in Reading Nonsense Words

	Normal Reading Adults				Dyslexic Adults			
	Number of Nonsense Errors				Number of Nonsense Errors			
PDP	0–10	11–20	21–50	Total	0–10	11–20	21–50	Total
.00–.30	53*	10	0	63	9	7	1	17
	(.84)	(.16)	(.00)		(.53)	(.41)	(.06)	
.31–.60	28	12	0	40	6	12	5	23
	(.70)	(.30)	(.00)		(.26)	(.52)	(.22)	
.61–1.00	2	4	0	6	0	5	10	15
	(.33)	(.67)	(.00)		(.00)	(.33)	(.67)	
Total	83	26	0	109	15	24	16	55
	(.76)	(.24)	(.00)		(.27)	(.44)	(.29)	

*Numbers in cells represent number and row percentage of subjects with stated values of PDP and nonsense errors.

nonsense words. Table II shows the relationship both for adults whom we have classified as normal readers and for adults whom we have classified as dyslexic. First of all, no normal readers made more than 20 errors in reading two nonsense passages, but even within that group 61% of those who made as many as 11 errors in reading nonsense passages had greater than 30% dysphonetic spelling errors. Within the group of dyslexic adults, 29% made as many as 21 errors in reading nonsense passages and of those, 63% had more than 60% dysphonetic errors. Thus, although there can be dissociations between the use of grapheme-to-phoneme and phoneme-to-grapheme rules in reading and spelling, we find here a high correlation between the two skills.

Using the proportion of dysphonetic errors, then, as a measure we asked about the degree to which affected parents and offspring are similar on this measure. In Table III are listed the median values of the proportion of dysphonetic errors and farther to the right the distributions of those proportions for dyslexic children according to the value of the proportion of dysphonetic errors of their affected parents. We can see from the table that the probability that a dyslexic child will be a dysphonetic speller increases as a function of the affected parent's value. That is, there is a parent-child likeness.

Another study that has examined intrafamilial likeness is that of Omenn and Weber (1978) who studied 21 dyslexic probands and their families. Diagnosis and subtyping of probands were based on data from school academic and test records, history as given by the parents, and Slingerland Screening Test and spelling test results. Diagnosis and subtyping of parents and sibs were based predominantly on historical data relating to school difficulties and in some cases on spelling test data. When the investigators considered the data to be insufficient for classification the individuals were considered "uncharacterized." Probands were classified as having predominantly visual problems if their history and test results showed characteristics such as phonetic

Table III

Medians and Distribution of Proportion Dysphonetic Errors (PDP) of Offspring of Reading Disabled Parents Cross Tabulated by Parental Value of PDP

PDP of Affected Parent	Median PDP of Offspring	PDP of Offspring				
		≤.24	.25–.49	.50–.74	≥.75	Total
≥.75	.76	0	2	1	4̲	7
.50–.74	.48	5	7	9̲	3	24
.25–.49	.33	1	4̲	1	1	7
≤.24	.25	4̲*	3	2	0	9

*Modal value for each row is underscored.
(From Finucci and Childs.)
Reprinted from *Genetic Aspects of Speech and Language Disorders* by permission of Academic Press.

spelling errors, poorer performance on the visual components of the Slingerland, and persistance of reversals. Probands were classified as having predominantly auditory problems if their history and test results showed characteristics such as dysphonetic spelling, greater difficulty in learning from oral presentations, and poorer performance on the auditory components of the Slingerland. If distinctive features of both were noted, subjects were classified as belonging to a "mixed" subtype.

Eleven probands were classified in the visual-predominant subtype, seven in the auditory-predominant subtype and three as in the mixed subtype. Information gathered on 54 first degree relatives of the probands were sufficient to classify 40 of them into one of the three subtypes. Thirty-two (80%) of those classified were assigned to the same subtype as the proband in the family. The investigators concluded that the distribution of subtypes among the relatives "provides very suggestive support for the hypothesis that the phenotypic subtypes reflect independent familial predispositions . . . visual-predominant dyslexia clustered in families of probands with that subtype, and auditory-predominant dyslexia clustered in families of probands with the auditory-predominant subtype" (p. 339). As the investigators themselves note, however, the observations on which the classifications were based include subjective data gained from clinical history. Thus, their conclusions should not be regarded as definitive.

A more objective approach was that taken by Decker and DeFries (1981). They applied a principal components analysis to the age-adjusted test scores of 1044 subjects: 125 reading-disabled children (probands), their parents and sibs, and 125 matched controls, and their parents and sibs. Three ability dimensions emerged which they described as reading (word recognition, reading comprehension, and spelling), spatial/reasoning (abstract reasoning and spatial visualization), and coding/speed (automatic symbolic encoding speed). Four subtypes, defined by whether scores on each dimension were below or above a specified cutoff point, were present among the probands. In all subtypes, scores on the reading dimension were below the cutoff, thus the subtypes were characterized by the scores on the other two dimensions: above the cutoff on both, below the cutoff on both, above on spatial and low on coding or vice versa. The most frequent subtype among the probands was that in which reading was below the cutoff and scores on the other two dimensions were above the cutoff, that is, spatial and coding scores were normal. To determine the degree of within-family homogeneity, affected parents and sibs were classified into subtypes according to the same criteria used for the probands. The probability of specific subtype membership of sibs and parents was assessed as a function of subtype membership of the proband. There was no evidence that affected parents were more likely to manifest the same profile as the proband than would be expected by chance. Among the sibs, the only subtype which showed a greater than chance probability of occurring when the proband was of that subtype was that in which the reading dimension was low and other two were high. Thus, the examination of within-family data provided only suggestive evidence for validity of one of the four subtypes.

New Directions

In general, then, although there is some evidence for within-family homogeneity on subtyping characteristics, there is not a perfect fit between the phenotypic description of the proband and the phenotypic description of other affected family members. Therefore, we might consider why we see this discordance and how we might improve our studies to uncover phenotypic resemblance which reflects genetic resemblance where it exists.

First, we might examine some of the reasons why we might not be finding familial resemblance on our measures. One possibility is that the measures examined are inappropriate to the task. That is, they may be too broad to pinpoint one or more impaired component processes of reading. For instance, if we show that a subject is unable to read 75 out of 100 words, but do not attend to the characteristics of the words he is unable to read in comparison to those he is able to read, we learn little about the nature of the impairment. Or, if we find that a subject is fairly accurate in word recognition but ignore the speed of recognition, we may be missing a crucial characteristic of subjects who have not developed automaticity in word recognition. Second, there may be phenotypic changes in the nature of the impairment either as the result of natural developmental changes or as a result of response to instruction. Thus, members of the same family who are at different stages of development or who have been exposed to different educational programs may manifest their impairments differently. Third, the measured characteristics may be unrelated to the presence of dyslexia; or fourth, some cases of dyslexia may not be genetically determined, even when more than one family member is affected.

Thus, our task needs to be to find measures of behavioral deficits that reflect basic deficits in processing for those familial cases that are genetically determined. I would suggest we need to do more intensive study of dyslexic subjects within the same family to enable us to make inferences about component processes of reading and/or spelling that are impaired. Such study would require measures that are less broad and that are sensitive enough to uncover subtle deficiencies that remain even if the characteristics of an impairment are modified by remediation or developmental change. We might start on a simple level by determining if a subject's primary deficits relate to difficulties in the use of a lexical or a nonlexical route to reading and spelling or whether there might be difficulties with both.

This has been the approach of several case studies of developmental dyslexia done recently, mainly by British neuropsychologists. The purpose of many of those studies has been to draw an analogy between types of acquired dyslexia and types of developmental dyslexia.

For example, Temple and Marshall (1983) likened H.M., a 17 year-old developmental dyslexic, to acquired cases of phonological dyslexia whose pattern of skills and deficits has been interpreted as resulting from a deficit (though not complete) in the phonological route; that is, the ability to apply grapheme-to-phoneme conversion rules has been largely lost but the direct route, converting visual form to phonological form or visual form to semantic form, then to phonological form, remains relatively intact. Similar to acquired cases of phonological dyslexia, H.M. was impaired in nonword reading in comparison to word reading, a large proportion of her reading errors are derivational or visual paralexias, she is not influenced by spelling to sound regularities and word length, and she made no semantic errors or errors of regularization.

In contrast, Coltheart and his colleagues (Coltheart, Masterson, Byng, Prior, and Riddoch 1983) presented a case of developmental dyslexia, C.D., whom they suggested was analogous to acquired cases of surface dyslexia. Surface dyslexics exhibit a pattern of skills and deficits that have been interpreted as resulting from partial impairment of a direct route to the lexicon for word recognition, resulting in over reliance upon phonological encoding for reading. C.D. was similar to surface dyslexics in that she read orthographically regular words better than irregular words and was better able to detect homophones among regular word pairs and regularly spelled nonword pairs than among pairs in which one word was irregularly spelled. She defined words in accordance with the way she read them. For instance, given the word *spare,* she said "a weapon, spear, *s p a r e.*" She did not, however, show over-reliance on phonological rules which Coltheart in his later paper said characterized the surface dyslexic. She did poorly on some nonword reading tasks and only about 60% of her spelling errors were phonologically appropriate. What was clear was that she seemed to lack adequate access to word-specific information about pronunciation of irregularly spelled words.

Despite these and similar reports of developmental analogues of acquired cases, we should not expect developmental cases to mirror exactly the characteristics of acquired cases. Although both are manifested as deficits in reading, the differences in etiology would be expected to be reflected in differences in behavior. For instance, among acquired cases we may find relatively high levels of those skills that are left intact, because an individual was an accomplished reader prior to injury. In contrast, developmental dyslexics may display no reading skills at an above average level because of the interdependence of lexical and non-lexical pathways in developing reading skill. Thus, developmental deficits in an indirect, non-lexical phonological pathway might have a depressing influence on the development of a large lexical store. On the other hand, because any neurological impairment or irregularity probably occurs very early in developmental dyslexia, there is greater opportunity for compensatory mechanisms to intervene so that the reading deficits of developmental cases are milder than those of acquired cases.

Finally, in regard to this last point, a study by Baddeley, Ellis, Miles, and Lewis (1982), although not a case study, addresses the issue of differences between acquired and developmental dyslexia. Their study responded to a report by Jorm (1979) in which he drew attention to similarities between developmental dyslexia and acquired deep dyslexia. Their purpose was to determine if two characteristics of acquired deep dyslexia were also characteristic of developmental dyslexia. One was the difficulty in using a phonological route and the second was a sensitivity to imageability. Although the dyslexics showed evidence of phonological encoding in a lexical decision task, in a reading task the dyslexics as a group were slower than reading-age controls in reading both words and nonwords, and they were significantly less accurate in reading nonwords. But it was noted that the impairment was not as great for the developmental dyslexics as for deep dyslexics. With respect to imageability of words, they showed a similar effect of that factor on both normal readers and developmental dyslexics and suggested that the effect may be more general than investigators of deep dyslexia have thought. This paper illustrates well that, rather than trying to fit developmental dyslexias into the mold of acquired dyslexias, we might simply use tasks which have been used in studies of acquired dyslexics to attempt to characterize the skills and deficits of developmental dyslexics. This is what we have attempted to do with the father-son pair described in the next section.

Case Studies of a Father-Son Pair

The father (M.J.) and son (M.J.S.) chosen for study were selected because of two characteristics that emerged in our standard testing of them in our family study—they were severely disabled and the majority of spelling errors for both were dysphonetic. Both were tested in several sessions approximately two years after their initial testing in an attempt to determine which of any other characteristics of their reading, spelling or language processing might also be similar.

The father, M.J., was 42 when first seen. His WAIS Full Scale IQ was 111, and his verbal and performance IQ scores were both 110. The only below average subtest score was a 7 on digit span, and there was little variance among his other subtest scores. His grade equivalent score on the Gray Oral Reading Test was 8.0 and on the WRAT spelling subtest was 5.2. However, on the Gates-MacGinitie Comprehension subtest, designed for tenth through twelfth graders, and which has very liberal time limits, he attempted all 52 items and answered 37 correctly for a grade equivalent score of 12.9 + . M.J. completed a B.A. in Business at a city college four years after his high school graduation. He is president of a large insurance and financial consulting firm.

His son, M.J.S., was 13½ years old and in grade 7 when first seen. After a year in first grade at a public elementary school, he entered the first grade of a private day school whose curriculum was designed for children with reading disabilities. His full scale, verbal and performance IQ scores on the WISC-R obtained when we first saw him were 96, 97, and 96, respectively. His only below average subtest scores were a 5 on Digit Span and a 7 on Coding. His grade equivalent scores on the Gray Oral and WRAT Spelling were 2.0 and 3.7 respectively, and he was unable to complete more than a few items on the seventh-grade level of the Gates-McGinitie comprehension test. After completing 8 grades at the private day school, he entered a private boarding school with a special program for dyslexics.

On the WRAT Spelling subtest the father misspelled 36 of 46 words attempted and 67% of those were rated as dysphonetic renderings. M.J.S. misspelled 17 of 22 words attempted and 71% of those were rated as dysphonetic misspellings. Examples of dysphonetic spelling errors of each are listed in Table IV.

At follow-up, M.J. was given two sets of about 200 words each for oral reading and written spelling, half of which were read first and the other half of which were spelled first. The first set included words that were varied in orthographic regularity, length, and frequency and for some imageability was varied. These were taken from experimental tasks of Coltheart, Besner, Jonasson and Davelaar (1979) and Glushko (1980). Regularity or consistency of spelling did not affect M.J.'s accuracy in reading or spelling those words, but frequency, as measured by the Thorndike-Lorge count, did. The words read correctly were about twice as frequent as those read incorrectly (48/1000 vs. 21/1000) and likewise words spelled correctly were about twice as frequent as those spelled incorrectly (54/1000 vs. 28/1000). About 85% of the words were read correctly and about 65% were spelled correctly, but over both sets of

Table IV
Examples of Dysphonetic Spelling Errors of M.J. and M.J.S.

M.J. (At age 42)		M.J.S. (At age 13.5)	
Dictated	Error	Dictated	Error
reverence	reverlence	correct	crect
quantity	quility	material	mitterl
executive	excetive	educate	ejcate
necessity	nessity	believe	bleve
anxiety	ansinty	institute	instoot
lucidity	lucity	literature	litchere
possession	possion	reverence	revensens
loquacious	locaious	illogical	illoicle

words, reading a word correctly was not predictive of spelling it correctly. The vast majority of M.J.'s reading errors result in real words. About 50% of M.J.'s misspellings of words were phonologically appropriate.

He read correctly 64 of a set of 100 nonwords, 91 of which were monosyllabic. His accuracy in reading nonwords was unaffected by the structure—that is, whether it began or ended with a consonant cluster rather than a single consonant, whether the nonword rhymed with several or few read words, whether the medial vowel segment was a single vowel or a vowel cluster, or whether the medial and final segments had consistent pronunciations. Thus, it does not appear that his approach to reading nonwords was either by a strict grapheme-to-phoneme strategy or by analogy to real words. But close to 50% of his errors in reading nonwords resulted in real words, although he knew they were nonwords. He was no better at reading nonwords that were pseudohomophones than nonwords that were not.

On one task, which we called disambiguated homophones, M.J. was given the definition of a homophonic word, then the word was spoken and his task was to spell the word. The test used very frequent words. For instance, the definition and word given might be "to be sick—ail" and he wrote *a l e*. Or "tossed or hurled—thrown" and he wrote *t h r o n e*. On this test of 94 items he had 59% correct spellings. While some of his misspellings were the incorrect homophones, more were homophonic nonwords and even more were non-homophonic nonwords. In the opposite task in which he was shown a homophonic word and asked to define it, he performed at about 90% accuracy. Most of his errors resulted from giving definitions for words homophonic to the stimulus.

M.J. also showed some difficulty in detecting rhyming or nonrhyming word pairs that were read to him. While normal adults would be expected to perform perfectly on such a task, he made one error out of 40 on one task, and four out of 40 on another. Finally, on a task in which he was to determine if regularly spelled word pairs, irregularly spelled word pairs, or nonword pairs (all monosyllabic, and read silently) were homophonic or not, he performed at 85% accuracy. There was no difference in accuracy between nonwords and irregularly spelled words or between regularly spelled and irregularly spelled words.

In sum then, M.J. shows deficits both in applying grapheme-to-phoneme and phoneme-to-grapheme translation rules and in accessing the lexicon via a direct pathway. For some high frequency words which are orthographically regular he has not stored word specific information needed for both reading and spelling and for nonwords of simple CVC structure he has no apparent strategy for either reading or spelling.

The question is whether M.J.S. also shows both of these deficits. When M.J.S. was retested he was in grade 9. He was given the Gray Oral again and he obtained a grade equivalent score of 1.7. On a smaller set of the words, taken from the list read by his father, he read 68% correctly and had poorer performance on irregular words than on regularly spelled words. On a set of 75 nonwords (different from those given his father) he read 87% correctly and when asked to spell 25 of them he spelled 88% correctly. Thus, he has fairly accurate use of grapheme-to-phoneme and phoneme-to-grapheme rules.

However, on the disambiguated homophone task, which was also given to his father, he performed more poorly than his father; he spelled only 43% of the words correctly. About half of his errors were homophonic words. His poor store of lexical semantic information was, however, demonstrated by the opposite task in which he was to read homophonic words and give a definition. His performance was only slightly above chance level.

He was like his father in making 5 errors in detecting rhyme in a set of 40 word pairs read to him, half of which rhymed and half of which didn't and in reading the pairs silently he was correct in discriminating rhyming and non-rhyming pairs in only 73%. His performance was poorest for nonrhyming pairs that were visually similar and rhyming pairs that were visually dissimilar. Finally, in all of the single word and passage reading tasks given M.J.S., his time to complete the tasks was compared with that of a same aged dyslexic subject whose *accuracy* in single word recognition is about the same and whose misspellings have always been primarily phonetic. The major difference between the two is reflected not in the nature of their efforts, but in the overall time required to complete the tasks. M.J.S.'s time on five tasks was always longer, varying from about twice as great on one task to six times as great on two tasks.

Thus, I propose that M.J.S.'s deficits are like his father's, that he shows difficulty in auditory rhyming, in accessing word specific lexical information directly as measured by the disambiguated homophone task and that, although he is able to use grapheme-to-phoneme and phoneme-to-grapheme correspondence rules, they are not automatic. After 9 years of intensive instruction, M.J.S.'s errors do not reflect the severe phonological deficits shown by his father, but I suggest that his slow rate of applying the rules still reflects his difficulty. That difficulty would have been better seen if we had used an individual item response time measure in our tasks.

In summary, I suggest that M.J. and M.J.S., who were one of the concordant pairs in Table III, illustrate why there are some mismatches in looking at within-family likeness. To uncover within-family homogeneity we need to use measures that tap underlying skill and that look at the nature and speed of the response.

Conclusion

An attempt has been made in this chapter to give an overview of research on subtypes of dyslexia and the traditional approaches to validation of the subtypes. No study has yet produced unequivocal evidence for the validity of subtypes, however. It is suggested that research should be directed toward the use of measures that will allow inferences to be made about component processes of reading and the neurological mechanism underlying them that are either impaired or intact in individuals. Furthermore, these measures should be applied to dyslexic members of the same family to test for within-family homogeneity and between-family heterogeneity.

References

Aaron, P. G., Grantham, S. L., and Campbell, N. 1982. Differential treatment of reading disability of diverse etiologies. *In* R. N. Malatesha and P. G. Aaron (eds.). *Reading Disorders: Varieties and Treatments*. New York: Academic Press.

Baddeley, A. D., Ellis, N. C., Miles, T. R., and Lewis, V. J. 1982. Developmental and acquired dyslexia: A comparison. *Cognition* 11:185–199.

Boder, E. 1971. Developmental dyslexia: Prevailing diagnostic concepts and a new diagnostic approach. *In* H. R. Myklebust (ed). *Progress in Learning Disabilities, Volume II*. New York: Grune and Stratton.

Boder, E. 1973. Developmental dyslexia: A diagnostic approach based on three atypical reading-spelling patterns. *Developmental Medicine and Child Neurology* 15:663–687.

Boder, E., and Jarrico, S. 1982. *The Boder Test of Reading-Spelling Patterns: A Diagnostic Screening Test for Subtypes of Reading Disability*. New York: Grune and Stratton.

Camp, B., and Dolcourt, J. 1977. Reading and spelling in good and poor readers. *Journal of Learning Disabilities* 10:300–307.

Childs, B., and Finucci, J. M. 1983. Genetics, epidemiology, and specific reading disability. *In* M. Rutter (ed.). *Developmental Neuropsychiatry*. New York: Guilford Press.

Coltheart, M., Besner, D., Jonasson, J., and Davelaar, E. 1979. Phonological encoding in the lexical decision task. *Quarterly Journal of Experimental Psychology* 31:489–508.

Coltheart, M., Masterson, J., Byng, S., Prior, M., and Riddoch, J. 1983. Surface dyslexia. *Quarterly Journal of Experimental Psychology* 35A:469–495.

Coltheart, M., Patterson, K., and Marshall, J. C. (eds.). 1980. *Deep Dyslexia*. London: Routledge and Kegan Paul.

Decker, S. N., and DeFries, J. C. 1981. Cognitive ability profiles in families of reading-disabled children. *Developmental Medicine and Child Neurology* 23:217–227.

DeFries, J. C., Singer, S. M., Foch, T. T., and Lewitter, F. I. 1978. Familial nature of reading disability. *British Journal of Psychiatry* 132:361–367.

Doehring, D. G. 1984. Subtyping of reading disorders: Implications for remediation. *Annals of Dyslexia* 34:205–216.

Doehring, D. G., and Hoshko, I. M. 1977. Classification of reading problems by the Q-technique of factor analysis. *Cortex* 13:281–294.

Doehring, D. G., Trites, R., Patel, P., and Fiedorowicz, C. A. M. 1981. *Reading Disabilities: The Interaction of Reading, Language and Neuropsychological Deficits*. New York: Academic Press.

Finucci, J. M., and Childs, B. 1983. Dyslexia: Family studies. *In* C. L. Ludlow and J. A. Cooper (eds). *Genetic Aspects of Speech and Language Disorders*. New York: Academic Press.

Finucci, J. M., Guthrie, J., Childs, A., Abbey, H., and Childs, B. 1976. The genetics of specific reading disability. *Annals of Human Genetics* 40:1–23.

Finucci, J. M., Isaacs, S. D., Whitehouse, C. C., and Childs, B. 1983. Classification of spelling errors and their relationship to reading ability, sex, grade placement, and intelligence. *Brain and Language* 20:340–355.

Fisher, J. 1905. Case of congenital word-blindness (inability to learn to read). *Ophthalmic Review* 24:315–318.

Fisk, J. L., and Rourke, B. P. 1979. Identification of subtypes of learning-disabled children at three age levels: A neuropsychological, multivariate approach. *Journal of Clinical Neuropsychology* 1:289–310.

Glushko, R. 1980. The organization and activation of orthographic knowledge in reading aloud. *Journal of Experimental Psychology: Human Perception and Performance*. 5:674–691.

Hallgren, B. 1950. Specific dyslexia ("congenital word blindness"): A clinical and genetic study. *Acta Psychiatrica et Neurologica Scandinavica*, Supplement No. 65.

Healy, J. M., 1982. The enigma of hyperlexia. *Reading Research Quarterly,* 17:319–338.

Huttenlocher, R. R., and Huttenlocher, J. 1973. A study of children with hyperlexia. *Neurology* 23:1107–1116.

Ingram, T. T. S. 1971. Specific learning difficulties in childhood: A medical point of view. *British Journal of Educational Psychology* 41:6–13.

Ingram, T. T. S., Mason, A. W., and Blackburn, I. 1970. A retrospective study of 82 children with reading disability. *Developmental Medicine and Child Neurology* 12:271–281.

Johnson, D. J., and Myklebust, H. R. 1967. *Learning Disabilities: Educational Practices and Principles*. New York: Grune and Stratton.

Jorm, A. F. 1979. The cognitive and neurological basis of developmental dyslexia: A theoretical framework and review. *Cognition* 7:19–33.

Kimberling, W. J., Fain, P. R., Ing, P. S., Smith, S. D., and Pennington, B. 1985. Genetic linkage studies of reading disability with chromosome 15 markers. Paper presented at meeting of the Behavior Genetics Association. June 1985.

Lovett, M. W. 1984a. A developmental perspective on reading dysfunction: Accuracy and rate criteria in the subtyping of dyslexic children. *Brain and Language* 22:67–91.

Lovett, M. W. 1984b. The search for subtypes of specific reading disability: Reflections from a cognitive perspective. *Annals of Dyslexia* 34:155–178.

Lyon, G. R. 1983. Learning-disabled readers: Identification of subgroups. *In* H. R. Myklebust (ed.). *Progress in Learning Disabilities*, Volume V. New York: Grune and Stratton.

Lyon, G. R., and Watson, B. 1981. Empirically derived subgroups of learning disabled readers: Diagnostic characteristics. *Journal of Learning Disabilities* 14:256–261.

Malatesha, R. N., and Dougan, D. R. 1982. Clinical subtypes of developmental dyslexia: Resolution of an irresolute problem. *In* R. N. Malatesha and P. G. Aaron (eds.). *Reading Disorders: Varieties and Treatments*. New York: Academic Press.

Marshall, J. C., and Newcombe, F. 1966. Syntactic and semantic errors in paralexia *Neuropsychologia* 4:169–176.

Mattis, S. 1978. Dyslexia syndromes: A working hypothesis that works. *In* A. L. Benton and D. Pearl (eds.). *Dyslexia: An Appraisal of Current Knowledge*. New York: Oxford University Press.

Mattis, S., French, J. H., and Rapin, I. 1975. Dyslexia in children and young adults: Three independent neuropsychological syndromes. *Developmental Medicine and Child Neurology* 17:150–163.

Myklebust, H. R. 1978. Toward a science of dyslexiology. *In* H. R. Myklebust (ed.). *Progress in Learning Disabilities, Volume IV*. New York: Grune and Stratton.

Omenn, G. S., and Weber, B. A. 1978. Dyslexia: Search for phenotypic and genetic heterogeneity. *American Journal of Medical Genetics* 1:333–342.

Owen, F., Adams, P., Forrest, T., Stolz, L., and Fisher, S. 1971. Learning disorders in children: Sibling studies. *Monographs of the Society for Research in Child Development* 36:No. 4.

Patterson, K. E. 1981. Neuropsychological approaches to the study of reading. *British Journal of Psychology* 72:151–174.

Petrauskas, R., and Rourke, B. P. 1979. Identification of subgroups of retarded readers: A neuropsychological multivariate approach. *Journal of Clinical Neuropsychology* 1:17–37.

Rosenthal, J. H., Boder, E., and Calloway, E. 1982. Typology of developmental dyslexia: Evidence for its construct validity. *In* R. N. Malatesha and P. G. Aaron (eds.). *Reading Disorders: Varieties and Treatments*. New York: Academic Press.

Satz, P., and Morris, R. 1981. Learning disability subtypes: A review. *In* F. J. Pirozzolo and M. C. Wittrock (eds.). *Neuropsychological and Cognitive Processes in Reading*. New York: Academic Press.

Smith, S. D., Kimberling, W. J., Pennington, B. F., and Lubs, M. A. 1983. Specific reading disability: Identification of an inherited form through linkage analysis. *Science* 219:1345–1347.

Temple, C. M. and Marshall, J. C. 1983. A case study of developmental phonological dyslexia. *British Journal of Psychology* 74:517-533.

Thomas, C. 1905. Congenital word-blindness and its treatment. *Ophthalmoscope* 3:380–385.

van den Bos, K. P. 1984. Letter processing in dyslexic subgroups. *Annals of Dyslexia* 34:179–193.

Walker, L., and Cole, E. M. 1965. Familial patterns of expression of specific reading disability and population sample. *Bulletin of the Orton Society* 15:12–24.

11

Applications of Recombinant DNA Techniques to Neurogenetic Disorders

David Housman, Shelley D. Smith, and David Pauls

*T*he recent development of techniques for the analysis of the structure of DNA molecules has had profound impact on human genetics. The observation that reading disabilities exhibit a hereditary transmission pattern in some families provides an approach to understanding the etiology of dyslexia through the use of these DNA techniques. In the discussion that follows, we will outline the principles underlying the DNA technology that can be applied toward the understanding of dyslexia and we will comment on the particular problems that a condition such as dyslexia present in the application of these methods.

Genetic Linkage as an Approach to Gene Identification

The program for the development of each human being is encoded in the molecules of DNA found in the cells of the body. Each cell contains a faithful copy of the genetic material (DNA) received from each parent. Information in the DNA is encoded in a linear fashion, like information on a computer tape. Demonstrating that a condition such as dyslexia is inherited has direct implications regarding the relationship between the structure of the DNA in the cells and the physiological basis for dyslexia.

A hereditary basis for dyslexia is indicated in certain families where dyslexia appears to be due to an altered form of the program in the DNA. Identification of differences in the information content of the DNA that distinguish individuals who exhibit dyslexia and those who do not would be the first step in determining the basic cause of this condition.

The technical difficulty in achieving this goal may be considered in the following context. The cells of each individual contain six billion base parts or units of DNA information. If we could compare the entire DNA information content of a large number of individuals with dyslexia and a large number of individuals who are not dyslexic, it might be possible to identify directly a common feature of the DNA responsible for the condition in dyslexic individuals. Despite the powerful nature of current DNA techniques, a direct comparison of this type is not technically feasible. However, a very powerful strategy, which requires considerably less scientific effort, can be applied to dyslexia. The strategy is based on the fact that genes (specific segments of DNA) are arranged within chromosomes in an orderly array. In almost all human beings, the same order of genes is found on each chromosome. When genes are passed on they are usually inherited as a unit. The association of genes during transmission through several generations in a family is the basis by which genes can be located on chromosomes.

To review, chromosomes are the structure that contain the DNA, which is the molecule that perpetuates the genetic code. The DNA can be thought of as an array of linear segments of information, genes, which come in discrete packages, chromosomes. Each gene has a specific position, or locus, in this array, and thus can be mapped to a particular chromosome. Each person has two copies of each chromosome, one of which came from the mother and one from the father. In turn, each child may inherit either maternally derived chromosomes or paternally derived chromosomes from each parent, which actually represent their grandmaternal or grandpaternal chromosomes, respectively.

If one knew that a gene was located on a particular chromosome, one could theoretically follow the inheritance of the gene from generation to generation along with that chromosome. Conversely, if one does not know which chromosome a gene is on, one could study the transmission of the gene along with the transmission of all of the chromosomes in a kindred. By identifying which chromosome was always transmitted with the gene, one could infer which chromosome carried the gene. This is the basis of gene localization, or mapping. However, several factors can complicate this technique. One is variable penetrance. Penetrance is defined as the probability that a specific genotype exhibits a particular phenotype. Penetrance values can range from 0 to 1. Thus, it is possible that not everyone who inherits a specific gene(s) will manifest the trait. This results in an apparent discrepancy in the observed co-occurence of the gene and the chromosome carrying it. Another complicating factor is that chromosomes are not transmitted intact from grandparent to parent to child. In the formation of the germ cells the two chromosomes of each pair (called homologs) intertwine and can exchange genetic material at random places along their length. This is termed crossing-over or recombination. As a result, a chromosome can be partially grandmaternal and partially grandpaternal. If one does not know that such an exchange has taken place, the gene and its chromosome will appear to have diverged in the family. In fact, knowledge of such cross-overs and their position can help to determine exactly where on the chromosome the gene is located.

Finally, one must have a method of distinguishing the four grandparental chromosomes, so they can be followed throughout the family. This has been done by using other genes known to be on the chromosomes as landmarks, or "markers." If the grandparental chromosomes differ at enough of these landmarks, each chromosome can be characterized by its own set of alleles at these markers. If there are enough landmarks, specific regions of each chromosome can be followed. The transmission of the landmarks can be compared with the transmission of a particular gene, and linkage analysis can produce probability estimates that the gene and a landmark are located on the same chromosome at a certain distance apart. By associating a particular region of a particular chromosome with a genetic condition, one can zero in on the location of the gene causing the condition.

Measuring Genetic Recombination

Recombination frequencies range from 0% recombination to 50% recombination or random assortment. The magnitude of recombination is a function of the distance between two genetic loci. If two loci are close together on a chromosome the recombination frequency will be close to 0 and the loci are said to be tightly linked. If the two loci are far apart or on different chromosomes the recombination frequency will be 0.5.

Several approaches are available for measuring the association within families between alleles at two loci. The most commonly used approach is the LOD score method. LOD scores are derived from the *log* of the *od*ds of the likelihoods for two hypotheses regarding the magnitude of recombination frequency. The LOD score reflects the probability that a given gene and a marker are linked. The usual procedure is to calculate log likelihoods for several recombination frequencies (e.g. 0.0, 0.05, 0.10, 0.15, 0.20, 0.25, 0.30, 0.35, 0.40, 0.45) and compare them with the log likelihood calculated under the assumption of independent assortment (i.e., recombination fraction equal to 0.50). LOD scores are simply the difference between the log likelihood for the hypothesis of no linkage (i.e., recombination frequency equal to 0.50) and the log likelihood for some specific recombination frequency less than 0.50. For each analysis a series of LOD scores are calculated so that it is possible to examine whether there is any evidence for linkage between the two genetic loci being examined. A LOD score of -2 or lower is equivalent to odds of 100:1 against linkage at that particular level of recombination, and a score of 3 or greater indicates odds of 1000:1 that the association between the two markers is not by chance and that, in fact, they are in proximity to each other.

Huntington's Disease: A Prototype for DNA Based Genetic Linkage Studies

Once a gene for a specific condition has been localized to a specific chromosome, one is then in a position to discover how the gene produces the disorder. In addition, this knowledge can be useful for genetic counseling. An example of such a disorder is Huntington's disease, and this will be used in the following discussion to illustrate the use of this technology. The symptoms of this disorder are quite stereotyped, and the diagnosis is usually straightforward. The onset is gradual, usually beginning in the fourth or fifth decade, although it may begin at any age. There is progressive impairment of muscle control with the development of choreiform movements, and there may be accompanying dementia. The duration of the disorder may be as long as 15–20 years. It has been recognized for many years that this disease is caused by a single autosomal dominant gene. Family studies have shown that almost exactly 50% of the children of affected individuals are themselves affected, indicating that this gene has very high penetrance. The late age of onset makes this a particularly tragic disease, since most at-risk individuals do not know if they actually carry the gene until after their child-rearing years, so they must make their decisions on career, relationships, and having a family with the uncertainty about their future health and with the knowledge that they may be passing the gene on to their children. The late age of onset has also complicated genetic studies attempting to identify the gene. Even when large families were identified with many individuals related by direct descent to individuals with Huntington's disease, many of those individuals were not useful in a genetic study because it could not be determined whether or not they carried the gene. There was no way to determine if an asymptomatic person was a gene carrier and was going to develop the disease later. Still, the disease is sufficiently prevalent to allow construction of very large family histories which could compensate for this lack of information. One of the largest families was studied by Dr. Nancy Wexler and colleagues in Venezuela. Over 1,200 blood samples were obtained from members of this kindred who all trace their ancestry back to one individual who immigrated to the Lake Marachibo region of Venezuela in the 19th century. It is this family that formed the basis for the work of Gusella, Wexler, Conneally and co-workers who localized the gene to chromosome 4 (Gusella et al. 1983). This example particularly illustrates the usefulness of the recombinant DNA techniques. Attempts had been made previously to see if the gene for Huntington's disease was located near other traditional genotyping markers, but as it happened there were no good markers on the specific region of chromosome 4 containing the gene.

The Principles of Restriction Fragment Length Polymorphisms Analysis

Recombinant DNA techniques are not dependent on expressed genes, but instead use variation in the actual DNA code as landmarks. The DNA code is specified by the sequence of the nucleotide bases adenine, guanine, thymine, and cytosine. It is as if all of the ''words'' in the code are written based on an alphabet of A, G, T, and C. A particular region of a chromosome can then be characterized by its unique base sequence, which is writing out the information for the genes in that region. The discovery of enzymes called restriction endonucleases has made these codes accessible. These enzymes each recognize a certain unit of DNA sequence that is four, five, or six bases in length. Wherever the enzyme detects its particular recognition sequence of bases it will cleave the DNA. If two different chromosomal homologs differ in their DNA sequence at a recognition site, one will be cleaved by the enzyme while the other will be left intact. This will cause a difference in the length of the DNA fragment that is created by the cleavage.

All of the DNA fragments created by the enzyme treatment can be separated using gel electrophoresis, so that differences in fragment length can be detected. If the DNA from a human being was the size of the DNA of a virus, we could simply look at the results of the electrophoresis and detect a difference in the location of the DNA on the gel. Human DNA, however, is much more complex than the DNA of a virus. Rejection of human DNA with a restriction enzyme produces so many fragments that only a smear of DNA running the length of the gel is observed. Therefore a powerful analytical technique is necessary to visualize a single restriction fragment of human DNA which consists of about one-millionth of the DNA present in a human cell. To do this, one can take advantage of the fact that the DNA is in the form of a double helix, the two halves of which fit together like a lock and key when the base sequences are matched. If the gene or the region of DNA that one wishes to study can be isolated, it can be tagged with radioactivity or a dye and then be added to the smear of DNA on the gel. This DNA "probe" will then anneal specifically to the fragment of DNA containing the same base sequence, thus "lighting up" its position on the gel. Differences between homologues in base sequences in the region of the probe sequence will then show up as different annealling patterns on the gel.

These patterns are reproducible, in that the DNA can be isolated from an individual a hundred times and the same pattern will result. They are also heritable, and can be followed from generation to generation, and many are quite polymorphic, meaning that variations are common. Thus, they make very good genetic landmarks. Availability of these markers has revolutionized the field of human linkage analysis. Whereas before, the limited number of markers meant that a good part of the genome was inaccessible to study, now the number and location of markers is merely dependent upon the number of investigators willing to look for them. The eventual development of a "screening battery" of several hundred markers spanning all of the chromosomes would ensure that any gene eventually would be detected. The limiting factor then becomes the informativeness of the families.

Increased Precision in Gene Localization

Once a gene is located on a chromosome how can its exact location be determined? The next step is to find new markers that are on either side of the gene, bracketing it. Using these as starting points, new markers can be generated by "walking" along the DNA. In a genetic "squeeze play" one can get closer and closer to the gene in the middle and essentially define the DNA fragment on which the gene resides. From there, the fragment can be analyzed to determine what the gene actually does to produce the phenotype in question.

There are limitations, however, to this process of precise gene localization. One limitation is defined precisely by the degree to which a large enough family can be located for study of the inheritance of the gene from generation to generation. The length of the smallest distance that can be analyzed between loci is inversely proportional to the size of the family; that is, the smaller the family, the larger the minimum detectable distance between the gene and a marker. This is because cross-overs that occur between loci define the limits of the localization. As the distance between loci shortens, cross-overs become more infrequent, and larger families are needed to allow detection of the few cross-overs that might occur.

Another limitation to linkage analysis, mentioned previously, is variable penetrance. A third limitation is etiological heterogeneity. That is, the disorder being studied may have different causes resulting in phenotypes that are clinically indistinguishable. In such cases studies of some families may indicate that the gene causing a disorder is linked to a given locus, while other families will apparently exclude that linkage because the disorder in those families is caused by a different gene or even by a non-genetic mechanism. Detection of heterogeneity also requires the study of large families, preferably from different ethnic backgrounds, so that detection and discrimination of linked and non-linked kindreds can be made with certainty. This requires statistical testing for heterogeneity of LOD scores. If LOD scores are not significantly heterogenious, one is not justified in separating "linked" and "unlinked" families unless a clear-cut phenotypic variable can be found that also consistently discriminates them. Further studies that discriminate families based on that variable would be necessary to confirm the linkage findings. Conversely, if LOD scores do show heterogeneity, the different types of families can be examined to detect underlying phenotypic differences. Neurofibromatosis is an example of a disorder in which linkage findings may support the splitting of the disease into two separate entities, classical neurofibromatosis and central neurofibromatosis with acoustic neuroma. Heterogeneity is likely to be a very important issue in complex behavioral disorders where the ultimate phenotype may be influenced by a variety of genetic and non-genetic pathways.

From Gene Location to Gene Action

Assuming that these limitations can be overcome and the gene is actually located and isolated, gene action can then be studied. In almost all cases genes code for proteins, and proteins are important in various aspects of metabolism and development. By determining what protein the gene makes, and the function of that protein, one can begin to answer the questions posed by neurogenetic disorders. How do they happen? What causes particular cells in the brain to start to degenerate? Why do particular cells in the brain follow an abnormal course of development? Why is it that a particular neurotransmitter is present at a reduced or increased level in a specific region of the brain?

There are several other neurological disorders that have a familial component and may be amenable to this type of analysis. One example is Alzheimer's disease, which is similar in many respects to Huntington's disease. Two factors make this disorder more difficult to study, however. One is that the age of onset is later, usually in the late 40's in the best of pedigrees. The other problem is that of heterogeneity, which has been discussed previously. In any disorder that is relatively frequent in the population, there is a good possibility that there are several causes, both genetic and non-genetic. About 5% of cases of Alzheimer's disease have pedigrees that are appropriate for genetic studies.

Duchenne muscular dystrophy is a degenerative neuromuscular disease for which the chromosomal location has been known for years. The pattern of inheritance indicates that the gene occurs on the X chromosome—it is "X-linked." Thus, studies on this disorder have taken the next step in bracketing and gradually isolating the gene itself. The markers can be used for carrier detection and prenatal diagnosis, but ultimately analysis of the gene itself will allow more precise detection of its presence and hopefully some way of counteracting its effects.

Application of DNA Technology for Dyslexia

The application of these techniques to dyslexia requires much additional work. Extensive family studies are needed so that it will be possible to categorize families reliably on the basis of clinical features, discriminate affected from unaffected individuals, and demonstrate a reliable pattern of transmission consistent with a relatively simple genetic mechanism. To those familiar with how dyslexia is manifest (the phenotypic variability in dyslexia), this may seem like an impossible task. However, some degree of phenotypic variability should be expected. It is certainly true that variable expression has been observed in disorders where the underlying genetic mechanism is clearly understood. For example, in Huntington's disease, there is variation in age of onset, clinical course, and symptomatology within the same family. Phenotypic variation between identical twins has been described (one of whom exhibits choreiform movements while the other shows the rigid form of the disease) also suggesting variable expression of the same gene. Nevertheless, reliable diagnostic criteria for dyslexia must be developed and applied consistently in family studies so that genetic hypotheses can be rigorously examined prior to the application of DNA techniques. (See Pennington in press, for a review). It is necessary to understand the mode of transmission prior to attempting to identify the gene responsible for expression of the disorder.

There has been one study in which linkage analysis with dyslexia has been attempted (Smith, Kimberling, Pennington, and Lubs 1983). Smith et al. ascertained families in which dyslexia appeared to be transmitted in an autosomal dominant pattern through several generations. All family members were given a battery of tests to compare reading ability with other academic abilities and children were termed dyslexic if their non-reading abilities were in the average range but their reading was at least two grade levels lower. This definition was not practical for adults, however, since women especially appeared to be able to compensate for earlier disabilities. Thus, the most important criterion for diagnosis in an adult was history of early and significant reading problems. In an adult who had apparently compensated, this history had to be corroborated by other family members.

This study was completed before DNA restriction fragment polymorphisms were available as markers, so standard genotyping markers and chromosomal heteromorphisms were used. A LOD score of 3.241 was obtained between dyslexia and heteromorphisms of the centromeric and short arm regions of chromosome 15, suggesting that there may be a gene on chromosome 15 that influences reading ability. There was some suggestion of heterogeneity in that one family had noticeably negative LOD scores. However, there was not statistical evidence that the LOD scores were heterogeneous, thus this family's scores were not removed from the total LOD score.

These studies are now continuing using the DNA techniques described above. Both the original families and new families are being studied to see if these preliminary results can be confirmed. Because it is critical that accurate diagnoses be made, more objective criteria have been developed by Pennington and McCabe which should allow a more precise determination of affected status (Pennington, McCabe, Smith, Kimberling, and Lubs in press). These new criteria include information about performance on achievement tests and take into account individual spelling characteristics. In addition, the history of reading disability in adults is measured by questionnaire. More detailed phenotypic studies in the context of family studies should facilitate development of reliable diagnostic criteria. These criteria then should be used in the study of a large number of families so that it would be possible to identify etiologically distinct subtypes of dyslexia. In conjunction with this work, families suitable for linkage studies should be collected so that both types of methodologies could be employed to help us understand etiologic factors important for the manifestation of this disability.

References

Gusella, J. F., Wexler, N. S., Conneally, P. M., Naylor, S. L., Anderson, M. A., Tanzi, R. E., Watkins, P. C., Ottina, K., Wallace, M. R., Sakaguchi, A. Y., Young, A. B., Shoulson, I., Bonilla, E., and Martin, J. B. 1983. A Polymorphic DNA marker genetically linked to Huntington's disease. *Nature* 306:234-238.

Pennington, B. F. (In Press) Issues in the diagnosis and phenotype analysis of dyslexia: Implications for family studies. *in* S. D. Smith (ed). *Genetics and Learning Disabilities*. San Diego: College-Hill Press.

Pennington, B. F., McCabe, L. L., Smith, S. D., Kimberling, W. J., and Lubs, H. A. (In Press) The spelling phenotype in a form of familial dyslexia. *Child Development*.

Smith, S. D., Kimberling, W. J., Pennington, B. F., and Lubs, H. A. 1983. Specific reading disability: Identification of an inherited form through linkage analysis. *Science* 219:1345-1347.

12

Linguistic Abilities and Spelling Proficiency in Kindergarteners and Adult Poor Spellers

Isabelle Y. Liberman, Hyla Rubin,
Susan Duquès, and Joanne Carlisle

*T*he research effort over the past several years by the Haskins Laboratories reading research group has bolstered our conviction that the problem of most beginners who have difficulties in acquiring literacy is basically linguistic in nature. That is, in our view, the problem is not visual or auditory or motor, as many have proposed, but lies rather in the ineffective use of phonologic strategies. We have found this linguistic deficiency in regard to two major requirements for reading proficiency—lexical access and representation in short-term memory. We have recently also begun to look more closely at spelling from the standpoint of linguistic sophistication. In this paper we will describe two recent studies we have done that are concerned with linguistic abilities and spelling—one in a group of kindergarteners and the other in an adult literacy class. But, first, since the nature of orthography is a central consideration in spelling, we should like to prepare the way by describing our assumptions about how the alphabetic orthography represents language, assumptions which are, in effect, the guiding principles of our research.

The introductory section of this paper ("Some Guiding Principles") is adapted from "A Language-Oriented View of Reading and its Disabilities" by Isabelle Y. Liberman, which appeared in H. Myklebust (ed.), 1983, *Progress in Learning Disabilities,* Vol. 5. New York: Grune and Stratton.

The research of the authors was supported by NICHD grant HD-01994 to Haskins Laboratories, New Haven, CT.

Special thanks for their generous cooperation in the kindergarten experiment are due to Jerome Spears, Director of Pupil Personnel of the Mansfield, CT school system, and, in the Annie E. Vinton School, to James Chilleri, principal and Anita Satriano, teacher of the kindergarten class and her pupils. For their thoughtful assistance in the adult literacy experiment, we are also indebted to Isobel Kaufman, Director, Adult and Community Education Services and to Thomas Rameaka, teacher and the students of the adult education class.

Some Guiding Principles

Everyone would agree, we believe, that an orthography represents a language, that languages are used to convey meaning, and that words are the basic units by which languages do that. What is often forgotten, however, is that whether one receives language by eye or by ear, one must get to the word before one can get to its meaning and that a word exists apart from its typically various meanings. Moreover, a word has a uniquely linguistic, complex, phonological structure that must be somehow apprehended before one can deal with a message conveyed by language, whether written or spoken. In the primary language functions of speaking and listening, a special processor copes with that phonological structure in operations that normally function naturally, quite automatically, and below the level of awareness. One does not need to understand how it works in order to speak and listen. In contrast, both the reader and writer must have some fundamental understanding of the structure. Indeed, they must become, to some degree, linguists of sorts, sufficiently aware of the phonology to be able to divide the spoken language into the constituent segments that the orthography represents. How easy or how difficult that is will depend largely on the nature of the linguistic segment that the orthography represents.

In the case of orthographies in which the segment represented is the word, as it is in the Chinese logography and the Japanese kanji, or the syllable, as it is in the Japanese kana,[1] we contend that the beginner's task is relatively simple. If what they need to do is separate the word or syllable from the speech stream for purposes of pairing it with its appropriate orthographic unit, they will find it to be readily isolable. This has been found to be true both here and abroad in a number of experiments with young children (Alegria and Content 1983; Fox and Routh 1975; Holden and MacGinitie 1972).

The problem faced by beginners in an alphabetic orthography is much more difficult. The essence of the problem can be put in this way: though it is often said that an alphabetic orthography represents speech (or ought to), it is, in fact, an abstraction from speech. Although it does bear a fairly regular relation to speech, the nature of that relation will be hard for a child, or indeed any beginner, young or old, to apprehend. To understand why that is so, we would remark briefly, first, on why it is misleading to say that the alphabetic orthography represents the sounds of speech; second, why it is also misleading to say that it does (or should) represent speech phonetically; and, finally, what it means to say that it is an abstraction from speech. Let us consider these remarks one at a time.

---

[1] The ways in which the individual characters in these orthographies represent their respective languages are more complex than can be described here. It should be noted that the segments represented by the characters in the Chinese logography and the Japanese kanji are more correctly defined as morphemes rather than words; similarly, the segments in the Japanese Kana are better described as moras than syllables. However, it is sufficient for our purposes, and sufficiently accurate, to speak of the word in the first case and the syllable in the second.

The Alphabet Does Not Represent the Sounds of Speech

The alphabetic orthography does not transcribe the sounds of speech. In the first place, the letters obviously do not portray acoustic events, as they might if they were bits of oscillograms or spectrograms. So in that rather trivial sense, the alphabet certainly does not represent the sounds of speech. However, there is a more significant sense in which the alphabet does not transcribe sounds. The point that needs to be made, and which is not trivial, is that the segmentation of the sound does not correspond to the segmentation of the letters. To take a simple example—it would be impossible to divide a recording of the spoken word, "big," into three parts, such that when played back, one part would be "buh," a second part "ih," and the last part "guh." That is because in the spoken syllable, "big," there is only one piece of sound and the three phonological segments we write with the letters B, I, and G are nearly simultaneously encoded into it.

Encoding several segments of the phonology into one segment of sound provides an important gain in efficiency for the listener, who, as we have said, has a built-in processor nicely equipped to deal with it automatically. But it has quite adverse consequences for the beginner dealing with the written language. One unfortunate consequence of the very odd relation between phonological structure and sound is that the phoneme, which is the segment represented by the alphabetic orthography, unlike the word and the syllable, is not easily separable from the speech stream. If we had not found this to be so in our research with children (Liberman, Shankweiler, Fischer, and Carter 1974), we should have suspected it from the history of writing systems; the system using an alphabetic unit was the last to be developed, long after logographies and syllabaries. Moreover, unlike those others, the basic unit of the alphabetic orthography, the phoneme, was apparently discovered only once and all other alphabets were later adapted from that original, brilliant discovery (Diringer 1948).

If readers and writers must be able to appreciate the relationship between the orthographic character and the linguistic unit it represents, as we believe they must, then beginning learners of an alphabetic system are put at a disadvantage initially. They will find it difficult to see the relation between spelling and sound. And it will even be difficult for teachers to demonstrate that relationship to them. If teachers wish to do this with even a simple word like "big," they will try to isolate three sounds and in the process will unavoidably produce, not three phonemes, but three syllables: "buh," "ih," and "guh." Put together, these form a nonsense trisyllable "buhihguh" and not the monosyllable "big" that comprises the three phonological segments we spell as B-I-G (see Liberman 1983, for a more complete discussion of this point and of the two sections that follow).

The Alphabet Does Not Represent the Phonetic Surface of Speech

If it is now evident that the alphabet is not a transcription of the sounds of speech, what about the alphabetic orthography as a phonetic transcription? It is, of course, possible to use an alphabet phonetically. Linguists do just that when they use a phonetic transcription to represent as precisely as possible what they perceive when they listen to speech. Unfortunately, the wealth of phonetic information that our natural speech-perceiving mechanisms can use creates serious problems when, as in reading and writing, we try to put all that information through the eye.

A phonetic transcription, such as the linguist uses, preserves much surface information that is not represented in any alphabetic orthography. It includes all the context-conditioned variations of speech both within words and across syllable and word boundaries. For example, in a phonetic transcription, the plural s in "cats" would be transcribed as *s* but its counterpart in "dogs" would be *z* to reflect its pronunciation in that context. To take another example, the final consonant in the word, "sit," would be transcribed as *t*, but what we ordinarily consider to be the same consonant in the related word, "sitter," would have to be changed from *t* to *d* to reflect accurately that manner of change in our pronunciation. Similarly, in American English, the contraction "what's" would be transcribed differently in the context of "What's he saying?" from its rendition in the context of "What's your idea?" where, because of context-conditioned effects, it would be coarticulated with "your" to produce "Wuchur" (idea)?"

In view of these confusing context-conditioned variations, one would suppose that it should be extremely difficult to apprehend messages conveyed by means of a strictly phonetic transcription. And so it is, in fact. To be sure, any literate adult can learn to decode a phonetic transcription more easily than s/he can decode the visual display of acoustic events in a spectrogram, but even highly trained phoneticians cannot read an unfamiliar text written phonetically as fluently as they would the same passage written in our English orthography. The representation of context-driven articulatory distinctions, to say nothing about differences in linguistic stress, emphasis, idiolect, and dialect, seriously detracts from the broader requirements of language representation. This is certainly a case in which, except for very specialized purposes, more is definitely not better.

The Alphabet Represents Phonological Structures

Given that reading the sounds of speech is hard and reading a phonetic transcription is only slightly less so, what is it that an alphabet should represent if reading is to be made as easy as possible? Presumably, in the ideal case, the representation should match the way words are organized in our heads, in what linguists refer to as our lexicons. It stands to reason that our lexicons must be organized in terms of phonological or morphophonological (see note 1 above) segments that are sufficiently abstract to stand above the many variations at the auditory and phonetic surfaces. We have described the difficulties we get into when, in trying to put language in by eye, we begin with the variable auditory and phonetic forms. To get around these problems, we would want, ideally, to have words spelled in a way that matches the abstract (morpho)phonological structures as they must be stored in the speaker's lexicon. But that is an ideal that is not easily achieved.

The problem is that there are undoubtedly great differences among speakers of the language in the way in which their lexicons are organized and in exactly how abstractly the items are entered. To take one example, for the would-be reader who understands that such pairs as heal/health, steal/stealth, and even weal/wealth are related, the individual members of those pairs might well be entered quite differently than they would be for the reader who has never noted those relationships. The entries of the former reader would in this instance be closer to the way English spelling deals with the language.

For better or worse, English spelling happens to be quite far out on the abstractness dimension, rising considerably above the phonetic surface variations to preserve the identities of lexical cognates. The spelling is, in this sense, morphophonological in nature. As such, it necessarily must strain the linguistic sophistication of many would-be readers and spellers. The young child is especially likely to lack even the tacit knowledge, what we have elsewhere called "phonological maturity" (Liberman, Liberman, Mattingly, and Shankweiler 1980), that is needed to rationalize so much of the spelling. For example, the use of the same alphabetic characters for phonological segments that are phonetically quite different, as in such pairs as muscle/muscular and magic/magician, preserves the morphemic relations of the words and thus may increase fluency and efficient comprehension for a mature reader[2] but would serve only as a roadblock to the young child who is trying to figure out how the system works.

In summary, the point that should be emphasized here is that no matter how abstract it may often be and how far or how close to a given reader's lexicon, the alphabetic orthography does represent the (morpho)phonological structure of the spoken word, not its sounds or its phonetic surface. Now we can consider how this characteristic of the orthography relates to the attainment of literacy.

Linguistic Awareness and Reading

It has been our contention that in addition to the obvious need to have some command of the spoken language and the ability to discriminate the graphic symbols, the first requirement for beginning readers is to acquire a certain degree of linguistic sophistication, beyond that required for speaking and listening. One important aspect of linguistic sophistication is what Mattingly (1972) of the Haskins research group has dubbed "linguistic awareness."

---

[2]The representation in the ideal speaker-hearer's lexicon is often morphophonological, that is, the word is represented as a sequence of systematic phonemes divided into its constituent morphemes. For example, the words *heal, health, healthful,* have the morphophonological representations /hēl/, /hēl + θ/, /hēl + θ + ful/, respectively (see Liberman et al. 1980 for a more complete discussion of the morphophonological nature of orthographies).

Though it could be taken to have a more general connotation, this term has been defined in a rather special way in the context of initial reading acquisition—to refer to the awareness of the units of speech that are represented by the orthography. In the alphabetic orthography, the phoneme, the unit of which the learner must become aware, is a constituent part of larger units, i.e., the word and the syllable, both of which have considerably more salience, as we have said. Awareness that these larger units have parts and the ability to identify those parts does not come easily and does not happen all at once. The ability to segment speech into its constituent units, of whatever size, has been found to show improvement from ages four to six or seven (Calfee, Chapman, and Venezky 1970; Liberman 1973; Treiman and Baron 1981). But in this developmental sequence, awareness of the phonemic unit is always harder, develops later, and is generally found to be a more sensitive predictor of reading skills in kindergarteners and first graders than the syllable or word. There is by now a long list of studies, originating both here and abroad, that have been strongly supportive of phoneme segmentation skill as a predictor of reading ability. Among the studies that come to mind (and there are surely others as well) are Blachman (1983), Helfgott (1976), Mann and Liberman (1984), Zifcak (1981) from our research group, Bradley and Bryant (1983) in England, Lundberg and associates (1980) in Sweden, Fox and Routh (1975) in the United States, and Bertelson's laboratory (Alegria and Content 1983) in Belgium.

Most of the previous research on linguistic awareness and the acquisition of literacy has been concerned with the attainment of reading skills. Recently, we have begun to look more closely at spelling from this vantage point. We should like to report on two of these investigations in this paper, one in which we examined the invented spellings of kindergarteners and the other in which we explored the virtually uncharted territory of linguistic factors in adult illiteracy.

Linguistic Abilities and the Invented Spellings of Kindergarteners

The first study we will describe looked into the linguistic abilities of kindergarteners in relation to their skill in invented spelling. Before reporting on our findings, we should take a moment to say what we mean by invented spellings. When spelling words in their spontaneous writings, preschoolers are, of course, limited by their meager orthographic knowledge, which in the beginning may include only the knowledge of names of letters ("bee" and "dee," for example). In his seminal work in the early seventies, Charles Read (1971) demonstrated that the invented spellings of preschoolers display a predictable pattern in their choice of the letter symbols used to represent the spoken language. Relying on their apparently quite acute perception of the phonetic, surface features of both the utterance to be recorded and the letter names they know, young children begin by devising what amounts to a primitive phonetic transcription, rather than the phonological representation of our spelling system.

To the extent that English is written abstractly, it assumes, as we said earlier, a user who has, to a considerable degree, what we have called "phonological maturity" (Liberman et al 1980). These younger children clearly do not have the requisite degree that our orthography demands. Given a word like "train," to borrow one of Read's examples, a preschooler might produce an *H* as the first letter of the word in an attempt to represent the first phone in their own spoken version of the word ("*ch*rain") by its closest counterpart in a letter name they know ("ait*ch*"). As the children begin to develop more sophisticated apprehensions of the phonology, the purely phonetic transcription becomes less prevalent in their spellings. They begin to assimilate the rules according to which our abstract spelling makes sense.

This growing awareness of the (morpho)phonological rule structure of words is implicit in their invented spelling productions. Therefore, if one is interested, as we are, in evaluating the level of linguistic sophistication in children's spellings, it is possible to do so by constructing a scoring system that is fashioned to reflect that awareness, rather than being limited to a consideration simply of right/wrong judgments. Louisa Cook Moats (1983), using an analytic scoring system of this kind, did a pioneering study in which she found the misspellings of dyslexic fourth through eighth graders to be quite similar linguistically to those of nondyslexic second graders.

We were curious to learn whether we could find possible precursors of linguistic deficiencies in the spelling of much younger children—those in a public school kindergarten class. Accordingly, we chose to examine the relationship between kindergarteners' proficiency in invented spelling and in their other linguistic abilities.

All the children in the kindergarten class were given a dictated, real word spelling test. A given word could receive a score from 0 (for simply random letters) to 6 (for a correct English spelling). In this scoring system, we measured the children's spelling proficiency along two dimensions—the number of phonemes that the child included in spelling the word and also the level of the orthographic representation. Thus, for the target word, "sick," increasing scores would be awarded for the following sequences of responses: one phoneme with conventional letters (s, c); more than one phoneme but not all (sk, ck); all phonemes with phonetically related letters (sec, sek); all phonemes with conventional letters (sic, sik); all with correct spelling (sick).

In addition to the spelling test, eight language-based tasks were administered to the class. We found that three of these made a difference statistically in a multiple regression analysis, accounting for 93% of the variance in invented spelling proficiency. Of these, a phoneme segmentation task patterned after Lundberg (1980) accounted for 67% of the variance in invented spelling performance and one that tested the ability to write letters to phoneme dictation accounted for an additional 20%. A phoneme deletion task ("Say meat without the 'm' "), adapted from Rosner's Test of Auditory Analysis Skills (Rosner 1975), added another 6%. A measure of expressive vocabulary, the Boston Naming Test (Kaplan, Goodglass, and Weintraub 1976), contributed 1%, but did not quite attain significance.

The four other language-based tasks in our study did not contribute to the variance of the invented spelling performance. They included a test of receptive vocabulary (the Peabody Picture Vocabulary Test, Dunn and Dunn 1981); a syllable deletion task ("Say cowboy without the 'cow' "), also adapted from Rosner's TAAS (1975); word repetition (correctly repeating words spoken by the examiner); naming letters and writing letters to dictation. Analysis of the children's performance on word repetition, letter naming, and letter writing revealed only developmentally appropriate errors such as slight infantilisms in articulation and occasional confusions of visually similar letters in writing. In regard to the latter type of error, it is of interest to note that letter reversals, though present in some protocols, were not found to be related to invented spelling ability. That is, children could be good invented spellers at the kindergarten level without having fully mastered the correct orientation of the reversible letters.

This study suggests that spelling skill develops systematically as young children master the ability to analyze words into their constituent phonemes. That conclusion is supported by the strength of phoneme segmentation ability, writing phonemes to dictation, and the deletion of phonemes as predictors of invented spelling ability. These three tasks all require a degree of explicit awareness of internal phonological word structure that is not tapped by the other language tasks. The other tasks all reflect certain aspects of language development but either do not include the analytic component at all (Peabody Picture Vocabulary, letter naming, letter writing, and word repetition) or tap it at a less abstract level, closer to the basic unit of articulation (syllable deletion).

Linguistic Abilities and Adult Poor Spellers

Among kindergarteners, then, we found that the children who were the best spellers in the class also exhibited better skills in analyzing the phonemic constituents of words. Recently, we examined a group of adults enrolled in a community literacy class with a view toward finding out whether their profiles would be similar to those of younger learners. The subjects in this study were nine men whose occupations ranged from lower-level management to semi-skilled labor, all of whom reported serious difficulties with spelling. Five of the men had repeated a grade in school, but only one had received remedial assistance.

Once again, as we had with the kindergarteners, we administered a number of tests of language ability as well as measures of spelling proficiency. To determine the kinds of spelling problems characteristic of adult illiterates, we used two dictated lists of spelling words. One list was taken from the spelling subtest of the Gallistel-Ellis Test of Coding Skills (1974), which includes real words of both regular and irregular orthographic construction. The other was a list of pseudowords taken from the reading subtest of the Gallistel-Ellis Test. In order to provide a comparison with their spelling proficiency in spontaneous writing, we also collected writing samples, using the stimulus pictures of the Test of Written Language (Hammill and Larsen 1978).

Four tests of language ability were included in the adult study. As a check on the possibility that gross problems in speech perception might be at the root of their difficulties, we examined the performance of the adults on the Sound Mimicry subtest of the Goldman-Fristoe-Woodcock Auditory Skills Test Battery (1974). In this subtest subjects are required to repeat taped nonsense words, one to three syllables in length.

In view of previous findings with children which have suggested that poor readers and spellers may have difficulty analyzing other aspects of internal structure of words (Carlisle 1984; Rubin 1984), we wished to measure the analytic abilities of the adults at both the phonemic and morphemic levels of language. The test used for phonemic analysis was the Sound Analysis subtest of the Goldman-Fristoe-Woodcock Auditory Skills Test Battery (1974). Here, monosyllabic nonsense words are presented on tape and the subject is required to identify the first, middle, or last phoneme in the word. To determine the subjects' ability to apply basic inflectional and derivational rules of morphology, they were also given the Berry-Talbott Test of Language (1966). Normal children have been found to develop the morphological abilities tapped by this test in a systematic progression from the easier items at the beginning to the more difficult ones at the end, with mastery expected by age seven or eight.

Finally, in addition to testing them on spelling and language tasks, we also measured the oral reading ability of our adult subjects. For this purpose, both single word and passage reading measures were used. The reading subtest of the Gallistel-Ellis Test of Coding Skills was chosen to assess reading of single words. This subtest includes real words of two types—those of irregular (unpredictable by the more common orthographic rules) construction, and those of regular construction that are presented in order of increasing difficulty by syllable type. The test also includes nonsense words that are arranged by syllable type as well. The Spache Diagnostic Reading Scales (1972) were used to assess oral passage reading.

We can turn now to the results of our study of adults and look first at their spelling performance. On the dictated spelling of real words, they did somewhat better on the irregular than on the regular words—63% as against 57% correct, reflecting, perhaps, the tendency to rely on the memory of the global appearance of words often found clinically in poor readers. This possibility is supported by the large drop to 38% correct in their performance on nonsense words often found clinically in poor readers. In order to appreciate the seriousness of the drop, it should be noted that whereas there is, of course, only one correct response for real words, whether of regular or irregular construction, there can be several acceptable spellings of each nonsense word. Consider the pseudoword "lete," for example. Four spellings—*lete, leet, leat, liet*—would all be scored as correct.

To be sure, even with this apparent advantage for the nonsense words, one might still expect some discrepancy in performance between the spelling of nonsense and real words, in favor of the real words. However, it was evident from the pattern of their results that our adult subjects had not mastered the basic phoneme-grapheme spelling patterns that would allow them consistently to produce even phonetically reasonable renditions of words they had not seen before. One striking example that occurred during the reading test comes to mind. When presented with the written word, *peg,* one of the adult subjects puzzled over the word for some time and finally said: "Pig? Well, I know it's not pig, because there's a *e* in the middle, but I guess I'll go with pig." (Letter discrimination was obviously not his problem.) It is relevant to remark at this point that our adults had little difficulty in the spoken repetition of the auditorily presented nonsense words, performing there with 92% success. This suggests that the problems they are having with spelling cannot be attributed to gross difficulties in speech perception (nor in articulation, for that matter, or some bias against using nonsense words).

Thus far we have reported only on spelling performances on dictated single words. The spelling of the adults on the spontaneous writing samples was somewhat better than on the dictated words—78% of the words were spelled correctly. But it was apparent that whatever improvement occurred here could probably be attributed to the tendency of the subjects to limit their productions to words that they thought they could spell correctly. A large proportion of one subject's output even included his copying of the wording of the printed test directions, for example.

An informal qualitative analysis of the errors made by the adults on the writing samples showed clearly that they had serious linguistic problems over and above their poor spelling. Approximately a third of the errors reflected grammatical weaknesses—difficulties with function words accounted for 12% of the errors, and omissions or substitutions of inflectional endings accounted for another 21%.

In the light of these findings, it is of interest to note that our adults passed only 63% of the items on the Berry-Talbott test which measures inflectional and derivational knowledge. In contrast, in a study recently completed by one of us (Rubin 1984), a group of 60 first graders was able to pass 57% of the same items. Moreover, the young children did well on the lower level items and less well on the higher, thus showing a systematic development of morphemic understanding. The adults, on the other hand, often performed poorly on even the simplest categories like plural and past tense inflections, though they were able to use them correctly in their spontaneous speech. It would seem that when they have to do even a moderate degree of analysis of their language, whether written or spoken, their linguistic abilities are strained to the point of breakdown.

In view of their performance on the morphemic analysis task, it was not surprising to find that language analysis at the phonemic level was especially trying for these adults. On our very simple phoneme analysis task, which is similar to those used in training kindergarteners and first graders in phonemic segmentation, only 58% of their responses were correct. Moreover, they found the task frustrating and unpleasant.

This inability of adults with literacy problems to perform well in a task requiring explicit understanding of the internal structure of words has also been found by other investigators (Byrne and Ledez 1983; Marcel 1980; Morais, Cary, Alegria, and Bertelson 1979; Charles Read, personal communication 1984). Particularly convincing in this connection is the finding by Morais and associates (1979) that the performance of first graders in the third month of school was slightly better in both phoneme deletion and addition tasks than that of the adult illiterates in their study.

We now turn to a comparison of the reading and spelling of our adult subjects. We found that their reading of single real words was better than their spelling, as would be expected in any comparison of recognition and production measures. But the pattern of performance was quite similar. Real words were read with greater accuracy than nonsense words, just as had been the case with spelling. But perhaps the most telling result was found in a direct comparison of reading and spelling as a function of word type. Whereas the reading of real words, as we have said, was generally better than the spelling, the situation was quite different in regard to the nonsense words. On nonsense words, for which a structural analytical approach is obligatory rather than optional as it may be in dealing with real words, the performance of the adults on both reading and spelling was virtually identical in quality and quite poor.

In short, the adult subjects, like the poorest invented spellers in the kindergarten study, appeared to have only the dimmest understanding of the phonemic structure of words. Qualitative analysis of their successes in reading suggested that memorizing words as global entities was a favored strategy. The analysis revealed, for example, that they often did well on words they had seen frequently before, even when the words were polysyllabic or irregular in construction. They might, for example, read correctly a ten-letter, trisyllabic word with uncommon spelling like *photograph,* but be at a loss to deal with a simple trigram like *peg* that they had never encountered before. The same kind of contrast between performance on complex practiced words and unknown but relatively simple words was also apparent in their spelling.

Their oral reading of connected text on the Spache test (1972) was clearly superior to their reading of single words, suggesting, as has been found in other studies of poor readers (Perfetti and Hogaboam 1975), that our adult subjects were relying heavily on context to assist them in apprehending familiar words. At all events, reading, like spelling, was patently a struggle for these men, generating once more grammatical errors not present in their everyday speech. Examination of their errors in oral passage reading revealed a pattern of incorrect use of inflectional morphemes and functors much like that noted in their spontaneous writing samples.

Educational Implications

In our introductory remarks, we have advanced our reasons for expecting that the acquisition of literacy would be related to a certain degree of linguistic sophistication, that is, to the ability to deal with the structure of language in an analytic manner. In the first study reported here we found that among kindergarteners, the better spellers, like the better readers among older children in previous investigations, have developed this ability to a higher degree than those who spell more poorly. In the other study, a group of adults in a community literacy class, who showed no serious deficiencies in everyday speaking and listening, were extremely poor spellers and at the same time were also deficient in various tasks requiring analytic linguistic skills. They found phonological segmentation tasks particularly troublesome.

The ability to stand back from one's language and analyze its structure apparently does not develop naturally as a result of cognitive maturation. It must be learned or taught. But there are several ways in which it can be learned or taught. Many children, as we have pointed out elsewhere (Liberman and Shankweiler 1977), will develop linguistic insights as a consequence of their experiences in learning to read an alphabetic orthography. But even for those children, the process might have been made easier and faster by giving them explicit instruction. For other children, including especially those who for whatever reason are at risk linguistically, more explicit instruction will be required if they are ever to attain true literacy; to be able, that is, to deal effectively with unknown or previously unlearned words, which is what an alphabetic orthography is all about. The adults in our community literacy class can still profit from explicit instruction in all aspects of the structure of language (phonological, syntactic, and morphological). But they would have been spared much grief and embarrassment if their deficits had been discovered and addressed in kindergarten instead.

Several investigations have now demonstrated that linguistic awareness can be trained (Bradley and Bryant 1983; Olofsson and Lundberg 1983; Vellutino and Scanlon this volume) and will make a difference in reading acquisition. Recent studies make it clear that phonological (Fischer, Shankweiler, and Liberman in press) and morphological knowledge (Carlisle 1984; Fischer et al. in press; Rubin 1984) make a difference in spelling proficiency. At all events, it now seems reasonable to suggest, in view of the present findings and in light of the characteristics of the alphabetic orthography and how it relates to language, that more and earlier training in all aspects of linguistic sensitivity may promote better spelling and should be encouraged. Kindergarten is not too soon to start.

References

Alegria, J., and Content, A. 1983. Explicit analysis of speech and learning to read: Some experimental studies. Paper presented at the Third Language and Language Acquisition Conference on Pragmatics and Education, March 1983, Gent.

Berry, M. 1966. *Berry-Talbott Language Test: Comprehension of Grammar*. Rockford, IL.

Blachman, B. A. 1983. Are we assessing the linguistic factors critical in early reading? *Annals of Dyslexia* 33:91–109.

Bradley, L, and Bryant, P. E. 1983. Categorizing sounds and learning to read: A causal connection. *Nature* 301(3):419–421.

Byrne, B., and Ledez, J. 1983. Phonological awareness in reading-disabled adults. *Australian Journal of Psychology* 35:185–197.

Calfee, R. C., Chapman, R. S., and Venezky, R. L. 1970. *How a Child Needs to Think To Learn To Read.* Madison, WI: Wisconsin Research and Development Center for Cognitive Learning, The University of Wisconsin.

Carlisle, J. F. 1984. The relationship between derivational morphology and spelling ability in 4th, 6th, and 8th graders. Ph.D. diss., University of Connecticut, Storrs.

Diringer, D. 1948. *The Alphabet: A Key to the History of Mankind.* New York: Hutchinsons.

Dunn, L. M., and Dunn, L. M. 1981. *Peabody Picture Vocabulary Test, Revised.* Circle Pines, MN: American Guidance Service.

Fischer, W., Shankweiler, D., and Liberman, I. Y. In press. Spelling proficiency and sensitivity to word-structure. *Journal of Verbal Learning and Verbal Behavior.*

Fox, B., and Routh, D. K. 1975. Analyzing spoken language into words, syllables, and phonemes: A developmental study. *Journal of Psycholinguistic Research* 4(4):331–342.

Gallistel, E., and Ellis, K. 1974. *Gallistel-Ellis Test of Coding Skills.* Hamden, CT: Montage Press.

Goldman, R., Fristoe, M., and Woodcock, R. W. 1974. *G-F-W Sound-Symbol Tests, Goldman-Fristoe-Woodcock Auditory Skills Test Battery.* Circle Pines, MN: American Guidance Service.

Hamill, D. D., and Larsen, S. C. 1978. *Test of Written Language.* Austin, TX: Pro-Ed.

Helfgott, J. 1976. Phonemic segmentation and blending skills of kindergarten children: Implications for beginning reading acquisition. *Contemporary Educational Psychology* 1:157–169.

Holden, M. H., and MacGinitie, W. H. 1972. Children's conceptions of word boundaries in speech and print. *Journal of Educational Psychology* 63:551–557.

Kaplan, E., Goodglass, H., and Weintraub, S. 1976. *Boston Naming Test.* Boston, MA: Boston University School of Medicine.

Liberman, I. Y. 1973. Segmentation of the spoken word and reading acquisition. *Bulletin of The Orton Society* 23.65–77.

Liberman, I. Y. 1983. A language-oriented view of reading and its disabilities. In H. R. Myklebust (ed.). *Progress in Learning Disabilities,* Vol. V. New York: Grune and Stratton.

Liberman, I. Y., Liberman, A. M., Mattingly, I. G., and Shankweiler, D. 1980. Orthography and the beginning reader. In J. F. Kavanagh and R. L. Venezky (eds.). *Orthography, Reading, and Dyslexia.* Baltimore, MD: University Park Press.

Liberman, I. Y., and Shankweiler, D. 1977. Speech, the alphabet, and teaching to read. In L. Resnick and P. Weaver (eds.). *Theory and Practice of Early Reading.* Hillsdale, NJ: Lawrence Erlbaum Associates.

Liberman, I. Y., Shankweiler, D., Fischer, F. W., and Carter, B. 1974. Explicit syllable and phoneme segmentation in the young child. *Journal of Experimental Child Psychology* 18:201 212.

Lundberg, I., Olafsson, A., and Wall, S. 1980. Reading and spelling skills in the first school years predicted from phonemic awareness skills in kindergarten. *Scandinavian Journal of Psychology* 21:159–173.

Mann, V. A., and Liberman, I. Y. 1984. Phonological awareness and verbal short-term memory. *Journal of Learning Disabilities* 17:592–599.

Marcel, A. 1980. Phonological awareness and phonological representation: Investigation of a specific spelling problem. In U. Frith (ed.). *Cognitive Processes in Spelling.* London: Academic Press.

Mattingly, I. G. 1972. Reading, the linguistic process, and linguistic awareness. In J. F. Kavanagh and I. G. Mattingly (eds.). *Language by Ear and by Eye.* Cambridge, MA: MIT Press.

Moats, L. C. 1983. A comparison of the spelling errors of older dyslexic and second-grade normal children. *Annals of Dyslexia* 33:121–140.

Morais, J., Cary, L., Alegria, J., and Bertelson, P. 1979. Does awareness of speech as a sequence of phones arise spontaneously? *Cognition* 7:323–331.

Olofsson, A., and Lundberg, I. 1983. Can phonemic awareness be trained in kindergarten? *Scandinavian Journal of Psychology* 24:35–44.

Perfetti, C. A., and Hogaboam, T. W. 1975. The relationship between single word decoding and reading comprehension skill. *Journal of Educational Psychology* 67:461–469.

Read, C. 1971. Pre-school children's knowledge of English phonology. *Harvard Education Review* 41(1):1–34.

Read, C. 1984. Personal communication, November 9, 1984.

Rosner, J. 1975. *Helping Children Overcome Learning Disabilities.* New York: Walker and Co.

Rubin, H. 1984. An investigation of the development of morphological knowledge and its relationship to early spelling ability. Ph.D. diss., University of Connecticut, Storrs.

Spache, G. D. 1972. *Diagnostic Reading Scales.* Monterey, CA: California Test Bureau.

Treiman, R., and Baron, J. 1981. Segmental analysis ability: Development and relation to reading ability. *In* G. E. McKinnon and T. G. Waller (eds.). *Reading Research: Advances in Theory and Practice,* Vol. 3. New York Academic Press.

Zifcak, M. 1981. Phonological awareness and reading acquisition. *Contemporary Educational Psychology* 6:117–126.

13

Verbal Memory in Poor and Normal Readers: Developmental Differences in the Use of Linguistic Codes

Frank R. Vellutino and Donna M. Scanlon

Introduction

*I*n this chapter we present results of studies we have recently completed contrasting verbal memory in poor and normal readers. Previous studies conducted in our laboratory (Vellutino 1979) had provided documentation that specific reading disability in young children is not caused by dysfunction in visual perception, cross modal transfer, and various other basic processes involved in learning to read. Moreover, the data from these studies, and research conducted elsewhere, prompted us to consider seriously the possibility that poor readers may be encumbered by limitations in the use of linguistic codes to store and retrieve information. On the other hand, the possibility remained that word identification problems result from the cross-referencing process itself, the implication being that poor readers are encumbered by specific dysfunction in integrating visual and verbal information. These latter alternatives were tested and the evidence to date favors the linguistic coding notion rather than the visual-verbal deficit notion. The results of these studies are presented in the sections that follow.

Subjects in each study were selected using essentially the same sampling criteria. Thus, poor readers were severely impaired and typically scored between the fourth and the tenth percentiles on an oral reading test. Normal readers were at or above grade level in reading and were randomly selected

Much of the research reported in this chapter was supported by Grant 2RO1HD09658 awarded by the National Institute of Child Health and Human Development, National Institutes of Health. The authors thank Mark Prockton and Linda Rupert for their help in data collection and data analysis and Melinda Taylor for her help in the preparation of this manuscript. We also express our sincere gratitude to the administrators, staff, and students from schools in the Albany, New York metropolitan area for their participation in the various studies.

from among those attending schools from which the poor readers were selected. All subjects were also of average or above average intelligence, having achieved an IQ of at least 90 on either the Verbal or Performance subtests of the WISC or WISC-R (Wechsler 1949, 1974) or in some instances on the Slosson's Intelligence Test (Slosson 1963). Each was free from sensory, physical, neurological, emotional, and socioeconomic handicaps. In addition, all groups were equated for sex ratios. Grade levels in the various studies we have conducted have ranged from two through eight, inclusive, but in the memory studies to be discussed, poor and normal reader groups were stratified at second and sixth grade. With our particular sampling criteria, this procedure has allowed us to compare reader groups matched for age and grade as well as for reading achievement (second grade normal and sixth grade poor readers).

Background Research

For over a decade, we and our colleagues have conducted research evaluating the nature and origin of word identification problems in poor readers, since this is perhaps the most pervasive of all of their difficulties in learning to read. We initially evaluated Orton's (1925) suggestion that, because of maturational delay resulting in failure to establish hemispheric dominance for language, these children were subject to a selective breakdown in visual processing, characterized by anomalous activation of mirror-image transforms of letters (b/d) and words (was/saw) they attempted to identify, and attendant confusion in orienting and sequencing these items. This idea later gave rise to the popular notion that poor readers literally perceive letters and words in reverse. Hermann (1959) later qualified this theory and suggested that such errors may *not* be due to maturational delay affecting hemispheric dominance, but to an inborn disposition toward spatial confusion. He, in fact, made special note of the common observation that poor readers seemed less able than normal readers to progress smoothly from left to right when reading connected text and interpreted this behavior as an indication of directional confusion.

In the first study conducted (Vellutino, Steger, and Kandel 1972), we attempted to test Orton's (1925) theory by teasing apart the visual and verbal encoding components of word identification. Thus, unstratified samples of poor and normal readers (grades 2 through 8) were given consecutive tachistoscopic presentations of scrambled letters, words, numerals, and geometric designs, and were asked to both name and copy these stimuli from visual memory. The poor readers were able to copy these stimuli much better than they could name them. Moreover, they performed about as well as the normal readers on the visual recall task, but not as well on the naming task. Essentially the same results were obtained in a second study (Vellutino, Smith, Steger, and Kaman 1975). What these findings seemed to indicate is that poor readers who see a *b* and call it "d" or *was* and call it "saw," do not actually perceive these stimuli in reverse, but misname them because they do not have ready access to the linguistic representations corresponding with each. Our data therefore cast serious doubt on the perceptual deficit explanation of reading disability.

Our skepticism was greatly reinforced by the results of a second series of studies (Vellutino, Pruzek, Steger, and Meshoulam 1973; Vellutino, Steger, Kaman, and DeSetto 1975) in which poor readers (grades 2 through 6) performed as well as normal readers on immediate visual recall of the letters in three, four, and five letter Hebrew words in correct order. However, neither group performed as well as children learning to read and write Hebrew, except in the case of three-letter words, which did not greatly tax visual memory. Moreover, when we counted the number of omission errors made in given letter locations, we found that poor and normal readers, who were unacquainted with Hebrew, made all of their errors at the right terminal positions of the words, whereas children learning to read and write Hebrew made all of their errors at the left terminal positions. These results were consistent with our previous findings and suggested that poor readers are not basically impaired in visual-spatial orientation, visual sequencing, or serial memory in general. They also suggested that when poor readers have difficulty in maintaining a left to right scan in reading, it is a consequence of reading disorder and not symptomatic of directional confusion that causes reading disorder.

We then turned our attention to Birch's (1962) cross-modal transfer theory of reading disability. According to this theory, many poor readers are impaired by an inability to cross-reference and integrate information represented in different sensory modalities, but may be relatively normal in processing information within a given modality. In an initial test of this theory, Birch and Belmont (1964) gave poor and normal readers (ages 9 and 10) auditory presentations of Morse-code-like patterns and had them match these patterns with their visual counterparts. Because the poor readers were not as proficient as normal readers on this task, the investigators concluded that reading disability in some children is caused by dysfunction in cross-modal transfer. A flurry of studies followed, most obtaining essentially the same results (Vellutino 1979). However, Blank and her colleagues (Blank and Bridger 1966; Blank, Weider, and Bridger 1968) presented poor and normal readers (grades 1 through 4) with similar pattern matching tests, both across and within the visual and auditory modalities, and by having subjects attempt to "remember out loud," they found that the poor readers were less inclined than the normal readers to use rehearsal and organization strategies and were also less proficient in generating verbal mnemonics to aid memory. The investigators suggested that results from the cross-modal transfer studies could be more parsimoniously explained by postulating verbal coding and organization deficits in poor readers rather than cross-modal transfer deficits.

We subsequently evaluated Birch's theory by using learning rather than pattern matching tasks to control for short term memory limits. Accordingly, poor and normal readers (grades 4 through 6) were given paired associates learning tasks using non-verbal as well as verbal associates (Vellutino, Steger, Harding, and Phillips 1975; Vellutino, Steger, and Pruzek 1973). The nonverbal learning tasks respectively compared reader groups on their ability to learn visual associates, auditory associates and visual-auditory associates. The verbal learning tasks (respectively) compared these groups on their ability to attach names to objects and letter strings.

We found no appreciable differences between reader groups on the non-verbal learning tasks, regardless of whether associates were presented within or across modalities. However, there were significant differences between poor and normal readers on both of the visual-verbal learning tasks. These results provided additional evidence against Birch's cross-modal deficit explanation of reading disability, and ruled out earlier suggestions that the problem might be caused by difficulties in associative learning (Brewer 1967; Gascon and Goodglass 1970). They also suggested, in agreement with Blank, that a basic source of reading disability may be dysfunction in verbal encoding. This inference was reinforced by the results of yet another study we conducted evaluating the possibility that poor readers may be impaired in their ability to abstract and generalize invariant units in patterned information (Rabinovitch 1959; Morrison and Manis 1982).

In this study (Vellutino, Harding, Phillips, and Steger 1975) poor and normal readers (grades four, five, and six) were randomly assigned either to a visual-verbal or visual-visual pattern learning condition. In each, subjects were presented with initial training and transfer learning subtests, both of which required that they learn paired associates containing units that corresponded invariantly. Invariant units were permuted on the transfer task to form ''new'' stimulus and response pairs. Poor readers performed below the level of the normal readers only on the visual-verbal learning task, suggesting that they have difficulty in learning to map alphabetic symbols to sound, because they are impaired by deficiencies in some aspect of verbal processing and not by deficiencies in their ability to detect and use invariance.

However, the possibility remained that such problems were caused by a specific breakdown in cross-referencing visual and verbal information and two alternatives were considered. One was suggested by research conducted by Sperry (1964) and his associates (Gazzaniga, Bogen, and Sperry 1965) who found that split brain patients could *not* identify printed words when visual half-field presentations stimulated the right hemisphere, but could identify these same words when such presentations stimulated the left hemisphere. Extrapolating from these results, we wondered whether the word identification problems observed in poor readers could possibly be due to dysfunction in interhemispheric transmission. In order to evaluate this possibility, we conducted a series of studies using the hemifield presentation technique used by Sperry (1964). Because of the way the visual system is connected to the hemispheres, visual presentations to the right visual field stimulate the left hemisphere and visual presentations to the left visual field stimulate the right hemisphere. Thus, in the first study (Vellutino, Bentley, and Phillips 1978), second and sixth grade poor and normal readers were given a paired associates learning task using Chinese idiographs as visual stimuli and common English words as verbal responses. If the visual-verbal learning difficulties observed in poor readers are caused by dysfunction in interhemispheric transmission, then reader group differences on the paired associates task should have been observed only on presentations to the left visual field (right hemisphere). However, poor readers performed below the level of normal readers on both visual field presentations and there were no reader-group-by-visual-field interactions. Moreover, these findings were duplicated in a second study using the same materials and experimental techniques with an independent sample (Vellutino, Scanlon, and Bentley 1983). The interhemispheric transmission explanation of reading disability was therefore rejected.

We alluded earlier to a second type of visual-verbal integration problem that might encumber poor readers, and we had in mind the possibility that there could yet be some breakdown in the cross-referencing of visual and verbal representations *within* the language hemisphere, if not between the hemispheres. However, this would be a more likely alternative if it were also found that poor and normal readers performed at comparable levels on verbal processing tasks that did *not* involve the association and integration of visual and verbal symbols. But, if group differences, favoring normal readers, were consistently found on such tasks, then deficiencies in visual-verbal integration would not be a viable explanation of reading disability. We, therefore, designed another series of studies that more directly evaluated these alternatives.

Research Evaluating Verbal Memory in Poor and Normal Readers

Linguistic Codes

Our conceptualization of specific reading disability is, in part, based on the assumption that facility in storing and retrieving words from the lexicon requires a functional acquaintance with their multiple attributes. In processing spoken words, one is especially dependent upon familiarity with their linguistic attributes, specifically their semantic, phonological, and syntactic features. In processing written words, one must also be familiar with their graphic and orthographic features. We also assume that the featural attributes of words are qualitatively and functionally distinct, and that one must be able to activate and cross-reference individual codes for lexical storage and retrieval.

Semantic codes are the linguistic representations of meaningful concepts, as encoded in both individual words and groups of words. The meanings embedded in given words and the words themselves come to exist in a complex network of interrelated associates that become increasingly more elaborate and better defined during the course of lexical development. It would seem to follow that the child with a more highly differentiated and more highly elaborated semantic network, as manifested in a rich vocabulary and a rich fund of world knowledge, is better able to rely on semantic encoding to assist in the storage and retrieval of words from lexical memory than the child with a less highly differentiated and less highly elaborated semantic network.

Phonological codes[1] are highly abstract representations of the auditory properties of given words in the form of "systematic phonemes" (Chomsky and Halle 1968) that transcend the surface or allophonic variations generated by unique pronunciations of those words. The term also has reference to a system of "rules" for ordering phones and phonemes in the language. However, when used in reference to printed words, it should be distinguished from *graphic codes*, which, more accurately, refer to visual representations of letters corresponding with the phonemes in given words, as well as from *orthographic codes*, which refer to visual representations of the structural characteristics of given words and to abstract rules for ordering the letters in words. We suggest, along with others (e.g., Liberman and Shankweiler 1979), that lexical storage and retrieval rely heavily upon one's ability to activate and access the phonological properties of printed words. There is, in fact, reason to believe that children who have difficulty in making functional use of phonological codes also have significant difficulty in remembering all verbally coded material. To the extent that such difficulty could impair the ability to remember the names of things, it could, theoretically, place limitations on one's vocabulary development as well.

Syntactic codes are highly abstract representations, in the form of grammatic "rules," which define the functional properties that words have in common with other words, and that constrain their use in sentences. When used in conjunction with free morphemes or words, the term refers to representations of the form class (e.g., nouns, verbs, etc.) from which given words are derived. When used in conjunction with bound morphemes (e.g., inflections such as "ed" and "ing"), it refers to representations that generate changes in grammatic properties (e.g., number, person, tense, and mood) that qualify the meanings of words. The term "syntactic codes" also refers to abstract rules for ordering words in the language and for representing structural differences in sentences in the language. We believe that the child who becomes increasingly adept at encoding grammatic distinctions among free and bound morphemes enhances his/her ability to store and retrieve these items from memory, and is better equipped to do so than the child who has difficulty in encoding such distinctions. Similarly, the child who is able to make grammatic distinctions among sentences is better equipped to comprehend them and, thereby, encode their meanings, than the child who has difficulty in making these distinctions.

It should be apparent that semantic codes have reference to the substantive properties of spoken and printed words, while syntactic and phonological codes have reference to their structural and formal properties, or what we have

---

[1]It has been a convention in the literature to use the term "phonological" to refer to morphophonological representations of speech that are derived at a deeper level of abstraction than input representations that are "phonetic," using the latter to refer to the surface features of linguistic stimuli. However, it is an open question whether linguistic units stored in working or short term memory are encoded only at the phonetic level or also at the more abstract phonological level. The question holds regardless of whether the linguistic stimuli are auditorily or visually presented. Thus, to avoid confusion, we shall use the term "phonological" to refer to linguistic units that are smaller than the syllable with no intent to imply by the use of the term any particular degree of abstractness.

elsewhere termed their "purely linguistic" properties (Vellutino and Scanlon, 1985b). As we have just indicated, each of these codes is qualitatively distinct, but equally important is the fact that each has a unique function in processing verbally encoded information. For example, in processing words for meaning, one might be attuned more to their semantic than to their phonological attributes, whereas in processing words for verbatim recall, one might be attuned at least as much to their phonological as to their semantic attributes. On the other hand, the syntactic attributes of given words seem to provide qualifying information that might affect the encoding of both their meanings and their surface characteristics and, depending on the task, one may be more or less attuned to these attributes. For example, sensitivity to syntactic codes is an obvious necessity when one processes connected text for meaning, but if the task requires verbatim recall of a list of common nouns, syntactic codes provide no edification and may not be readily activated. On the other hand, if the list consists of words representing different parts of speech, then attention to syntactic codes would have more utility and may well be activated.

If one assumes the validity of the foregoing distinctions, then it becomes reasonable to suggest that reading disability in otherwise normal children may be due in significant measure to difficulties they may encounter in using language to code information. If this is the case, then such difficulties should be apparent, not only on word identification and other reading tasks, but on any measure that involves memory for linguistically coded material. By logical extension, poor readers should perform below the level of normal readers on verbal memory tasks involving auditory presentations of words and sentences. This possibility is suggested in our consistent observation that poor readers performed below the level of normal readers only on paired associates learning tasks that involved verbal processing. It is also suggested in research conducted elsewhere.

Concretely, Liberman, Shankweiler, Liberman, Fowler, and Fischer (1977) compared second grade poor and normal readers on recall of visually presented rhyming versus non-rhyming letters and found that while normal readers generally performed better than poor readers, they were disrupted more than the poor readers by rhyming letters. Shankweiler, Liberman, Mark, Fowler, and Fischer (1979) obtained essentially the same results with second grade reader groups using auditory presentations of the same stimuli. Byrne and Shea (1979) also tested second grade reader groups using a continuous recognition task involving antecedents and distractors that were either semantically or phonologically similar and found that false recognition errors in the poor readers were prompted much more by the semantic than by the phonological distractors. However, in the normal readers, such errors were more evenly distributed across both types of distractors, suggesting that they were more sensitive than the poor readers to phonological codes. (See also Mark, Shankweiler, Liberman, and Fowler, 1977; and Mann, Liberman, and Shankweiler 1980).

The results of these studies provide initial documentation that poor readers may be deficient in verbal memory. However, none of them systematically contrasted poor and normal readers on memory for verbal material that varied with respect to reliance on particular linguistic codes, and none allowed contrasts of these two groups at different levels of reading skills development, since each evaluated children in second grade or below. In view of our characterizations earlier of the qualitative and functional differences in the respective roles played by linguistic codes in lexical memory, both types of contrast would seem to be important. Accordingly, a series of studies was designed that systematically varied the featural attributes of words presented on verbal memory tasks, contrasting poor and normal reader groups matched for age and grade as well as for reading ability.

Semantic Memory in Poor and Normal Readers

Free Recall of Concrete and Abstract Words.   In the first investigation in this series, (Vellutino and Scanlon 1985b) we varied degree of reliance on substantive (semantic) versus purely linguistic (phonological and syntactic) codes in memory encoding by constructing two lists of words, dichotomized as to degree of abstractness. This procedure was motivated by previous research conducted by Paivio and his associates (Paivio 1971; Paivio and Begg 1971a, 1971b) who have documented that abstract words are more difficult to remember than are concrete words, not only because they are less imbued with referential imagery, but also because they are linguistically more complex. For example, many abstract words derive meaning primarily from their functional relationship with other words appearing in connected text (e.g., functor words such as *if, but, because*, etc.), while others are derivatives from concrete words or other abstract words (e.g., *judge ⟶ justice ⟶ judicial*). Many also require an implicit knowledge of complex syntactic and phonological rules for comprehension and correct usage, as with derived words that acquire their meanings by virtue of morphological prefixing and suffixing (*judicial ⟶ prejudicial; judge ⟶ judgment*). Abstract words are therefore more diffuse and less easily discriminated than are concrete words and facility in encoding and retrieving them would seem to make greater demands on one's linguistic abilities than would encoding and retrieving concrete words.

Thus, if it is true that poor readers have limited facility in using linguistic codes to store and retrieve information, then they should perform significantly below normal readers on recall of abstract words, but should be closer to the normal readers on recall of concrete words.

This hypothesis was evaluated in two separate experiments, both using a standard free recall paradigm, with all stimuli being presented by ear. In the first experiment, concrete and abstract words were co-mingled on random presentations of the entire stimulus set (N = 20 items), while in the second experiment these stimuli were presented in homogeneous blocks counter-balanced for order of presentation. The major findings from these studies are presented in Figure 1.

It can be seen that the predicted interaction between word type and reader group emerged in second grade contrasts on both randomized (Panel A) and blocked (Panel B) presentations. That is, reader group discrepancies at the

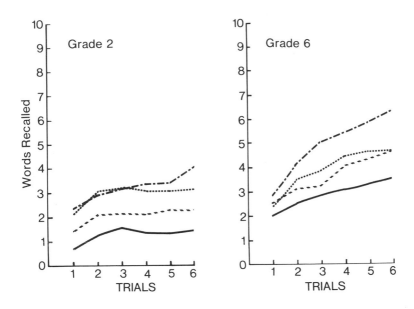

PANEL A : EXPERIMENT I
Random Presentations

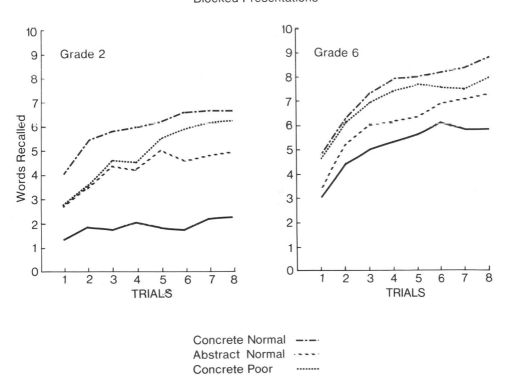

PANEL B : EXPERIMENT II
Blocked Presentations

Concrete Normal —·—·
Abstract Normal ·—·—·
Concrete Poor ··········
Abstract Poor ——————

Figure 1.   Mean number of concrete and abstract words recalled on each trial for poor and normal
readers in second and sixth grade.

second grade level were much greater on abstract than on concrete words. These results are consistent with our suggestion that poor readers would be especially encumbered by linguistic coding deficits in recall of abstract words and less so in recall of concrete words. However, a linguistic coding deficit could not be the sole explanation for reader group differences observed at the sixth grade level, because, at this level, the poor readers performed as far below the normal readers on the concrete words as they did on the abstract words. Thus, our data provide only partial support for the differential coding hypothesis tested in this experiment.

In keeping with our earlier suggestion that deficiencies in semantic coding could also impair performance on verbal processing tasks, we thought that a more plausible explanation of group differences at the sixth grade level might be that the older poor readers, in part because of long standing reading disorder, may have been impeded by acquired and cumulative deficiencies in semantic and lexical development. That is, a poorly elaborated and less well developed semantic network could result in comparatively poor performance on recall of a given word list, regardless of whether the words on that list happened to be high on either the concrete or abstract dimensions. In this connection, we also wondered whether deficiencies in semantic coding were the primary cause of reader group differences on the two word lists, the question being whether the sixth grade reader groups were less disparate than the second grade groups in their sensitivity to the structural properties of the stimulus words.

To evaluate these questions, we performed a qualitative analysis of the different types of intrusion errors made by each respective reader group, so as to gain insight into the types of coding strategies utilized by subjects in a given group. Accordingly, frequency counts were made of errors that were prompted either by the meaning or by the structural characteristics of given words. Intrusion errors such as "king" for "queen" or "thinking" for "thought" were taken as evidence that the subject was more attuned to the semantic than to the phonological and syntactic characteristics (respectively) of the stimulus words, while errors such as "fought" for "thought" or "though" for "thought" were taken as evidence that he/she was more attuned to their phonological and orthographic components.[2] We also recorded intrusion errors that were judged to be the result of the cross-referencing and synthesis of more than one featural attribute, for example, "soap," combining associates prompted by the stimulus words "bath" and "hope." These were called featural synthesis errors. The results of this analysis appear in Table I.

As is evident, second grade poor readers were inclined to make more meaning than structural errors, while second grade normal readers made both types of errors in approximately equal measure. The second grade poor readers also made fewer featural synthesis errors than did the second grade normal readers. In contrast to their second grade counterparts, the sixth grade poor

---

[2]Orthographic errors are those that we inferred were promoted by the visual features of given stimulus words rather than by its phonologic features. Ehri (1980) has shown that orthographic representations of spoken words may be activated and help to mediate recall even if the word is presented auditorily.

Table I

Proportions of Intrusion Errors Falling into Meaning, Structural and Featural Synthesis
Categories Following Randomized Presentations of Concrete and Abstract Words

		Meaning	Structural	Featural Synthesis	Unrateable
Grade 2 Poor	X̄	.49	.16	.15	.11
	(SD)	(.37)	(.29)	(.27)	(.22)
Grade 2 Normal	X̄	.33	.27	.29	.09
	(SD)	(.32)	(.28)	(.37)	(.20)
	Adjusted	.27	.30	.34	.07
Grade 6 Poor	X̄	.26	.34	.25	.09
	(SD)	(.32)	(.38)	(.33)	(.19)
Grade 6 Normal	X̄	.45	.26	.26	.02
	(SD)	(.46)	(.38)	(.37)	(.07)

Because one of the second grade normal readers made an unusual number of errors (N = 36),
the proportions were recalculated dropping this subject from the group. These appear in the row
labeled "adjusted" under the second grade normal data. It should be noted that given proportions
may not always sum to 1.00 both because of rounding error and because, in most instances, several
extraneous intrusions were made that were not tabled, for example, intrusions prompted by
directions given to the subjects.

readers made approximately as many structural as meaning errors and, in fact,
slightly more structural errors than the sixth grade normal readers. Indeed, the
sixth grade normals were considerably more inclined to make meaning than to
make structural errors. Moreover, the number of featural synthesis errors was
roughly equivalent in both groups. These results suggest that the second grade
poor readers were more attuned to the semantic than to the phonological,
syntactic and orthographic attributes of the word stimuli, while the second
grade normal readers were more evenly attuned to each of these attributes.
They, therefore, complement the quantitative analyses and are entirely consistent with our suggestion that the performance patterns observed at this level
are due largely to the differential use of meaning and structural (linguistic)
codes for lexical storage and retrieval. However, the results for sixth graders
suggest that the poor readers at this level were at least as sensitive to structural
codes as the normal readers and less sensitive than the normal readers to
meaning codes, thus favoring the semantic development interpretation of
reader group differences at the sixth grade level.

    In connection with these points, we would like to draw the reader's
attention to the striking similarities in the pattern of intrusion errors made by the
second grade normal and sixth grade poor readers, suggesting that subjects in
these two groups adopted similar encoding strategies. Yet, inspection of Figure
1 will indicate that the older poor readers performed better than the younger
normal readers on both lists and, in fact, these differences were found to be
statistically significant.[3] At the same time, these two groups were also found to
perform at comparable levels on the oral reading and pseudoword decoding

---

[3]Throughout this chapter, an alpha of .05 has been used as the level of significance.

tests that were administered during sample selection (data not shown). If one couples these findings with the pattern of results observed in contrasts of the age and grade matched groups, certain conclusions seem warranted.

First, one may have additional confidence in our suggestion that reader group differences that emerged on the lexical memory tasks at the sixth grade level were due more to group differences in semantic development than to group differences in linguistic coding. Second, it would also seem that a probable cause of observed differences between the second normal and sixth poor readers, on the lexical memory tasks, was group differences in semantic development and thus semantic encoding. Third, one might reasonably conclude from this pattern of results that facility in structural encoding is as important a determinant of skill in beginning reading as facility in semantic encoding, if not more important. That is, if second grade normal and sixth grade poor readers did have comparable ability in linguistic coding, as suggested in our qualitative analyses, and if the sixth grade poor readers were better developed lexically and semantically than the second grade normal readers, as suggested in performance differences between these groups on the lexical memory tasks, then it may be reasonably inferred from their comparable abilities in oral reading and pseudoword decoding that the ability to learn to read leans heavily on facility in linguistic coding ability.

Finally, the data provide us with a working hypothesis as to the nature of reader group differences at different developmental levels, specifically, that individual differences on reading and other lexical processing tasks will be determined as much or more by facility in the use of structural or purely linguistic codes as by facility in the use of meaning or semantic codes at the beginning stages of skills acquisition and somewhat more by facility in the use of meaning codes at later stages of acquisition. This hypothesis incorporates the twofold assumption that, owing to some degree of maturation and/or experience, older poor readers have more facility in linguistic coding than they had at earlier stages of development, but because of cumulative deficits fostered, in part, by long standing reading disorder, these children fall increasingly behind their age matched peers in lexical development and, perhaps, in language development in general. These possibilities were further evaluated in a second study we conducted contrasting poor and normal readers on lexical memory tasks (Vellutino, Scanlon, and Tanzman 1985).

Cued and Non-cued Recall. To add substance to the developmental hypothesis just articulated, we used a memory paradigm employed successfully in the study of memory processes in normal adults (Tulving and Pearlstone 1966) and normally developing children (Halperin 1974). This paradigm specifically evaluates one's ability to utilize taxonomic structure as an aid to recall under conditions that allow direct comparisons of encoding versus retrieval operations. These two processes have been traditionally evaluated by contrasting subjects on memory for a list of words in taxonomic categories under conditions of (a) cued presentation, where they are given category "names" during acquisition trials to alert them to the semantic similarities among the words on a stimulus list and (b) constrained retrieval, where they are given category names immediately before recall of items in each respective category, to control for a random search of memory. Performance under the constrained retrieval condition relies more heavily on degree of semantic development, since this condition places greater demands on one's ability to organize spontaneously a list containing semantically related words and the ability to do so implies that semantic categories are more widely represented, more highly elaborated and thus, more readily apprehended in subjects who are the better performers. On the other hand, performance under cued presentation conditions relies more heavily upon the availability and use of structural or purely linguistic codes, since this condition minimizes the effects of semantic organization ability, and retrieval therefore depends on one's ability to encode the linguistic attributes of both category cues and words on the list proper during acquisition trials.

Using a variant of the cueing paradigm employed by Halperin (1974), second and sixth grade reader groups were presented with four lists of taxonomically related words under four different conditions: (1) cued acquisition/non-cued retrieval (CN), (2) non-cued acquisition/cued retrieval (NC); (3) cued acquisition and cued retrieval (CC), and (4) non-cued acquisition and non-cued retrieval (NN). In the CN condition, subjects were given category words in homogeneous blocks on acquisition trials and each block was preceded by the name of the superordinate category associated with the words in that block. However, on retrieval trials, the words were recalled freely with no category cues. In the NC condition, subjects were given no category cues and random presentations on acquisition trials, but were given category cues and were required to recall items in blocks on retrieval trials. In the CC condition, subjects were given category cues on both acquisition and retrieval trials. The NN condition was a baseline condition wherein subjects were given random presentations of words from the entire list on acquisition trials and were required to recall these words freely on retrieval trials. Subjects were given five trials for each condition. In all instances, the NN (control) condition was presented first, followed by the experimental conditions in counterbalanced order across subjects. Testing sessions were given at four week intervals.

The four stimulus lists used in this study were taken from the category norms compiled by Battig and Montague (1969). Each list consisted of five exemplars from each of six conceptual categories, for a total of thirty words per list. All four lists were equated for category potency and frequency of items within categories.

In accord with the distinctions we made earlier, group differences favoring the normal readers under the CN condition would be consistent with linguistic coding difficulties in the poor readers, given that variability that might be occasioned by group differences in the ability to encode taxonomic similarity on acquisition trials is greatly reduced. Performance under this condition therefore leaned heavily on one's ability to encode the phonological[4] as well as

---

[4]Because the word lists consisted primarily of concrete nouns, it would seem that syntactic coding would have little relevance. Therefore, linguistic coding, in this study, is assumed to have been primarily phonological in nature.

the semantic attributes of both category cues and words subsumed under those categories. Conversely, group differences under the NC condition would imply semantic coding problems in the poor readers, insofar as variability that might be occasioned by a random search of memory on retrieval trials is eliminated by constrained recall. Thus, performance in this condition was determined largely by one's ability to detect taxonomic similarity in list words and organize these words for later recall. Differences between poor and normal readers under the CC condition provides the strongest indication of possible group differences in phonological encoding, given that the probability of encoding and retrieving semantic categories represented in the word list is maximized.

The NN or control condition, of course, provides a baseline against which to evaluate performance in the three experimental conditions, and is quite likely influenced both by one's implicit ability to detect semantic similarities in taxonomically related words as well as by one's ability to store, cross reference, and retrieve linguistic codes. To the extent that young children are less well developed semantically than are older children and therefore less inclined toward spontaneous organization of list words into semantic categories (Cole, Frankel and Sharp 1971; Halperin 1974; Moely, Olson, Halwes and Flavell 1969), it would seem likely that variability among second graders under the NN condition would depend more heavily upon the ability to encode the phonological attributes of the stimulus words than upon the ability to note similarities in word meanings, while the reverse should be true for sixth graders.

Figure 2 presents the trial means for total number of words recalled for reader group, grade level, and treatment conditions. As is evident, the normal readers at both grade levels generally performed better than the poor readers, under each of the experimental conditions. However, as anticipated, the treatments had differential effects on the two reader groups, depending on level of development. The largest reader group difference at the second grade level occurred in the double cuing (CC) condition and the smallest difference occurred in the noncued (NN) condition. Group differences in the cued presentation (CN) and cued retrieval (NC) conditions were intermediate to those observed in the CC and NN conditions and were of comparable magnitude. At the sixth grade level, the largest reader group differences occurred in the two conditions that presented subjects with no category cues during acquisition trials (NN and NC), while the smallest differences between reader groups were manifested in those conditions that presented subjects with category cues during acquisition trials (CN and CC).

These results are consistent with the developmental hypothesis we advanced earlier and suggest that reader group differences in semantic encoding were a more influential source of lexical memory differences that emerged at the sixth grade level than were group differences in phonological encoding, while reader group differences in phonological encoding contributed to lexical memory differences at the second grade level as much as or more than group differences in semantic encoding. That semantic encoding ability was a more influential source of reader group differences at the sixth grade level than was phonological encoding ability is suggested in the fact that the largest differ-

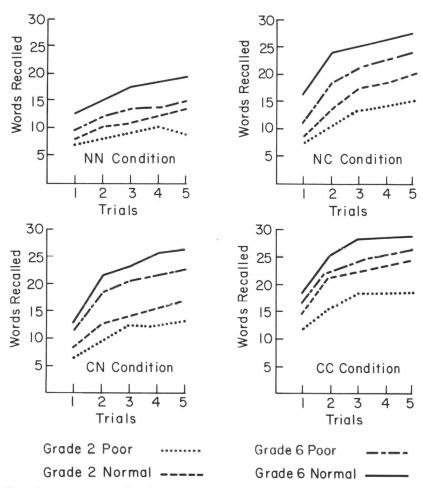

Figure 2.   Mean number of words recalled by poor and normal readers in second and sixth grade under four different cuing conditions.

ences between the poor and normal readers occurred under conditions (NN and NC) which made the greatest demands on one's ability to organize the word lists into semantic categories to aid recall, while the smallest difference occurred under the condition (CC) that minimized these demands. That phonological encoding ability was a more influential source of group differences at the second grade level than was semantic encoding ability is suggested in the fact that the largest differences between reader groups occurred under the condition (CC) which made the smallest demands on semantic organization ability, while the smallest difference between these groups occurred under the condition (NN) which maximized reliance on this ability. Indeed, since young children are not inclined to organize a list spontaneously into semantic categories, it is doubtful that group differences in semantic encoding ability accounted for the largest proportion of the variance under the NN condition. Thus, we infer that because of list complexity and list length, phonological encoding of the stimulus words was a more taxing enterprise for the second graders under the NN condition and group differences, although statistically significant, were not very large. However, under the CC condition, the additional structure imposed by the double cuing procedure increased efficiency in encoding the phonological attributes of the stimulus words, which therefore allowed the normal readers to increase their advantage.

Implied in the results presented thus far is the possibility that observed differences between poor and normal reader groups on the lexical memory tasks were determined by group differences in both linguistic coding and semantic organization ability, but in unequal proportions at the two grade levels. This possibility is further documented in another relevant finding. As we suggested earlier, it would seem that reader group differences under the NN condition would be determined more by the ability to encode the semantic attributes of the stimulus words than by the ability to encode their phonological attributes in the case of contrasts at the sixth grade level, while group differences at the second grade level should be determined primarily by the ability to encode their phonological attributes. If this is true, and if performance under the NN condition is used as a covariate, then any group differences that remain statistically significant after partialing out the effects of NN recall scores should primarily reflect differences in phonological coding ability on sixth grade contrasts and differences in semantic coding ability on second grade contrasts. In fact, we found that residual effects were evident only under the NC condition at the sixth grade level and only under the CC condition at the second grade level, consistent with our developmental hypothesis.

Finally, it is interesting to note that our second grade normal and sixth grade poor readers, who, by our sampling criteria, were matched for oral reading and pseudoword decoding ability (data not shown), were much closer together under the NN and CC conditions than they were under the NC and CN conditions. This pattern of results becomes coherent if we assume that the second grade normal readers, because of limited lexical and semantic development, were less proficient than the sixth grade poor readers in semantic coding ability while comparable to the sixth graders in phonological coding ability. Thus, the groups were more disparate under the NC and CN conditions, quite likely because the older subjects were more facile than the younger subjects in utilizing category cues to aid recall. However, this advantage was reduced under both the NN and CC conditions — under the former condition because of the absence of category cues, and under the latter condition because category cuing was maximized. And if it is true, as we suggest, that these two groups were in close approximation on phonological coding ability, then the fact that they were closer together under the NN and CC conditions would also be explained.

Selective Reminding vs. Free Recall.   One problem with memory tasks such as those employed in the studies just discussed is that they provide no adequate basis for distinguishing between list items that may have been in temporary or ''working'' memory at the time of retrieval and those that may have been in a more permanent or long term storage (Atkinson and Shiffrin

1968; Norman 1972). In both cases, any given item recalled may or may not have existed as a lexical unit in the permanent memory of the learner. Thus, a list item retrieved from working memory is presumed to have been in a short duration, limited capacity system and, by definition, had not yet been encoded or "tagged," in some way, as an item on the list being learned. Conversely, an item retrieved from long term storage, whether it had been a new item or one that had already existed in permanent memory, is presumed to have been in short term storage only long enough to be encoded as an item on that particular list. However, free and cued recall paradigms do not allow one to distinguish between items retrieved from short term memory and those retrieved from long term memory because, on each acquisition trial, subjects are always presented with *all* items on the list to be learned. This is an important distinction to make in the present context for there is considerable documentation that the ability to maintain linguistically codeable information in working memory depends, in large measure, upon one's ability to activate and maintain phonological codes (Baddeley and Hitch 1974; Conrad 1972; Kleiman 1975; Perfetti and McCutchen 1982), while the ability to store (or tag) and retrieve information in permanent memory depends, in addition, on the degree to which an item can be assimilated to existing knowledge embodied in the semantic network (Gardiner, Craik, and Birtwistle 1972, Halperin 1974; Tulving and Pearlstone 1966; Watkins and Watkins 1975).

Applying these distinctions to the present problem, it may be inferred, from the results discussed thus far, that limitations in processing information in short term storage would be a more important source of reader group differences on lexical memory tasks at younger than at older age levels, while limitations in processing information in long term storage would be a more important source of group differences at older age levels. To evaluate the validity of these inferences, we used a procedure devised by Buschke (1973, 1975) that, on any given trial, allows one to distinguish between items retrieved from short and long term memory, as well as between long term storage and long term retrieval (Vellutino and Scanlon 1985a). This procedure, termed "selective reminding," involves presentation of all words on a given list in random order on the first trial, but on any given trial after the first one, subjects are "reminded" of only those words that were not recalled on the trial immediately preceding that trial. *Short term retrieval* (STR) is defined as the total number of items recalled on a given trial that had not been recalled without reminding on any preceding trial and are not recalled spontaneously on the next trial. *Long term storage* (LTS) is defined as the total number of items recalled at least once without reminding. *Long term retrieval* (LTR) is defined as the total number of items stored in long term storage (LTS), that are actually recalled on a given trial.

It should be apparent that by presenting subjects with increasingly fewer list items across trials, the selective reminding procedure greatly reduces the load on short term memory, compared with the standard free recall paradigm, and therefore allows for more efficient processing of these items. As a result, items not yet identified as list items should be more readily tagged as such in long term storage, and most items recalled can be regarded as taken from long term rather than short term memory.

In the study using the selective reminding procedure, poor and normal readers in second and sixth grade were presented with both related and unrelated concrete words (nouns) in counterbalanced order. There were fifteen words on each list and most were of high or moderately high frequency (Battig and Montague 1969; Palermo and Jenkins 1964). A comparably selected sample of second and sixth grade poor and normal readers were presented with the same word lists using the standard free recall paradigm. It was expected, in accord with our developmental hypothesis, that the selective reminding task would greatly reduce or eliminate group differences in lexical retrieval at the second grade level, but less so at the sixth grade level. However, we anticipated that *within* reader groups at both grade levels, performance levels under the selective reminding condition would be substantially greater than performance levels under the free recall condition.

Figure 3 presents mean raw scores for total number recalled for the two studies employing these respective procedures. The first thing to note is that reader group differences under the selective reminding condition are negligible at the second grade level, but significant at the sixth grade level, as expected. However, also as expected, group differences at both grade levels are substantial under the free recall condition. Moreover, for reader groups at both grade levels, performance levels under the selective reminding condition are, generally, much higher than performance levels under the free recall conditon.

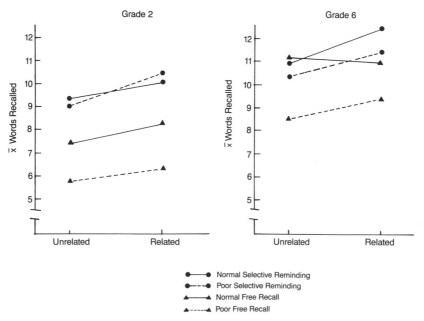

Figure 3.   Mean number of related and unrelated words recalled by poor and normal readers under selective reminding and free recall conditions.

The only exception occurs in the sixth grade normal readers, where memory for unrelated words was as good under the free recall condition as it was under the selective reminding condition. These results support our suggestion that limitations in short term memory processing contribute more to reader group differences at the second than at the sixth grade level, while limitations in long term memory processing contribute more to group differences at the sixth than at the second grade level. They also support our suggestion that these respective disparities emanate primarily from linguistic coding deficits in younger poor readers and semantic coding deficits in older poor readers. If the free recall procedure places greater demands on short term memory than does selective reminding, and if phonological coding ability is especially important for short term memory processing and semantic coding ability is especially important for long term memory processing, then the differential performance patterns yielded by these two conditions can be taken as evidence for both claims. Still more evidence comes from results on the short and long term memory measures yielded by the selective reminding procedure.

We should first point out that there were no significant reader group differences in number of items retrieved from short term memory, either at the second or at the sixth grade levels. However, performance patterns at the two grade levels are discordant on the long term memory measures. Figure 4 indicates that poor and normal readers at the second grade level do not differ substantially on either the long term storage or long term retrieval measures. In contrast, group differences on these measures are substantial at the sixth grade level. However, it should be noted that, at this grade level, the ratio of the number of items retrieved from long term memory to the number of items stored in long term memory is the same for both reader groups (proportions not shown). This would imply that the poor readers were impaired in storing

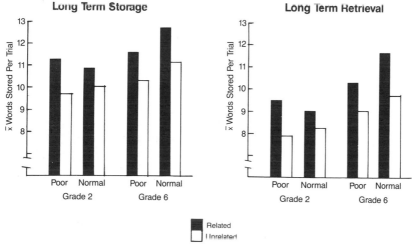

Figure 4.   Mean number of related and unrelated words stored in and retrieved from long term memory by poor and normal readers in second and sixth grade.

information in long term memory and, perhaps, unimpaired in retrieving information from long term memory. These findings add weight to our position, insofar as they are consistent with our suggestion that reader group differences at the second grade level are determined primarily by group differences in phonological coding ability, while group differences at the sixth grade level are determined primarily by group differences in semantic coding ability.

It is interesting to note that under both the free recall and selective reminding conditions, the sixth grade poor readers performed better than the second grade normal readers, as indicated on the measures of total recall, long term storage and long term retrieval. In contrast, these groups did not differ on the measure of short term retrieval, suggesting that they were comparable in short term memory processing. These findings are similar to results reported in the two lexical memory studies discussed in the foregoing sections, and provide still more support for our suggestion that the second grade normal and sixth grade poor readers are comparable in linguistic coding ability, but more disparate with respect to semantic coding ability and semantic development in general. Here it should be pointed out that, in the present studies, as in those discussed previously, second grade normal and sixth grade poor readers were matched for oral reading and pseudoword decoding ability. When coupled with the strong suggestion, in the results thus far discussed, that these two groups are comparable in their sensitivity to and functional use of structural or purely linguistic codes, then it may be tentatively suggested that achievement in the beginning and intermediate stages of reading is determined in large measure by linguistic coding ability. In the next section, we report results that provide more direct support for this possibility.

Linguistic Coding in Poor and Normal Readers

Phonological Coding, Phonemic Awareness, and Code Acquisition. In the study described in this section, we specifically evaluated Liberman and Shankweiler's (1979) suggestion that reading disability results from the failure to become consciously aware that spoken words are composed of phoneme size units (Vellutino and Scanlon, 1984). As pointed out in a previous section, this notion emanates from a more general theory of reading disability, which suggests that poor readers are basically impaired in using phonological codes in memory processing and that such impairment should be apparent not only on reading tasks such as word identification and reading comprehension, but on all tasks requiring the use of language to store and retrieve information. However, while a few studies have provided direct support for a causal relationship between phonemic segmentation and word identification ability, that is, by demonstrating that training in phonemic segmentation can significantly improve reading ability (e.g., Bradley and Bryant 1983; Treiman and Baron 1983), they did not provide independent evidence that inadequate ability to segment spoken and printed words phonemically is an outgrowth of basic deficits in phonological coding.

In an attempt to demonstrate a causal connection between phonological coding and word identification ability, poor and normal readers in second and sixth grade were compared on code acquisition tasks that simulated printed word identification, after they had received alternative treatments designed to facilitate learning. The study was rather complex and involved three different phases. In the first phase, all subjects were given a test of phonemic segmentation ability to evaluate the reliability of previous findings, which had suggested that poor readers are deficient in phoneme analysis (Liberman and Shankweiler 1979). The second phase was the experiment proper and consisted of five different treatments to which subjects in each group were randomly assigned: three experimental conditions and two control conditions.

In one condition—*phonemic segmentation training* (PST)—subjects received five or six consecutive days of training (one-half hour per day) in structural analysis, which consisted of a number of exercises designed to facilitate eduction of phoneme level units using both words and pseudowords presented auditorily and visually. These exercises included counting and vocalizing phonemes as well as locating their positions in given words. Following such practice, subjects were given extensive practice in grapheme-phoneme conversion. This entailed structural analysis of four phonetically redundant pseudowords composed of novel alphabetic characters and nonsense syllables (see Figure 5, Panel A) containing phonemes that corresponded invariantly with each of the characters. Subjects were then presented with permuted versions of these stimuli and attempted to learn the new responses.

After no more than a two day hiatus, each subject was given the code acquisition task, which consisted of two subtests: initial training and transfer learning. On the initial training subtest, subjects were given a new set of pseudowords, composed of a different set of novel alphabetic characters that were again in one-to-one correspondence with the phonemes in four new nonsense syllables (see Figure 5, Panel B). During this phase, subjects were given a maximum of twenty acquisition/test paired associates trials, which required that they produce whole word responses. Our purpose in using stimuli different from those used during segmentation training was to evaluate the degree to which subjects who had received such training could adopt an "analytic attitude" that would allow them to abstract and generalize graphemes-phoneme units. Because they were always required to give whole word responses, they had to detect these units implicitly.

The transfer subtest was administered on the following day. During this phase of code acquisition, subjects were presented with four "new" pseudowords, constructed by reversing the order of the characters in the training set (Figure 5, Panel B), and each was administered twenty more paired associates trials using the same presentation format used on initial training.

In a second condition—*verbal response acquisition* (RA)—subjects received no instruction in phonemic segmentation, but were given extensive practice in remembering the verbal responses subsequently used on the training subtest of code acquisition. Thus, on the first day of testing, each was given

A. <u>Stimuli Used on the Coding Portion of the Phonemic Segmentation Training Program</u>

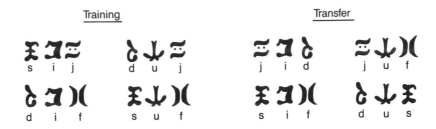

B. <u>Stimuli Used on the Training and Transfer Subtests of Code Acquisition</u>

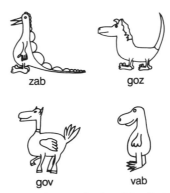

C. <u>Stimuli Used in the Picture-Syllable Portion of the Response Acquisition Treatment</u>

zab   goz

gov   vab

Figure 5.   Stimuli employed in the experiment evaluating of the effects of phonemic segmentation and response acquisition training on code acquisition. Adapted from Vellutino and Scanlon, 1986.

twenty free recall trials and after a five minute break, each was administered an association learning task in which the same nonsense syllables presented on the free recall task were paired with cartoon-like animal pictures for another fifteen trials (see Figure 5, Panel C). The acquisition/test format was used for both subtests. The free recall test served as our operational definition of phonological coding ability, inasmuch as it required the encoding and retrieval of phonetically redundant strings devoid of uniform meanings. The picture-syllable task simulated object naming and thus provided an independent measure of visual-verbal association learning. The code acquisition phase of the experiment was initiated on the following day, using the same materials and presentation procedure used on the code acquisition tasks administered to subjects in the PST condition. The RA condition was designed to familiarize subjects with the verbal responses used in code acquisition and to confer meaning on those responses. It also allowed us to evaluate the effects of verbal response learning on code acquisition.

The third and final experimental condition was the *phonemic segmentation and response acquisition combined* condition (PSTRA). In this condition subjects were presented with segmentation training followed by response training, combining those materials and treatments used in the PST and RA conditions respectively. The PSTRA allowed us to compare the effects of both segmentation training and response training on the code acquisition subtests. It also allowed us to compare the effects of segmentation training on free recall of nonsense syllables. The fourth and fifth conditions were control conditions. One (Control 1) involved administration of both the training and transfer subtests of code acquisition and the other (Control 2) involved only the transfer subtest.

In the third and final phase of the experiment, subjects were administered an alternate form of the phonemic segmentation test given prior to the experiment proper to further evaluate treatment effects.

Several important findings emerged from this study. First, at each grade level, poor readers performed significantly below the normal readers on both the pre- and post-experimental tests of phonemic segmentation ability (see Table II). This, of course, replicates previous results, but also documents the fact that subjects in our sample were significantly impaired in phoneme analysis. Secondly, poor readers at both grade levels performed significantly below the level of normal readers on the free recall (Figure 6) as well as on the picture-syllable subtests (Figure 7) of response acquisition. The finding of reader group differences on the free recall test is important because it indicates that poor readers are less proficient than normal readers in storing and retrieving phonological descriptions of auditorily presented syllables from which it may be inferred that they are generally less proficient in phonological coding. It is also important because it answers the question we raised earlier (see Background Research section), of whether or not previously observed differences between poor and normal readers on visual-verbal learning tasks (Vellutino, Steger, Harding, and Phillips 1975) are due to impairment, in poor readers, in the ability to integrate visual and verbal representations or to impairment in verbal response learning. Since the poor readers performed below the normal readers on the free recall as well as on the picture-syllable subtests, it seems reasonable to infer that their difficulties on word identification and other visual-verbal learning tasks were due to dysfunction in remembering the verbal

Table II
Means and Standard Deviations for Percentage Correct on Pre- and Post-Treatment Measures of Phonemic Segmentation Ability

		Grade 2 Poor		Grade 2 Normal		Grade 6 Poor		Grade 6 Normal	
		Pre	Post	Pre	Post	Pre	Post	Pre	Post
PSTRA	$\overline{X}$	43.46	53.21	63.21	76.05	57.78	75.55	76.05	88.27
	SD	(10.98)	(10.64)	(14.31)	(15.26)	(18.00)	(11.23)	(14.22)	(6.05)
PST	$\overline{X}$	46.05	54.81	57.65	69.75	62.35	76.79	70.99	85.55
	SD	(6.71)	(10.54)	(18.77)	(18.72)	(14.66)	(11.69)	(15.96)	(8.32)
RA	$\overline{X}$	45.31	45.43	57.41	60.00	60.25	61.23	75.43	80.74
	SD	(8.28)	(9.72)	(15.53)	(13.03)	(11.48)	(16.38)	(12.59)	(16.00)
C-1	$\overline{X}$	41.98	44.81	56.54	64.32	59.26	65.80	75.55	86.19
	SD	(7.69)	(6.31)	(15.82)	(13.74)	(14.24)	(12.40)	(15.27)	(10.28)
C-2	$\overline{X}$	45.19	51.73	54.32	63.58	59.51	63.58	73.21	78.27
	SD	(11.26)	(12.07)	(12.80)	(13.58)	(11.88)	(13.35)	(12.02)	(12.93)

Reprinted from Vellutino and Scanlon, 1986 by permission of Heinemann Educational Books, Inc.

RESPONSE ACQUISITION
FREE RECALL

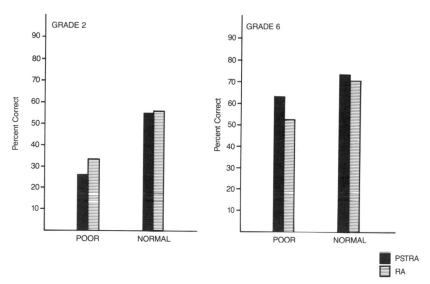

Figure 6.   Mean proportion of correct responses on the task requiring free recall of nonsense syllables. Adapted from Vellutino and Scanlon, 1984.

RESPONSE ACQUISITION
PICTURE SYLLABLE ASSOCIATION

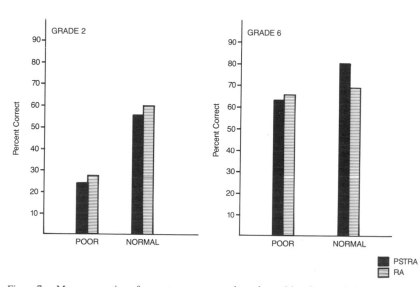

Figure 7.   Mean proportion of correct responses on the task requiring the association of nonsense syllables with novel animal characters. Adapted from Vellutino and Scanlon, 1984.

response counterparts of visual-verbal associates rather than to dysfunction in visual-verbal integration. This interpretation is further reinforced by the fact that at both grade levels and within both reader groups, performance on the free recall test was significantly correlated with performance on both the picture-syllable test and the code acquisition subtests (data not shown).

The third finding of note is that in all treatment groups, poor readers at each grade level performed below the level of normal readers on both the training and transfer subtests of code acquisition (Figures 8 and 9). This finding is consistent with previous results obtained in our laboratory (Vellutino, Harding, Phillips, and Steger 1975) and, when coupled with the observation of reader group differences on the free recall and phonemic segmentation tests, it suggests that group differences on code acquisition tasks and (printed) word identification tasks in general, are causally related to difficulties encountered by poor readers in phonological coding and phonemic segmentation. This possibility is more directly supported by the fact that subjects who received either phonemic segmentation training (PST) or verbal response training (RA) performed better than control group (C-1) subjects on the training subtests of code acquisition. Moreover, with the exception of the second grade poor readers, the groups that received both segmentation and response training (PSTRA) performed substantially better than those that received only one or the other of these treatments, suggesting that the ability to analyze the internal structures of printed words and the ability to remember their verbal response counterparts are both important determinants of successful learning in the initial stages of code acquisition.

However, results on the transfer subtest of code acquisition make it clear that skill in verbal response learning does not, by itself, guarantee successful generalization learning. Figure 9 indicates that subjects in the groups that received segmentation training (PST and PSTRA) performed considerably better than those that did not receive segmentation training. In addition, those who received only segmentation training (PST) performed about as well as those who received both segmentation and response training (PSTRA). In contrast, subjects who received only response training (RA) did not perform much better than control group subjects on the transfer subtest, and generally performed below the level they had achieved on the training subtest.

These findings suggest that phoneme analysis is especially important for success in learning to generalize the grapheme-phoneme units embedded in printed words. They also suggest that those who do not adopt an analytic attitude in learning to identify printed words will be relatively insensitive to grapheme-phoneme invariance and will therefore be vulnerable to such miseries as generalization error and proactive interference from words previously encountered. A particularly compelling illustration of this possibility is provided in another finding yielded by group contrasts on the transfer task. Some researchers have suggested that reversal errors—so often observed in poor readers (e.g., was/saw—are the result of spatial and directional confusion in these children [Orton 1925; Hermann 1959]). We have long maintained that such errors are secondary manifestations of the failure to make the fine-grained

CODE ACQUISITION
TRAINING

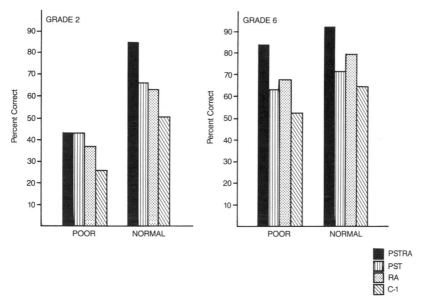

Figure 8. Mean proportion of correct responses for code acquisition training for second and sixth grade poor and normal readers. Adapted from Vellutino and Scanlon, 1984.

CODE ACQUISITION
TRANSFER

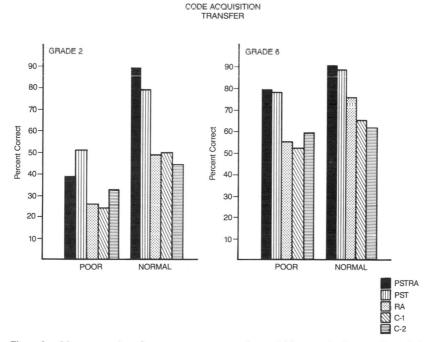

Figure 9. Mean proportion of correct responses on code acquisition transfer for second and sixth grade poor and normal readers. Adapted from Vellutino and Scanlon, 1984.

discriminations that accompany successful acquisition of grapheme-phoneme correspondence rules. In other words, reversal errors are the result of dysfunction in verbal mediation rather than dysfunction in visual processing. Since the paired associates used on the transfer task were reversed derivatives of those used on the training task (see Figure 5, Panel B), we had a good opportunity to test this hypothesis and the results are supportive. As can be seen in Figure 10, poor readers in general made no more reversal errors than did normal readers. More important is the fact that, in both groups, reversal errors were at a minimum in subjects exposed to segmentation training. In contrast, they were plentiful in those who did not receive this training, poor and normal readers alike. To our knowledge, these results constitute the only *direct* evidence available that reversal errors accrue because of the failure to adopt an analytic attitude in word identification, and not because of perceptual deficiencies.

Finally, results on the post-experimental segmentation test (see Table II) indicate that phonemic segmentation training generally improved performance in segmentation analysis in both poor and normal readers, whereas response training had no such effect.

Of the results reviewed thus far, those yielded by the present study provide perhaps the most compelling and most direct support for the view that linguistic coding deficits are causally related to reading disability and, in particular, implicate phonological coding deficits as a major cause of both word identification and verbal memory problems in disabled readers. The data also add substance to the developmental hypothesis of interest here. If one examines the age-matched reader group means on the various experimental measures reported, it will become evident that on all contrasts, with no exceptions, the magnitude of group mean differences are considerably less at the sixth grade level than at the second grade level. Given that these measures more directly evaluated skill in phonological processing, it seems reasonable to infer that older poor readers are not as seriously impaired as younger poor readers in their ability to use phonological codes to store and retrieve information and are perhaps closer to normal readers of the same age and grade, in this ability, than they were at an earlier point in their development. And in this connection, we would also like to draw the reader's attention to the striking similarity, on all measures, between the second grade normal readers and the sixth grade poor readers, who, it will be recalled, were matched for oral reading ability. In light of the fact that these groups were also found to be comparable on the test of pseudoword decoding ability, which was administered after they were chosen for inclusion in the study (data not shown), this degree of concordance is impressive. The combined results provide still more support for our suggestion that the child's level of phonological coding ability is a major determinant of reading ability at an early point in skills development and may well set upper limits on the acquisition of various reading subskills.

However, although we have assumed that linguistic coding ability, as a construct, has reference to the use of syntactic as well as phonological codes in storing and retrieving spoken and written words, the fact remains that we have produced only indirect evidence that poor and normal readers differ in syntactic

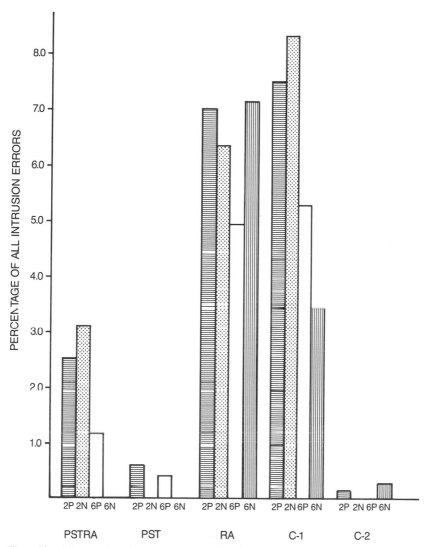

Figure 10.   Mean number of reversal errors made under each condition on the transfer subtest of
code acquisition by poor and normal readers in second and sixth grade. Adapted from
Vellutino and Scanlon, 1984.

coding ability. In the final study we wish to discuss, we report more direct
evidence for reader group differences in syntactic coding.

Sensitivity to Syntactic, Phonological, and Semantic Codes.   Vellutino,
Scanlon, and Greenberg (1985) evaluated the degree to which poor and normal
readers are sensitive to structural and meaning codes using a continuous
recognition procedure similar to that used by Byrne and Shea (1979). This
procedure gives subjects repeated presentations of antecedent words, as well as
distractor words that are similar to the antecedents, on a critical featural
dimension. These stimuli are intermingled with control words that are matched

with the distractors on all but the critical featural dimension(s). Antecedents are each presented twice and are followed by single presentations of the distractors and their associated controls. By varying the degree to which distractor words have particular features in common with antecedent words and by making note of the types of recognition errors made by given subjects, the experimenter is able to evaluate individual differences in sensitivity to particular word features. Saying "old" to words not encountered before (false positives) or saying "new" to words that had been encountered (false negatives) are the two general types of errors that are possible on this task.

Subjects were exposed to three experimental conditions in counter-balanced order, but the results of only two of those conditions are reported here. In one (Condition 1), subjects were presented with three kinds of distractor words; those that were *phonologically* (P) similar to antecedents (e.g. *train* vs. *cane*), those that were *semantically* (S) similar to antecedents (*train* vs. *car*), and those that were both phonologically and semantically (PS) similar to antecedents (*train* vs. *plane*). A second condition (Condition 2) was specifically designed to evaluate reader group differences in sensitivity to inflectional morphemes, and antecedent words, therefore, consisted of root and bound morphemes (e.g., *boy* + *s* = *boys*). Accordingly, phonologically (P) similar distractors rhymed with antecedents, but were not composed of root and bound morphemes (*boys* vs. *noise*). Syntactically (S) similar distractors were composed of root morphemes that were semantically and phonologically different from the root morphemes contained in antecedent words, and bound morphemes that were identical to those contained in the antecedents (*boys* vs. *dogs*). Phonologically and syntactically (PS) similar distractors consisted of root and bound morphemes that were phonologically and syntactically similar to antecedents (*boy* + *s* vs. *joy* + *s*). Subjects were second and sixth grade poor and normal readers, selected in accord with the sampling criteria used in earlier studies.

Table III presents the reader-group means for (total) recognition accuracy scores for each of the experimental conditions. It is apparent that, at both grade levels, the recognition accuracy scores of normal readers are substantially above those of poor readers, indicating that short term memory encoding was considerably better in the normal than in the poor readers. These results add substance to our suggestion that poor readers at both grade levels are deficient in linguistic coding ability, that is, assuming that verbatim memory for items stored in short term memory relies heavily upon structural coding, and especially upon phonological coding, as suggested earlier. Noteworthy in this connection is the fact that the size of age-matched reader group differences is larger at the second than at the sixth grade level under both conditions, consistent with our developmental hypothesis. Note also that the second grade normal and sixth grade poor readers—our reading ability matched groups—are closer together in recognition accuracy than our age matched groups.

Turning now to the false recognition data, Figure 11 presents difference means for false positive errors (distractor minus control words) for the par-

Table III

Mean Number of Total Recognition Errors for Each Condition in the Study of
Reader Group Differences in Encoding Various Word Features*

	Condition 1	Condition 2
Grade 2 Poor	32.95	36.05
Grade 2 Normal	17.29	18.19
Grade 6 Poor	22.33	23.29
Grade 6 Normal	13.95	14.45

*Total possible correct = 150

ticular types of distractors used in each condition. The graph for second grade
contrasts (Condition 1) makes it clear that the normal readers were disrupted
more by the rhyming words than were the poor readers, as manifested in
significantly greater difference means in the normal than in the poor readers, for
P and PS distractors. In contrast, the difference means for the semantic

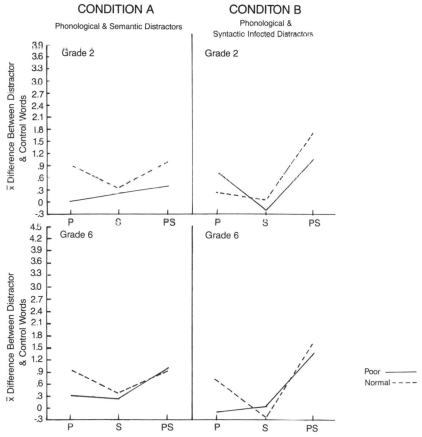

Figure 11. Mean differences between false positive errors on distractors versus control words
under two conditions of featural overlap between distractors and antecedents.

distractors were in close accord in the two groups. At the same time, there was no significant main effect for type of distractor and no significant interactions, indicating that while the normal readers were more sensitive to a word's phonological attributes than were the poor readers, *within* reader groups, subjects were about equally attuned to phonological and semantic attributes. This represents a slight deviation from Byrne and Shea's (1979) findings, insofar as their subjects produced more false positives to semantic distractors than did our subjects. However, Byrne and Shea used distractors that were highly associated with antecedents (i.e., synonyms and antonyms), while our words were only moderately associated with the antecedents. Nevertheless, the results are generally consistent with their findings and add weight to the idea that young poor readers are less sensitive to the phonological attributes of spoken words than are their normal reading peers.

Results at the sixth grade level are somewhat different. The normal readers appeared to be more inclined than the poor readers to make false positive errors on phonologically similar distractors, but this difference was not significant. Moreover, the two groups were in close accord on the proportion of false positive errors made on the semantic and phonologic/semantic distractors. In contrast, the main effect for type of distractor was highly significant ($p < .01$) indicating that phonological distractors prompted many more false positive errors than did the semantic distractors. These results are consistent with those of Olson (this volume), who reports that older poor readers are more sensitive to phonological attributes than are young poor readers and are comparable to normals in such sensitivity (see also Olson, Davidson, Kliegl, and Davies 1984; Siegel and Linder 1984). When combined with the results for second grade contrasts, they provide strong support for both our linguistic coding and our developmental hypotheses.

Still more support for these hypotheses are provided by the false recognition data yielded by Condition 2, which more directly measured differential sensitivity to the structural (phonological and syntactic) attributes of spoken words. The first finding of note (Figure 11) is the striking similarity in the reader group difference means for the identically inflected but different root morpheme type distractors, indicating that subjects in all groups made very few false positive errors on these stimuli. Thus, it is clear that when words differ in meaning and overall sound structure, inflectional similarities are not salient features of those words and therefore do not become a source of confusion.

The second finding of note is that overall differences between reader groups at both grade levels were not large and, in fact, the group main effect was not statistically significant at either grade level. On the other hand, the main effect for distractor type was significant at both grade levels and it is clear from the graphs that poor and normal readers were differentially responsive to the phonologically (P) similar versus the phonologically and syntactically similar distractors (PS). At the second grade level the relative number of false positive errors on P distractors is negligible in normal readers and is even somewhat lower than that made by the poor readers. In contrast, the relative number of false positives made by the normal readers on the PS distractors was significantly greater than that made on the P distractors, while in the poor readers, the difference between these two types of distractors was not statistically significant. At the sixth grade level, the difference between P and PS distractors was statistically significant in the poor as well as in the normal readers, but in this instance, the relative difference between P type distractors and control words is somewhat greater in the normal readers.

It should also be noted that for all subjects except the second grade poor readers, the relative number of false positive errors on the P type distractors is less under Condition 2 than under Condition 1, which is interesting since the P distractors in both conditions were rhyming words. How then do we account for these different response patterns? Our surmise here is that in all groups, save for the second grade poor readers, subjects were encoding the syntactic differences between antecedent words and P type distractors in Condition 2, as well as the syntactic similarities between antecedents and PS distractors in this condition. In other words, we suggest that except for the second grade poor readers, subjects were inclined to encode root and bound morphemes (e.g., boy + s) separately, giving semi-autonomous status to the two structures. Such a strategy would account for observed differences between false positive errors on the P and PS distractors. It would also account for the fact that all but the second grade poor readers tended to make fewer false positives on P type distractors under Condition 2 than on P distractors under Condition 1. This difference is especially striking in second grade normal readers who demonstrated a comparatively strong tendency toward false positives on P distractors under Condition 1.

It is interesting to note that the second grade poor readers were inclined to make more false positive errors on rhyming distractors under Condition 2 than on rhyming distractors under Condition 1. This finding may be an indication that poor readers are more sensitive to the phonological similarities of distractor words on a continuous recognition task, when distractors that are similar in meaning are excluded from the task. Moreover, it lends credence to a suggestion made by Byrne and Shea (1979), which is that poor readers are primarily attuned to word meanings as a preferred processing strategy and become attuned to their structural characteristics only when there is utility in doing so. This may well be the case, but it is also possible that attention to meaning as a preferred strategy is, itself, a consequence of deficits in linguistic coding that may be rather basic. These two possibilities are not mutually exclusive and it remains for future research to determine the pre-eminence of one or the other.

Finally, to provide additional support for the developmental hypothesis we have advanced, we draw the reader's attention to the overall similarity between the second grade normal and sixth grade poor readers in the number and type of false positive errors they manifested under the two experimental conditions used in this study (Figure 11). This pattern of results accords quite well with the fact that these groups were also comparable on the total number of recognition errors they made (Table III) and the combined results add more substance to the suggestion that subjects, who are at roughly the same level of ability in word identification are also similar in the ways in which they encode linguistic stimuli.

Summary and Conclusions

In this chapter we addressed the question of whether the difficulties encountered by poor readers in learning to identify printed words are due primarily to limitations in verbal memory associated with verbal coding deficits. To evaluate this question, we conducted a series of studies comparing second and sixth grade poor and normal readers on verbal memory tasks that were differentially reliant on one's ability to encode particular attributes of given words. A basic premise at the outset was that poor readers have more difficulty in using the phonological and syntactic (purely linguistic) attributes of spoken words, to store and retrieve those words, than in using their meaning or semantic attributes to do so.

Our studies provide strong documentation for the idea that poor readers are less proficient than normal readers in word storage and retrieval and the results constitute direct as well as indirect evidence that such ineptitude may be causally related to the problems they encounter in learning to identify printed words. However, as regards our suggestion that poor readers should be less facile in using structural than in using meaning codes to help remember spoken words, our results are not as straightforward. The data provide confirmatory support for this hypothesis in the case of poor readers in the second grade, but serve to qualify the hypothesis for poor readers in the sixth grade. While poor readers in second grade had significant difficulty in encoding the structural properties of spoken words and especially their phonological properties, sixth grade poor readers were less impaired in encoding word structures than were their second grade counterparts. Moreover, there was a good deal less disparity in structural encoding between poor and normal readers at the sixth grade level than between poor and normal readers at the second grade level. And whereas reader group differences in second grade were greater on verbal learning and verbal memory tasks that relied more heavily on the encoding of word structures than on the encoding of word meanings, reader group differences in sixth grade were greater on verbal learning and verbal memory tasks that relied more heavily on the encoding of word meanings than on the encoding of word structures.

Combining these results with those obtained elsewhere (Olson this volume; Olson et al. 1984; Siegel and Linder 1984), it seems reasonable to hypothesize that difficulties in learning to read, as measured by deficiencies in word identification, may be caused primarily by limitations in coding the structural or purely linguistic attributes of spoken and printed words. By this hypothesis, linguistic coding problems, in severely impaired readers such as those we have been studying, contribute to dysfunction in storing and retrieving the verbal response counterparts of printed words as wholes as well as to dysfunction in analyzing their phonemic structures, and, thus, to problems in learning to decode them phonetically. From all indications, such children more closely approximate normal readers in lexical and semantic development and are therefore closer to the normals in using semantic codes to store and retrieve information, although they are not equally effective in doing so.

However, because of the cumulative deficits that inevitably accrue as a result of long standing reading disorder, they fall increasingly below normal readers in semantic development and their ability to code information semantically decreases accordingly. But because of some degree of maturation and/or because of increased experience with spoken and written language (Ehri 1980), many poor readers become increasingly adept at coding the structural components of language. They should consequently be closer to age matched normals and equivalent to reading ability matched (younger) normals in structural coding, as may be manifested in performance on verbal learning and verbal memory tasks that do not rely heavily on semantic coding ability, for example, phoneme analysis, pseudoword decoding, and memory for nonsense words. They should, however, be a good deal less proficient than age matched normal readers, while somewhat more proficient than (younger) reading ability matched normals on tasks that rely heavily on semantic development and semantic coding ability, for example, lexical memory tasks as well as reading and listening comprehension.

Finally, the present hypothesis allows for different causes of word identification problems in developing readers and can accommodate both constitutional and environmental origins of these problems. It, therefore, allows for the possibility of etiological subtypes. That is, it is conceivable that some poor readers have difficulties in learning to identify printed words because of specific deficits that impair either whole word identification or phonetic decoding but not both. Thus, some of these children may be impaired in whole word identification either because of deficiencies in phonological processing that lead to dysfunction in name code retrieval (Denckla and Rudel 1976a, 1976b; Wolf 1982) or because of limited experience that leads to deficient lexical and semantic development and, thus, to difficulties in using a meaning based approach to word identification. At the same time, such children may have adequate ability to learn to map alphabetic symbols to sound and may therefore rely heavily on the latter approach to word identification.

However, because of environmental influences that limit metalinguistic analysis, other children may have difficulty in learning to identify words phonetically, but may have reasonably good lexical and semantic development and perfectly normal ability to store and retrieve name codes. Such children would no doubt rely heavily on a meaning based or holistic approach to word identification. Yet, our data suggest that exclusive reliance on one or the other of these approaches would lead to significant difficulties in word identification and reading in general. The severely impaired readers we have been studying appear to have difficulty in using both strategies for identification and there is reason to believe that they are impaired in all language domains, though to a greater or lesser degree depending on their age and experience. Thus, our etiological and developmental hypotheses are best applied to these children.

References

Atkinson, R. C., and Shiffrin, R. M. 1968. Human memory: A proposed system and its control processes. *In* K. W. Spence and J. T. Spence (eds.). *The Psychology of Learning and Motivation Advances in Research and Theory, Vol. 11.* New York: Academic Press.

Baddeley, A. D., and Hitch, G. 1974. Working memory. *In* G. H. Bower (ed.). *The Psychology of Learning and Motivation, Vol. 8.* New York: Academic Press.

Battig, W. F., and Montague, W. E. 1969. Category norms for verbal items in 56 categories. *Journal of Experimental Psychology Monograph* 80:1–46.

Birch, H. G. 1962. Dyslexia and maturation of visual function. *In* J. Money (ed.). *Reading Disability: Progress and Research Needs in Dyslexics.* Baltimore: Johns Hopkins Press.

Birch, H. G., and Belmont, L. 1964. Auditory-visual integration in normal and retarded readers. *American Journal of Orthopsychiatry* 34:852–861.

Blank, M., and Bridger, W. H. 1966. Deficiencies in verbal labeling in retarded readers. *American Journal of Orthopsychiatry* 36:840–847.

Blank, M., Weider, S., and Bridger, W. 1968. Verbal deficiencies in abstract thinking in early reading retardation. *American Journal of Orthopsychiatry* 38:823–834.

Bradley, L., and Bryant, P. E. 1983. Categorizing sounds and learning to read—A causal connection. *Nature* 303:419–421.

Brewer, W. F. 1967. Paired-associate learning of dyslexic children. Unpublished doctoral dissertation, University of Iowa.

Buschke, H. 1973. Selective reminding for analysis of memory and learning. *Journal of Verbal Learning and Verbal Behavior* 12:543–550.

Buschke, H. 1975. Short-term retention, learning, and retrieval from long-term memory. *In* D. Deutsch and J. Deutsch (eds.). *Short-term Memory.* New York: Academic Press.

Byrne, B., and Shea, P. 1979. Semantic and phonetic memory codes in beginning readers. *Memory and Cognition* 7:333–338.

Chomsky, N., and Halle, M. 1968. *The Sound Pattern of English.* New York: Harper and Row.

Cole, M., Frankel, F., and Sharp, D. 1971. Development of free recall learning in children. *Developmental Psychology* 4:109–123.

Conrad, R. 1972. Speech and reading. *In* J. F. Kavanagh and J. G. Mattingly (eds.). *Language by Ear and by Eye: The Relationship between Speech and Reading.* Cambridge, MA: MIT Press.

Denckla, M. B., and Rudel, R. 1976a. Naming of pictured objects by dyslexic and other learning disabled children. *Brain and Language* 39:1–15.

Denckla, M. B., and Rudel, R. 1976b. Rapid 'automatized' naming (R.A.N.): Dyslexia differentiated from other learning disabilities. *Neuropsychologia* 14:471–479.

Ehri, L. 1980. The role of orthographic images in learning printed words. *In* J. F. Kavanagh and R. L. Venezky (eds.). *Orthography, Reading and Dyslexia.* Baltimore: University Park Press.

Gardiner, J. M., Craik, F. I., and Birtwistle, J. 1972. Retrieval cues and release from proactive inhibition. *Journal of Verbal Learning and Verbal Behavior* 11:778–783.

Gascon, G., and Goodglass, H. 1970. Reading retardation and the information content of stimuli in paired associate learning. *Crotex* 6:417–429.

Gazzaniga, M. S., Bogen, J. E., and Sperry, R. W. 1965. Observations on visual perception after disconnection of the cerebral hemisphere in man. *Brain* 88:221–236.

Halperin, M. S. 1974. Developmental changes in the recall and recognition of categorized word lists. *Child Development* 45:144–151.

Hermann, K. 1959. *Reading disability.* Copenhagen: Munksgaard.

Kleiman, G. M. 1975. Speech recoding in reading. *Journal of Verbal Learning and Verbal Behavior* 14:323–340.

Liberman, I. Y., and Shankweiler, D. 1979. Speech, the alphabet and teaching to read. *In* L. Resnick and P. Weaver (eds.). *Theory and Practice of Early Reading Volume II.* Hillsdale, NJ: Lawrence Erlbaum Associates.

Liberman, I. Y., Shankweiler, D., Liberman, A. M., Fowler, C., and Fisher, F. W. 1977. Phonetic segmentation and recoding in the beginning reader. *In* A. S. Reber and D. L. Scarborough (eds.). *Toward a psychology of reading—The proceedings of the CUNY conferences.* Hillsdale, NJ: Lawrence Erlbaum Associates.

Mann, V. A., Liberman, I. Y., and Shankweiler, D. 1980. Children's memory for sentences and word storage in relation to reading ability. *Memory and Cognition* 8:329–335.

Mark, L. S., Shankweiler, D., Liberman, I. Y., and Fowler, C. A. 1977. Phonetic recoding and reading difficulty in beginning readers. *Memory and Cognition* 5:623–629.

Moely, B. F., Olson, F. A., Halwes, T. G., and Flavell, J. H. 1969. Production deficiency in young children's clustered recall. *Developmental Psychology* 1:26–34.

Morrison, F. J., and Manis, F. R. 1982. Cognitive processes and reading disability: A critique and proposal. *In* C. J. Brainerd and M. Pressley (eds.). *Verbal Processes in Children.* New York: Springer-Verlag.

Norman, D. A. 1972. The role of memory in the understanding of language. *In* J. F. Kavanagh and I. G. Mattingly (eds.). *Language by Ear and by Eye: The Relationships between Speech and Reading.* Cambridge, MA: MIT Press.

Olson, R. K., Davidson, B. J., Kliegl, R., and Davies, S. E. 1984. Development of phonetic memory in disabled and normal readers. *Journal of Experimental Child Psychology* 37:187–206.

Orton, S. T. 1925. "Word-blindness" in school children. *Archives of Neurology and Psychiatry* 14:581–615.

Paivio, A. 1971. *Imagery and Verbal Processes.* New York: Holt, Rhinehart and Winston.

Paivio, A., and Begg, I. 1971a. Imagery and comprehension latencies as a function of sentence concreteness and structure. *Preception and Psychophysics* 10:408–412.

Paivio, A., and Begg, I. 1971b. Imagery and associative overlap in short-term memory. *Journal of Experimental Psychology* 89:40–45.

Palermo, D. S., and Jenkins, J. J. 1964. *Word Association Norms—Grade School through College.* Minneapolis: University of Minnesota Press.

Perfetti, C. A., and McCutchen, D. 1982. Speech processes in reading. *In* N. Lass (ed.). *Speech and Language: Advances in Basic Research and Practice Volume 7.* New York: Academic Press.

Rabinovitch, R. D. 1959. Reading and learning disabilities. *In* S. Arieti (ed.). *American Handbook of Psychiatry.* New York: Basic Books.

Shankweiler, D., Liberman, I. Y., Mark, L. S., Fowler, C. A., and Fischer, F. W. 1979. The speech code and learning to read. *Journal of Experimental Psychology: Human Learning and Memory* 5:531–545.

Siegel, L. S., and Linder, B. A. 1984. Short-term memory processes in children with reading and arithmetic learning disabilities. *Developmental Psychology* 20:200–207.

Slosson, R. L. 1963. *Slosson Intelligence Test.* East Aurora, NY: Slosson Educational Publications.

Sperry, R. W. 1964. The great cerebral commissure. *Scientific American* 210:42–52.

Treiman, R. A., and Baron, J. 1983. Phonemic-analysis training helps children benefit from spelling-sound rules. *Memory and Cognition* 11:382–389.

Tulving, E., and Pearlstone, Z. 1966. Availability versus accessibility of information in memory for words. *Journal of Verbal Learning and Verbal Behavior* 5:381–391.

Vellutino, F. R. 1979. *Dyslexia: Theory and Research.* Cambridge, MA: MIT Press.

Vellutino, F. R., Bentley, W. L., and Phillips, F. 1978. Inter- versus intra-hemispheric learning in dyslexic and normal readers. *Developmental Medicine and Child Neurology* 20:71–80.

Vellutino, F. R., Harding, C. J., Phillips, F., and Steger, J. A. 1975. Differential transfer in poor and normal readers. *Journal of Genetic Psychology* 126.3–18.

Vellutino, F. R., Pruzek, R. M., Steger, J. A., and Meshoulam, U. 1973. Immediate visual recall in poor and normal readers as a function of orthographic-linguistic familiarity. *Cortex* 9:368–384.

Vellutino, F. R., and Scanlon, D. M. 1985a. Evaluation of short and long term memory processes in poor and normal readers using two different memory paradigms. Manuscript in preparation.

Vellutino, F. R., and Scanlon, D. M. 1985b. Free recall of concrete and abstract words in poor and normal readers. *Journal of Experimental Child Psychology* 39:363–380.

Vellutino, F. R., and Scanlon, D. M. 1984. Phonological coding, phonemic segmentation training and code acquisition in poor and normal readers. Paper presented at a Special Conference on the Biobehavioral Measures of Dyslexia sponsored by the National Institute of Child Health and Human Development, September, 1984, Bethesda, Maryland.

Vellutino, F. R., and Scanlon, D. M. (1986) Linguistic coding and metalinguistic awareness: Their relationship to verbal memory and code acquisition in poor and normal readers. *In* D. B. Yaden and W. S. Templeton (eds.). *Metalinguistic Awareness and Beginning Literacy.* Exeter, NH: Heinemann Educational Books, Inc.

Vellutino, F. R., Scanlon, D. M., and Bentley, W. L. 1983. Interhemispheric learning and speed of hemispheric transmission in dyslexic and normal readers: A replication of previous results and additional findings. *Journal of Applied Psycholinguistics* 4:209–228.

Vellutino, F. R., Scanlon, D. M., and Greenberg, S. 1985. Differential sensitivity to phonological, syntactic and semantic codes in poor and normal readers. Manuscript in preparation.

Vellutino, F. R., Scanlon, D. M., and Tanzman, M. 1985. Effects of category cuing at time of presentation and retrieval on memory performance in poor and normal readers. Manuscript in preparation.

Vellutino, F. R., Smith, H., Steger, J. A., and Kaman, M. 1975. Reading disability: Age differences and the perceptual deficit hypothesis. *Child Development* 46:487–493.

Vellutino, F. R., Steger, J. A., Harding, C. J., and Phillips, F. 1975. Verbal vs. non verbal paired-associates learning in poor and normal readers. *Neuropsychologia* 13:75–82.

Vellutino, F. R., Steger, J. A., Kaman, M., and DeSetto, L. 1975. Visual form perception in deficient and normal readers as a function of age and orthographic linguistic familiarity. *Cortex* 11:22–30.

Vellutino, F. R., Steger, J. A., and Kandel, G. 1972. Reading disability: An investigation of the perceptual deficit hypothesis. *Cortex* 8:106–118.

Vellutino, F. R., Steger, J. A., and Pruzek, R. 1973. Inter vs. intrasensory deficit in paired associate learning in poor and normal readers. *Canadian Journal of Behavioral Science* 5:111–123.

Watkins, O. C., and Watkins, M. J. 1975. Buildup of proactive inhibition as a cue-overload effect. *Journal of Experimental Psychology: Human Learning and Memory* 104:442–452.

Wechsler, D. 1949. *Wechsler Intelligence Scale for Children*. New York: Psychological Corporation.

Wechsler, D. 1974. *Wechsler Intelligence Scale for Children-Revised*. New York: Psychological Corporation.

Wolf, M. 1982. The word-retrieval process and reading in children and aphasics. *In* K. Nelson (ed.). *Children's Language, Volume III*. New York: Gardner Press.

14

Disabled Reading Processes and Cognitive Profiles

Richard K. Olson

Introduction

$\mathcal{R}$esearch on reading disability over the past decade has paid increasing attention to the manner in which disabled readers read, in addition to how well they read. A basic premise of this research is that reading involves the interaction of several component processes which draw upon different cognitive resources (Carr 1981). In this chapter I will review some between-group and within-group differences in reading processes that were found for 140 disabled and 140 normal readers tested during the first phase of our program project.[1] I will describe the relations between these reading-process profiles and measures of the subjects' perceptual and language skills in nonreading tasks. This comparison will help clarify the etiological significance of different specific cognitive deficits in disabled readers. I will also describe some developmental changes in reading disability that were observed across the sample's 7.8 to 16.8 year age range.

Previous between-group comparisons of disabled and normal readers have clearly demonstrated the presence of a variety of linguistic deficits in the disabled groups (for reviews see Frith 1981; Liberman 1985; Vellutino 1979). Some of the strongest deficits have been found in the disabled groups' ability to analyze the component phonemes in spoken words (Bradley and Bryant 1981; Fox and Routh 1980; Liberman 1973). Other group studies have compared disabled and normal reading-process profiles. Although the results of these studies have not been entirely consistent, most have shown that phonetic coding, the component reading process that demands the most analytic linguistic skills, is uniquely deficient in the reading-disabled group. I will summarize

[1]This research was supported by USPHS program project grant HDMH11681-01A1. Brian Davidson and Reinhold Kliegl shared in the design and execution of the research. A broad overview of the complete study is presented in Olson, Kliegl, Davidson and Foltz (1985). I thank Jan Keenan and Barbara Wise for their comments on an earlier draft.

215

some results from our program project that provide strong support for a specific phonetic coding deficit, rather than a general developmental delay or lag in reading processes, for most disabled readers.

Previous within-group comparisons of individual disabled readers have concluded that reading disability is a heterogeneous disorder, but there has been little consensus on the exact nature and importance of this heterogeneity (for reviews see Doehring 1984; McKinney 1984; Satz and Morris 1981). As we might expect from the group studies cited above, the majority of disabled readers show varying degrees and patterns of deficit in language skills (Denckla 1979). In the present sample of disabled readers we will see that there were trade-offs between different language skills in the determination of reading ability measured by a standardized reading test, and reading style measured by eye movement patterns in text. Several within-group studies have documented a significant minority of disabled readers with visual-spatial deficits (cf. Lyon and Watson 1981; Mattis 1978). We will see that these visual-spatial processing deficits are of doubtful etiological significance for reading disability.

The chapter is organized in four main sections. The theoretical background for our componential analysis of the reading process is outlined in the first section. In the second section, differences in the component reading processes will be described between older disabled and younger normal subjects matched in reading level. Developmental differences in the component processes and their changing relations to reading ability across age will also be considered. In the third section I will show that there are substantial individual differences in reading and spelling processes within the disabled sample after controlling for reading ability. The fourth section considers the etiology of individual differences in reading processes and presents some preliminary behavior genetic data.

Models of Reading and Individual Differences

Our theoretical approach at the beginning of the project was influenced by previous studies of individual differences in disabled reading and spelling styles (Boder 1973; Ingram, Mason, and Blackburn 1970), and by the dual-process model of reading (Coltheart 1978; Huey 1908). Boder described two distinct subtypes of disabled readers based on her clinical analyses of their reading and spelling errors. The largest subtype, called "dysphonetic," was able to read familiar words by "sight," but this subtype was unable to sound out unfamiliar words and their spelling errors were phonetically dissimilar from the target words. A smaller group of disabled readers was able to read and spell words phonetically that followed the common grapheme-phoneme-conversion (GPC) rules, but this "dyseidetic" subtype was not able to read words by "sight." Several recent studies have made similar distinctions among disabled or poor readers (Baron 1979; Mitterer 1982; Treiman 1984).

The "dual-process" model of reading provided the theoretical framework for our studies of individual differences in reading and spelling processes. In this model, there are separate phonetic and orthographic pathways between print and the lexicon.[2] The phonetic path may be used to determine the sound of a letter string which can be subsequently compared to words in the reader's oral vocabulary. There is still much debate about whether this path plays an important role in skilled reading (Henderson 1982). A number of researchers have argued that the phonetic path is primarily used in reading unfamiliar words and by beginning readers (Backman, Bruck, Hebert, and Seidenberg in press; McCusker, Hillinger, and Bias 1981; Reitsma 1984).

The other route to the lexicon in the dual-process model is the direct orthographic path. This path involves direct access to the lexicon for a familiar word through its unique pattern of letter identities, without necessarily depending on the sound of the word. The orthographic or direct path is thought to be dominant in normal adult readers (Singer 1980), and it may be functional in early reading development after only a few exposures to a word (Ehri 1980; Reitsma 1983). Most dual-process theorists argue that the phonetic and orthographic coding paths typically operate in parallel, although task demands, word familiarity, and developmental differences might influence readers' relative dependence on the two paths (cf. Crowder 1982; Ellis 1984).

Recently two important criticisms have been directed toward the dual-process model. First, the traditional view of how phonetic coding operates in the dual-process model has been that grapheme-phoneme-conversion (GPC) rules are applied to "sound out" letter patterns which are then blended to form the word. The strong version of this theory holds that the operation of GPC rules is completely independent from lexical knowledge (cf. Coltheart 1978), although Venezky's (1970) formulation of these rules included some lexical influences. Henderson (1982) has argued persuasively that GPC rules without lexical influence would be inadequate for reading many of the most common English words. The second criticism is that word decoding in the phonetic path does not necessarily have to employ GPC rules. For example, the sound of an unfamiliar word or nonword could be decoded by analogy to words in the reader's lexicon that have similar orthographic patterns (Baron 1977). Glushko (1979) and Henderson (1982) have taken the extreme position that reading occurs *only* by analogy to words in the lexicon. However, there are a number of problems with the exclusive-analogy view (Massaro and Venezky 1983; Olson and Keenan in press), including the fact that there are significant individual and developmental differences in the processing unit used in reading (Vellutino 1984).

Some theorists have argued for a model of reading wherein the orthography of words and nonwords may be simultaneously segmented for orthographic and phonetic coding at multiple, interacting levels ranging from the single grapheme to the whole word (Baron 1977; Humphreys and Evett in press; Shallice, Warrington, and McCarthy 1983). The model of reading used in the present study incorporates this multiple-level segmentation approach and it

---

[2]Lexical access refers here to the contact of a letter string with a memory representation that allows its identification as a word. In ordinary reading this would include access to the meaning and sound of the word.

retains a distinction, emphasized in the dual-process model, that reading may involve both the decoding of words indirectly through their phonetic codes derived from various levels of segmentation and directly through their orthographic codes.

There are three basic ways in which readers could differ in the above model. First, they could vary in their ability to decode the sound of a word or nonword in order to "hear" if it matches a word in their oral vocabulary (phonetic coding). Second, they could differ in their ability to recognize words directly through the orthographic path (orthographic coding), without relying on phonetic coding. (Ordinarily phonetic and orthographic coding are assumed to proceed in parallel, but two tasks to be described in the following section were used to separate these two coding skills. Results from this study indicate that phonetic coding best distinguishes disabled and normal readers.)

A third way in which readers could differ is in the level of segmentation that they use in reading. This has further implications for the relative use of the phonetic and orthographic paths. For example, in phonetic coding, subjects could use relatively small orthographic processing units and GPC rules to decode the sound of a word or nonword, or they could use larger unit analogies to words in their lexicon. Both approaches could be equally successful in determining the sound of a letter string, and ordinarily they would proceed in parallel. However, readers may differ in their relative use of large and small processing units in phonetic coding. The further implication of processing units for the subjects' relative use of the phonetic and orthographic paths is that larger orthographic processing units may be more compatible with the direct orthographic route, while smaller units may be more compatible with the indirect phonetic process. The section on individual differences among disabled readers presents evidence for a dimension of individual variation in the size of the processing unit used in reading and in the relative use of phonetic and orthographic coding. The following section describes some group differences between disabled and normal readers that were found for phonetic and orthographic coding.

Group and Developmental Differences in Phonetic and Orthographic Coding

The Sample of Normal and Disabled Readers

The sample consisted of 140 pairs of disabled and normal readers referred from Boulder area schools who scored at least 90 on either the verbal or performance subscales of the Revised Weschler Intelligence Scale for Children (WISC-R). The disabled-normal pairs were matched on sex and age within six months. Children with overt signs of brain damage, educational deficits, sensory deficits, or emotional problems were excluded from the sample. The sex distribution of the reading disabled sample that met our selection criteria was 111 boys and 29 girls. Peabody Individual Achievement Test (PIAT) word recognition grade-levels for the disabled and normal groups are presented in

Table I. Additional psychometric data for the normal and disabled groups are presented in DeFries (this volume).

Developmental differences in reading and spelling processes were evaluated by dividing the sample into three age ranges with mean ages of 10.1, 12.8, and 15.3 years (see Table I). This age division also allowed for the comparison of disabled readers with normal readers at similar levels of word recognition. The mean PIAT word recognition levels were not significantly different between the older group of disabled readers and the younger group of normal readers (see Table I). This made it possible to see if there were significant differences in reading-process profiles between disabled and normal readers that were independent from their general level of word recognition.

Phonetic and Orthographic Coding Tasks

Two tasks were designed to assess independently the subjects' skill in phonetic and orthographic coding. The complete methods and results of these tasks are presented in Davidson, Olson, and Kliegl (Note 1). In the phonetic coding task, subjects compared 40 pairs of nonwords (e.g., kake/dake; shurt/shart; derty/dorty). They were asked to press a button on the side of the letter string that would sound like a word in their vocabulary if pronounced aloud. The correct responses were phonetically identical to common words that would be in a first grader's oral vocabulary.

In the orthographic task, subjects compared 40 pairs of phonetically identical letter strings and designated the letter string that was actually a word (e.g., rain/rane; deep/deap; hurt/hert). Phonetic coding would not help the subjects make a decision in this task since both the word and nonword sound the same when they are pronounced. However, it is likely that phonetic codes are generated automatically when subjects perform the orthographic task. In ordinary reading, automatically generated phonetic codes may support the post-lexical storage of words in memory (Kleiman 1975; Perfetti and McCutchen 1982). Liberman (in press) has argued persuasively that reading in the orthographic path necessarily involves the access of abstract phonological codes that are associated with specific orthographic patterns.

The only distinctions I wish to make at this point about coding in the phonetic and orthographic tasks are that successful performance in the orthographic task requires the accurate representation of a word's specific ortho-

Table I
PIAT Word Recognition Grade Levels for Disabled and Normal Readers
in Three Age Groups

| Age Range | 7.8–11.4 yrs. | 11.5–14.1 yrs. | 14.2–16.8 yrs. |
Mean Age	10.1 yrs.	12.8 yrs.	15.3 yrs.
Normal			
Word Rec.	7.0	9.7	11.5
Disabled			
Word Rec.	3.3	5.0	6.7

Note: The values are mean PIAT grade levels based on the national norms.

graphic pattern, and that the task does not allow the use of phonetic coding to make a correct decision. In contrast, the phonetic task requires the use of phonetic coding to make a correct decision.

Phonetic and Orthographic Coding in Reading-Matched Groups

Disabled and normal readers' error rates in the phonetic and orthographic coding tasks are presented in Figure 1 for the three age groups. There are significant differences between the groups at each age level for the two tasks, as would be expected from the substantial group differences in reading ability at each age level shown in Table I.

One of the most informative ways of looking at group differences in reading processes between disabled and normal readers is to compare older disabled with younger normal subjects who are reading at the same grade level (cf. Bradley and Bryant 1978). For the oldest third of the disabled readers and the youngest third of the normal readers, there was no significant difference between their mean PIAT word recognition grade-levels (see Table I). If there were no significant differences in the component phonetic and orthographic coding processes between the younger normal and older disabled groups, it would suggest that the disabled readers suffered from a general developmental lag in their reading processes. If, on the other hand, specific component reading processes in the disabled group were either better or worse than those of the normal group, it would indicate that there were qualitative group differences between disabled and normal readers in their component reading processes.

A significant difference in phonetic coding was found between the reading-level matched groups. The older disabled group made 30% errors in the phonetic task compared to 18% errors for the younger normal subjects (chance performance would be 50% errors). In contrast, the disabled and normal error

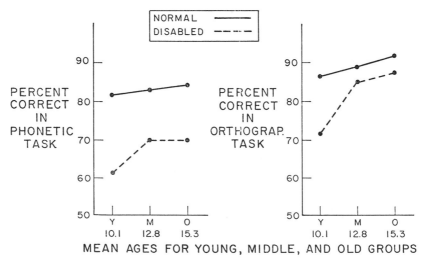

Figure 1.   Disabled and normal readers' performance in the phonetic and orthographic coding tasks for three age groups.

rates in the orthographic task were not significantly different (12.4% and 13.4% respectively). This highly significant cross-over interaction is plotted in the left side of Figure 2. It clearly indicates a qualitative phonetic coding deficit in the disabled sample. (Although the reading-level matched groups were not significantly different in the orthographic task, we will see in the within-group analyses of disabled readers that orthographic coding ability is not simply equivalent to reading ability.)

Other researchers have studied oral nonword reading in older disabled and younger normal groups matched in reading level. Although oral nonword reading requires an overt oral response and does not require lexical access through the phonetic path as does the present phonetic coding task, it seems likely that oral nonword reading and phonetic coding tap some similar processes. Consistent with the present results, most studies of oral nonword reading found a group deficit for their disabled samples. (Baddeley, Ellis, Miles, and Lewis 1982; Bradley and Bryant 1978; Kochnower, Richardson, and DiBenedetto 1983; Seymour and Porpodas 1980; Snowling 1981; Siegel and Ryan Note 2). However, three recent studies have not found differences between reading-level-matched disabled and normal readers in oral nonword reading (Beech and Harding 1984; Seidenberg, Bruck, Fornarlo, and Backman Note 3; Treiman and Hirsh-Pasek Note 4). In the Beech and Harding study, there may have been sample differences that accounted for their null results. Many of their disabled readers were from poor education and social backgrounds; this could be the primary reason for their reading failure. These subjects' reading problems would not fit the common definition of specific reading disability used for the present subjects and in other studies that have shown nonword deficits in reading-matched groups. When reading failure occurs in the context of normal education and social background, specific

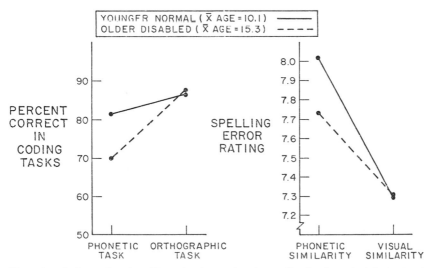

Figure 2.   Coding task and spelling rating interactions for reading-level matched disabled and normal readers.

deficits in phonetic coding may be more frequent and may be a symptom of underlying linguistic deficits that are the ultimate cause of specific reading disability. The null results of Treiman and Hirsh-Pasek (Note 4) may not be due to sampling differences. Their general description of the criteria for disabled and normal readers seemed similar to the criteria for the present sample. They suggested that their nonwords may not have been difficult enough to detect a phonetic coding deficit, but their general conclusion was that disabled reading is best viewed as a developmental lag in all component reading processes. Further research is needed to understand the basis for these conflicting results.

Developmental Asymptotes in Phonetic Coding

Developmental analyses indicated that a phonetic coding deficit may be a permanent aspect of the disabled group's reading process profile and that they are unlikely ever to catch up with the normal readers.[3] The left side of Figure 1 shows the disabled readers' performance in the phonetic task for the younger, middle, and oldest age groups. There was a significant increase in phonetic coding accuracy from the younger to the middle group, but there was no improvement from the middle to the older group, indicating an asymptote around 12 years of age. Analyses of the normal readers' phonetic coding accuracy revealed that they had reached an asymptote at least by the age of the youngest group (10 years) and there were no significant differences between the age groups. However, both the normal and disabled readers showed significant gains in word recognition beyond their asymptotes in phonetic coding (see Table I). Since the disabled readers had reached an asymptote in phonetic coding by the middle age group, their continued improvement in word recognition must have been due primarily to the accumulation and increase in precision of orthographic codes with reading experience. Snowling (1980) has reported a similar developmental asymptote in phonetic coding and continued improvement in word recognition for disabled readers.

Conclusions on Phonetic and Orthographic Coding in Disabled and Normal Groups

There was a substantial group deficit in phonetic coding for the disabled readers, and the disabled readers seemed to have reached an asymptote in phonetic coding by about 12 years of age. This suggests that weakness in this specific reading process may play a major causal role in reading disability. In the final section, I will consider some language processes that may be etiologically significant for the phonetic coding deficit.

It is encouraging to note that some previously disabled adults have achieved normal levels of word recognition even though their phonetic coding skills remained substantially below normal (Ellis and Miles 1981; Miles 1983;

---

[3]Conclusions about the development of phonetic coding and reading skills in the present disabled readers must be qualified by the fact that the comparisons are cross-sectional. The validity of the comparisons is strengthened by the fact that nearly all of the older disabled subjects were identified as reading disabled in a previous study under the same criteria when they were in the same age range as the present younger group (see DeFries this volume).

Rudel 1981). In the present study, a dissociation between phonetic coding and word recognition was observed for the oldest disabled sample. There was substantial variation in phonetic coding and word recognition within this group, but phonetic coding was not significantly correlated with level of word recognition ($r = .23$). In contrast, the correlation between word recognition and phonetic coding within the youngest disabled group ($r = .61$) was significantly larger ($p < .05$, by Fisher's z transformation for comparisons between independent rs). Similar reliabilities and variances for phonetic coding and word recognition in the two age groups justified the comparison of the correlations.

Firth (1972) has reported a nearly perfect relation between oral nonword reading and word recognition in first-grade normal readers. Younger readers may be more dependent on phonetic coding processes because their orthographic codes for words are still relatively weak (cf. Reitsma 1984). As the reading process shifts away from phonetic coding in older disabled readers, other factors may become more important in determining a particular child's reading ability. One of these factors may simply be the amount of reading the child does and the consequent familiarity with different orthographic patterns. We are now following the younger disabled readers in a longitudinal study. It will be interesting to see how their within-group differences in reading process profiles and cognitive profiles presented in the following section are related to changes in reading ability across age.

I have focused most of the preceding discussion on the phonetic deficit because it was significant for the reading-level matched groups. Orthographic coding levels were similar for the reading-level matched groups, but the older disabled subjects were significantly worse than the older normal subjects (see Figure 1). Venezky and Massaro (1979) have suggested that good phonetic coding skills may help orient the reader to the details of orthographic structure in words. These orthographic codes may then be used independently from phonetic coding for the recognition of familiar words. It is possible that the disabled readers' severe phonetic coding deficit contributed in this way to their relatively weak orthographic codes for the easy words in this task. However, the fact that the disabled readers' phonetic and orthographic coding were not equally deficient suggests that there are functionally independent skills involved in these two tasks. In the following section we will see that within the disabled sample, phonetic and orthographic coding are not consistently correlated, and they relate in *opposite* directions to other measures of reading and spelling processes.

Individual Differences in Disabled Readers' Process Profiles

There was substantial variance in the orthographic and phonetic coding tasks even after the disabled subjects' scores were adjusted for their word recognition on the PIAT. What needs to be demonstrated is that this variance represents meaningful individual differences in reading-process profiles rather than simple error variance in the tasks.[4] In this section, I will validate the disabled readers' different process profiles through correlations among their phonetic coding, orthographic coding, phonetic spelling errors, and eye-movement patterns in reading. I will briefly comment on differences in the spelling and eye-movement results between the reading-level-matched disabled and normal groups.

It is important to note that in the within-group correlational analyses, the primary interest was in individual differences in reading and spelling processes that were independent from the subjects' general reading skill. Therefore, because there was substantial variation in reading skill among the disabled readers within each age group, variance in word recognition scores on the PIAT was partialed out of the correlations.

All of the correlations reported in this section were computed within the previously described age groups. There were two reasons for this approach. First, there were nonlinearities in some of the variables across age that would have violated the linearity assumptions of correlational analyses (for examples, see Figure 1). The second reason for the age divisions is that there were significant developmental differences in the correlations between some of the variables. Most of the correlations presented in this section are from the youngest group of disabled readers. Contrasting results from the older disabled readers are discussed in the final section.

I will begin the discussion of within-group differences by comparing correlations between phonetic and orthographic coding within the disabled and normal samples. We will see that there was a greater dissociation between the coding skills in the disabled sample. The validity and implications of within-group variation in disabled readers' phonetic and orthographic coding skills will be subsequently clarified by correlations with their spelling and eye-movement data.

Correlations Between Phonetic and Orthographic Coding

Earlier I argued that phonetic and orthographic coding processes typically operate in an integrated fashion during reading, and that at least in normal readers, we would expect the two coding skills to be positively correlated. Table II shows that this expectation was confirmed for the normal readers in all three age groups, but the correlations for the youngest and oldest groups of disabled readers were not significant, and they were significantly lower than the correlations for the corresponding normal age groups. The correlation for the middle group of disabled readers was also lower, but it was not significantly different from the middle normal group. As in the group analyses described in the previous section, the most informative comparison is between the correlations for the older disabled ($r = .07$), and younger normal readers ($r = .55$),

---

[4]The phonetic and orthographic tasks each contained 40 forced-choice trials. Some or all of the variance in performance in these tasks after controlling for word recognition could be due to guessing when the subjects did not know the correct answer. Subjects would vary in their luck on these guesses and this would influence their final score. However, the variance due to luck should not be systematically correlated with the other measures of reading and spelling processes.

Table II

Correlations Between Phonetic and Orthographic Coding Within the Disabled and Normal Groups at Three Age Levels

Mean Age	10.1 yrs.	12.8 yrs.	15.3 yrs.
Normal	.55**	.69**	.62**
Readers	(N = 47)	(N = 42)	(N = 46)
Disabled	− .17	.51**	.07
Readers	(N = 41)	(N = 43)	(N = 50)
Normal-Disabled			
Difference z	3.57**	1.27	3.10**

Note: Correlations are partialed on PIAT word recognition. The number of subjects for each correlation who had complete data in the phonetic and orthographic tasks are given in parentheses. z scores for the difference between normal and disabled correlations are based on Fisher's z transformation. ** = $p < .01$.

who were similar in reading level on the PIAT. Here the correlation was significantly lower for the disabled readers ($p < .01$).

The interpretation of the within-group correlations between phonetic and orthographic coding is not entirely straightforward. At least part of the correlated variance may have been associated with the subjects' general adaptation to the similar methods of these two tasks (e.g. button pushing, accuracy criteria, etc.). If it is assumed that the disabled and normal readers were equally influenced by common adaptation to the two tasks, the lower correlations for the disabled readers are quite interesting. They suggest that there was a greater dissociation between phonetic and orthographic coding skills for the disabled readers. These results are consistent with the view that good reading depends on the integrated use of phonetic and orthographic coding processes, and poor reading is more likely to be associated with less integration of these processes. Now we will see how the disabled readers' variance in the phonetic and orthographic coding tasks is related to individual differences in their spelling processes.

Spelling Error Correlations With the Coding Tasks

Elena Boder (1973) was one of the first researchers to use spelling errors as a diagnostic aid in differentiating subtypes of disabled readers. Her approach has achieved considerable popularity and she has recently published a test manual (Boder and Jarrico 1982). The differential diagnosis of this test is supposed to reveal the etiology and appropriate remediation for each disabled reader. Earlier I mentioned Boder's distinction between dysphonetic and dyseidetic subtypes of disabled readers. Dysphonetic subjects could spell highly familiar words accurately by relying on whole-word images, but their spelling errors for unfamiliar words were phonetically bizarre. Dyseidetic subjects apparently had weak whole-word images, but they were able to use their relatively strong phoneme-grapheme-correspondence (PGC) rules to spell some words correctly. As a result, the dyseidetics' spelling errors were phonetically similar to the target words. Dyseidetic subjects were presumed to be constitutionally deficient in the visual-spatial skills necessary for the

"Gestalt" processing of whole words, and the dysphonetic subjects were thought to be deficient in language skills measured by the WISC-R verbal subscale. We will see that there is some validity in using spelling errors to define a dimension of individual differences in reading and spelling styles among younger disabled readers, but these individual differences did not fall into the distinct subtype clusters that Boder (1973) described, and they did not show the correlations with perceptual and verbal skills that she predicted.

The Spelling Test and Error Coding. The subjects in the present study were given a spelling test (Camp and McCabe Note 5), that was modeled after Boder's (1973) general description of her test. After assessing the subjects' reading level with a word recognition test, twenty spelling words were selected for difficulty so that the subjects read about 65% and spelled about 45% of the words correctly. This asymmetry between correct reading and spelling was typical of both disabled and normal readers. It is probably associated with an asymmetry in the predictive relations from spelling to sound and from sound to spelling (Henderson and Chard 1980).

The subjects' spellings were examined for several different types of errors such as letter reversals and mistakes in the beginning and end letters (details of the spelling test and error analyses are reported in Davidson, Olson, and Kliegl Note 1). In addition to these objective measures, each error was rated on a ten point scale separately for the phonetic and visual similarity of the error to the target word. The phonetic similarity rating was based on the rater's subjective impression of the similarity between a phonetic rendition of the spelling error and the sound of the target word. Spelling errors that could be pronounced the same as the target word according to phonetic rules were given a score of ten, and errors with no phonetic overlap with the target were scored as one on the ten point scale. The visual similarity ratings represented the rater's subjective impression of the overall visual similarity between the error and the target word. This impression was based on factors such as the number of letters in the spelling, the placement of ascending and descending letters, and the number of letters in common. Of course the phonetic and visual ratings were correlated, but the group differences in phonetic and visual ratings described below for the older disabled and younger normal readers indicate that they represent slightly different aspects of the subjects spelling processes.

Differences in Phonetic Spelling Between Disabled and Normal Readers. Before discussing individual differences within the disabled group, I will briefly comment on a significant difference in phonetic ratings between the reading-matched older disabled and younger normal subjects. Finucci, Isaacs, Whitehouse, and Childs (1983) reported that disabled readers' spelling errors were phonetically less similar to the target word than were the spelling errors of normal readers. However, the Finucci et al. disabled and normal groups differed in reading level, so we cannot be sure that there are qualitative differences between disabled and normal readers in phonetic spelling. This question was addressed in the present study by comparing the phonetic spelling ratings for the older disabled and younger normal groups that were similar in

PIAT word recognition. The mean phonetic rating for the disabled readers was significantly lower than the mean phonetic rating for the normal readers (7.7 vs. 8.0, $p < .05$). In contrast to the phonetic similarity ratings, the visual similarity ratings were not significantly different between the disabled and normal groups. The significant interaction between group and rating type is presented in the right side of Figure 2. The spelling interaction appears similar to the interaction between group and coding task presented in the left side of Figure 2. This suggests that in spelling as well as reading, it is the phonetic process that is most uniquely deficient in disabled readers.

Pennington et al. (Note 6) found a similar interaction between reading-level matched groups of disabled and normal readers and spelling error ratings that were based on a more objective coding scheme. Their phonetic rating was based on essentially the same information as in the present study, but they did not use a general visual similarity rating. Instead, they rated the spellings on their orthographic acceptability. It appeared that they were more successful in separating two aspects of the spelling process by this method, since their phonetic and orthographic ratings were not as highly correlated ($r = .5$) as the phonetic and visual ratings in the present study ($r = .74$ in the younger disabled group).

The significant interaction between reader group and type of spelling rating in the present study indicated that the phonetic and visual ratings were tapping different spelling processes to some degree, but the high correlation between the two ratings limited their usefulness as independent measures in the analyses described below. In fact, the two variables were similarly correlated with the measures of reading processes, although the correlations with the phonetic spelling ratings tended to be a bit stronger. For the sake of simplicity in reporting the spelling results, only the correlations with phonetic similarity ratings will be presented here.

Phonetic Ratings and Spelling Accuracy. The younger disabled readers' phonetic spelling ratings were not significantly correlated with the number of words spelled correctly (see Table III). This result shows that correct spelling depends on more than the ability to derive a phonetically acceptable response. The reason is that sound is not a very good predictor for spelling in English. Different spellings may often represent the same sound. The ambiguity of sound-spelling relations has been demonstrated by the fact that elaborate phoneme-to-grapheme rule systems can only spell 50% to 75% of common words (Hanna, Hanna, Hodges, and Rudorf 1966; Simon and Simon 1973). Many disabled readers can do better than this. Thus, it is clear that a representation of the specific *orthographic* structure of words is also important for spelling accuracy (Henderson 1982).

The absence of a significant correlation between the disabled readers' phonetic spelling ratings and their spelling accuracy is consistent with Boder's (1973) hypothesis. The dysphonetic subjects (with their strong orthographic codes and weak phonetic codes) might spell the same number of words correctly as the dyseidetic subjects (with their weak orthographic codes and strong phonetic codes), but the dyseidetic subjects' phonetic similarity ratings for their spelling errors should be higher. The latter prediction is confirmed in the following analyses.

Phonetic Spelling and Phonetic Coding.   Earlier I discussed a model wherein phonetic codes in reading could be derived interactively from several levels of orthographic segmentation, ranging from single letters to whole words. Similarly, in the phonetic coding task that involved the reading of nonwords, the correct phonetic code could be derived from GPC rules and/or from analogies to words in the lexicon. However, young disabled readers may not have had sufficient exposure to printed words to develop the lexical entries that support a strong analogy process in phonetic coding; therefore their nonword reading in the phonetic coding task may have depended, at least to some extent, on their ability to use GPC rules. Following Boder's (1973) hypothesis that higher phonetic ratings of spelling errors indicate the use of small-unit correspondence rules in both reading and spelling, the positive correlation between phonetic coding accuracy and the phonetic spelling ratings shown in Table III would be expected.

Phonetic Spelling and Orthographic Coding.   Accuracy in the orthographic task may also be related to individual differences in the unit of processing in reading and spelling. Relatively good performance in the orthographic task may depend on the use of orthographic representations for whole words, since the letter strings in this choice task were phonetically identical (e.g., rain/rane). Thus, subjects who do relatively well in the orthographic task relative to their PIAT reading level may tend to use relatively large processing units in reading and spelling. Recall that in Boder's (1973) theory, the dysphonetic subjects' use of whole-word representations was associated with spelling errors that were phonetically dissimilar from the target word. This would predict that there should be a negative correlation between orthographic coding and the phonetic spelling ratings. In fact, this correlation was $r = -.48$ (see Table III).

The pattern of correlations between phonetic coding, orthographic coding, and phonetic spelling suggests that the younger disabled readers varied

Table III
Correlations of Spelling Scores With Phonetic and Orthographic Coding

	Phonetic Spelling Rating	Phonetic Coding Correct	Orthographic Coding Correct
Number Spelled Correct	.01	.13	−.12
Phonetic Spelling Rating		.29*	−.48**
Phonetic Coding Correct			−.08

Note: The correlations are for 38 of the youngest disabled group who had complete spelling data. The correlations were partialed on PIAT word recognition. * = $p < .05$, ** = $p < .01$.

systematically in their preferred processing unit for reading and spelling. An independent index of the disabled subjects' unit of processing in reading is needed to confirm this hypothesis. For the purpose of ecological validity, this index should be based on a task that is as similar as possible to normal reading. Analyses of the subjects' eye movements while they were reading text for comprehension provided the desired measure of processing unit size.

Eye Movements in Text

Eye movements may provide a useful index of individual differences in reading processes (see McConkie this volume). The present subjects' eye movements were examined in several reading and nonreading tasks. I will briefly mention the results of some group comparisons between disabled and normal readers before turning to the within-group analyses.

Differences Between Disabled and Normal Readers' Eye Movements. Many eye movement studies over the past fifty years have found that when normal and disabled readers of the same age are compared using a text that is at a level of difficulty appropriate to the normal readers, the disabled readers show more frequent fixations, slightly longer fixation durations, and a higher percentage of regressive eye movements (see Tinker 1958, for a review). Some researchers have argued that erratic eye movements may be a primary cause of reading failure because they found that disabled readers also show more frequent fixations and regressions in nonreading tasks (cf. Pavlidis 1981, 1985). However, several studies, including one with the present subjects, have not found differences in eye movements between disabled and normal readers in nonreading tasks (Olson, Kliegl, and Davidson 1983a). We concurred with Tinker that the disabled readers' more frequent fixations and regressive move ments in text are a result, rather than a cause, of their difficulties in reading. Consistent with this view, when the present disabled and normal subjects read text that had been adjusted in difficulty for their level of word recognition, there were only minor eye-movement differences between the groups (Olson, Kliegl, and Davidson 1983b). Moreover, when the older disabled and younger normal subjects were matched in word recognition, and their eye movements were measured in the *same* text, there were no significant differences between the groups on variables such as the percentage of regressions, average saccade length, frequency of fixations, or fixation duration (Kliegl, Olson, and David-son Note 7).[5] However, we will see that there were significant within-group

---

[5]The only significant exception to similar eye movements for the reading-matched groups was found when the subjects read the difficult words from the Camp and McCabe test (Note 5). In this test, the words were presented one at a time. When each word appeared, the subjects shifted their eyes to the word from a fixation point ten spaces to the left of the word. Disabled and normal readers were similar in their average first fixation position on the words, which was usually just to the left of the word center. However, the disabled readers were more likely to regress to the beginning of the word on the second fixation. This difference was greatest when the subjects were slow in giving an oral response (longer than two seconds), and were incorrect. In this case, the disabled subjects regressed to the beginning of the word on 58% of their second fixations, compared to 18% for the normal readers. Disabled readers, because of their phonetic coding deficit, may prefer to deal with the beginnings of words they do not know because it is easier to decode phonetically initial phonemes that are not embedded.

differences in disabled readers' eye movements that were related to their reading, spelling, and cognitive profiles.

The Reading Task and Eye Movement Variables. The subjects' eye movements were monitored while they read two stories. The first story was read aloud and the second was read silently. The passages were selected from Spache's (1963) reading test based on the subjects' word recognition scores so that they would be neither trivially easy nor too difficult. The stories were approximately 200 words in length and the average disabled subject read each story in about three minutes. The subjects were told that they would be asked questions about the story when they were finished.

The subjects' eye fixations were mapped onto the text so that the percentages of different word fixation patterns could be computed. These percentages included forward saccades between adjacent words, word-skipping forward saccades, within-word forward saccades, within-word backward saccades, between-word backward saccades, and line switches. Frequencies, durations, and average lengths of forward and backward saccades were also computed. The complete results for all of these variables are presented in Kliegl et al. (Note 7). In the present discussion I will focus on the four eye-movement variables that were most strongly related to the other measures of reading and spelling processes. These were the four variables included in Table IV; the percentages of between-word regressions, within-word forward saccades, word-skipping forward saccades, and mean forward saccade length. Also included in Table IV are correlations with a composite eye-movement variable that we have called the "plodder-explorer" dimension. This dimension was based on the addition of the subjects' z scores for the percentages of their regressive and word-skipping saccades. Subjects who were high on this dimension showed an exploratory pattern in reading, with more frequent word-skipping and regressive eye movements. Subjects who were low on the dimension showed a more sequential pattern of forward saccades within and between words, and few regressions or word-skipping movements. We found that subjects at opposite ends of this dimension might read the text in the same amount of time and attain similar comprehension levels, but their reading styles were strikingly different (Kliegl et al. Note 7; Olson, Kliegl, Davidson, and Foltz 1985).

To simplify the presentation of the eye movement data, only the correlations from the oral stories are included in Table IV. The pattern of results was quite similar for the silent reading condition. Correlations that were significant in the silent condition at $p < .05$ are underlined in Table IV.

Eye Movements, Phonetic Coding, Phonetic Spelling, and Orthographic Coding. The correlations between orthographic coding, phonetic coding, and phonetic spelling described earlier suggested that some disabled readers read and spell using small units while others use larger units or whole words. How would the subjects' eye movements in reading be related to these differences? We hypothesized that a small-unit phonetic coding strategy would be associated with shorter forward saccades within and between words as the subjects visually attended to the word segments. Large-unit orthographic coding would

Table IV
Eye-Movement Correlations with the Coding Tasks, Phonetic Spelling,
and Verbal Intelligence

	Phonetic Coding Correct	Orthographic Coding Correct	Phonetic Spelling Rating	Verbal Intelligence
Between-word Regressions (17%, SD = 3.7%)	− .15	.39**	− .45**	.42**
Within-word forward Sac. (20%, SD = 4.7%)	.27	− .46**	.29*	− .42**
Word-Skipping forward Sac. (9%, SD = 3.2%)	− .26	.50**	− .31*	.51**
Forward Saccade Length (4.8, SD = .9)	− .29*	.45**	− .36*	.53**
Plodder-Explorer Dimension	.25	.54**	− .46*	.56**

Note: Correlations are for 37 of the youngest disabled readers with complete eye-movement data in the oral reading condition. Variance related to the subjects' PIAT word recognition was partialed out. Mean percentages and standard deviations for the different types of eye movements are in parentheses. Forward saccade length is measured in character spaces. The underlined correlations were significant in the silent reading condition at least at $p < .05$.
For the oral reading correlations presented here, * = $p < .05$, ** = $p < .01$.

be associated with longer saccades and fewer within-word progressive movements. We also hypothesized that more frequent regressive eye movements would be associated with large-unit coding. These regressions might arise from the need to refixate words when orthographic coding initially failed in lexical access. The correlations of the eye-movement variables with orthographic coding, phonetic coding, and phonetic spelling were remarkably consistent with our hypotheses.

The pattern of eye movement correlations with phonetic coding and phonetic spelling were quite similar, although they were stronger and more consistently significant with phonetic spelling (see Table IV). Disabled readers who were relatively strong in phonetic coding and phonetic spelling compared to their level of word recognition showed less frequent between-word regressions and word-skipping forward saccades, and more within-word forward saccades. Therefore, the better phonetic coders and spellers tended to be on the "plodder" end of the composite eye-movement dimension. The consistently weaker correlations with phonetic coding may be due to the fact that correct phonetic codes could be achieved through small-unit GPC rules or through large-unit analogies to words. Good phonetic spelling may be more consistently dependent on the use of small-unit rules in this younger disabled sample. In the final section, I will discuss some developmental changes in this relation.

The pattern of eye-movement correlations with orthographic coding was exactly opposite from the above patterns with phonetic coding and spelling. Disabled readers who were relatively strong in orthographic coding compared to their level of word recognition showed more frequent between-word regressions and word-skipping forward saccades, and fewer within-word forward saccades. Thus, the better orthographic coders tended to be on the "explorer" end of the composite eye-movement dimension.

Recall that orthographic coding and phonetic spelling were negatively correlated with each other ($r = -.48$). Since there was a substantial amount of uncorrelated variance, it is possible that the two variables were accounting for different variance in the subjects' eye movements. On the other hand, if the coding and spelling tasks were tapping the same underlying dimension of individual differences in word coding processes, they should account for essentially the same variance in eye movements. The latter view was supported by two hierarchical regression models. After entering either one of the variables first, the second variable did not account for a significant amount of additional variance in the plodder-explorer dimension.

The eye-movement patterns and their correlations with the other measures of reading and spelling processes provided strong support for the hypothesis that young disabled readers vary in their use of small- and large-unit codes. There are some important issues pertaining to the distribution, development, and etiology of these individual differences that I will discuss in the final section, but first we need to consider the disabled readers' correlations between verbal intelligence and eye movements in text.

Eye Movements and Verbal Intelligence.   The subjects were tested with the WISC-R IQ test, which includes a number of subtests. In Kaufman's (1975) factor analysis of the WISC-R, he found that four subtests formed a verbal factor (Vocabulary, Reasoning, Information, and Similarities). In the present study, an unweighted combination of scores from these verbal subtests was significantly correlated with all of the eye-movement variables in Table IV. For example, the more verbally intelligent disabled readers tended to show larger forward saccades that skipped words, and more frequent regressions (an explorer pattern). Moreover, the relation of verbal intelligence with eye movements in reading was statistically independent from the relations with orthographic coding and phonetic spelling. Removing variance in eye movements associated with either one of these tasks did not significantly reduce the remaining variance associated with verbal intelligence. Entry of both orthographic coding and verbal intelligence in a regression model resulted in a multiple R of .7, predicting 49% of the variance on the plodder-explorer dimension!

What is the basis for the eye-movement correlations with verbal intelligence? Verbal intelligence correlated positively with orthographic coding ($r = .21, p < .1$), negatively with phonetic spelling rating ($r = -.35, p < .05$), and negatively with phonetic coding ($r = -.23, p < .1$) in the younger disabled group when word recognition was partialed out. This suggests that the more verbally intelligent subjects may tend to use slightly larger processing units and less phonetic coding in these tasks. The eye-movement data suggest that the tendency to use larger processing units and less phonetic coding may be magnified when the more verbally intelligent disabled readers read text. Word decoding in text may benefit from the use of contextual information, particularly in poor readers (Perfetti and Roth 1981; Stanovich 1981). The more verbally intelligent subjects have better oral vocabularies and general reasoning abilities. Thus, they may depend more on context and their slightly stronger orthographic codes, and less on phonetic coding, when reading continuous text. Their explorer pattern of eye movements was consistent with this strategy.

The eye-movement correlations provided converging evidence that young disabled readers differ systematically in their reading and spelling processes. Several important questions about these individual differences are considered in the following section: How do these differences fit with the traditional dual-process model of reading, are there developmental differences in their expression, and what is their etiology?

Theoretical, Developmental, and Etiological Issues

Individual Differences and the Dual-Process Model

Phonetic coding in the nonword lexical decision task was strongly related to word recognition among the younger disabled subjects ($r = .61$), but it was only weakly related to individual differences in their unit of processing in reading and spelling. Recent revisions of the dual-process model allow for phonetic coding at different levels of orthographic segmentation (cf. Humphreys and Evett in press), and the level of segmentation may have been the most important individual difference within the disabled sample after reading level was controlled. In the multilevel theory described in the introduction, words and nonwords may be segmented at levels ranging from the grapheme to the whole word. Thus, some subjects might tend to derive phonetic codes for nonwords through the use of GPC rules, while others achieve equal success through the use of larger units and analogies to words in their lexion. Accuracy in the phonetic coding task may not have been very sensitive to these differences in the unit of processing. However, evidence from the other measures suggests that subjects may vary widely in their use of phonetic coding.

The use of small orthographic units in reading seems more likely to be associated with the assembly of a phonetic code for lexical access. The use of larger units or whole words could involve prelexical phonetic coding, but they also allow for direct lexical access. Subjects who have relatively good orthographic representations for whole words may be less likely to depend on prelexical phonetic coding. Mitterer (1982) has supported this hypothesis by showing that his "whole-word" poor readers were less disrupted in a lexical decision task than "recoding" poor readers when they had to count aloud during the task.

A final theoretical issue concerns the link between spelling and reading processes. Phonetic coding, orthographic coding, and eye movements were correlated with the phonetic similarity of spelling errors. While this supports a link between reading and spelling processes for some subjects, it does not imply that all subjects show this relation (or any of the other relations based on moderate correlations). A few subjects were above the mean for both phonetic spelling and orthographic coding. In the present study it was possible that these deviations from the group trends were due to error variance in the tasks, but other research has shown that there are reliable dissociations between phonetic reading and phonetic spelling in certain individuals (Ellis 1984; Frith 1980, 1984). As we will see below, the combination of large-unit reading and phonetic spelling may be more common among the older disabled readers, resulting in the weakening of the older disabled group's correlations between reading and spelling processes.

Developmental Issues

The young disabled readers showed more systematic variation in their reading-process profiles than the older disabled readers. Most of the correlations between the spelling ratings, phonetic coding, orthographic coding, and the eye-movement variables declined to lower but still significant levels for the middle age group, and most were not significant in the oldest group. Several of the declines in correlations between the youngest and oldest groups were significant by Fishers' z test. For example, the correlation between orthographic coding and the phonetic spelling ratings was $-.48$ for the youngest group and .15 for the oldest group ($p < .01$).

Two different factors may have contributed to the above declines in the correlations between different reading and spelling processes. The first factor pertains to the greater flexibility of younger disabled readers, and the second involves the increasing dominance of orthographic coding in older disabled readers.

Children in the early stages of reading development may be more susceptible to various influences that would modify their reading and spelling styles. The reading process is not yet fully automated so that different strategies could arise from relatively minor environmental and/or constitutional differences. For example, it has been shown in normal readers that the influence of teaching method on reading and spelling styles is particularly strong in the first and second grades (Barr 1974). Francis (1982) has described several case studies of normal first and second graders learning to read. The reading style differences, which Francis ascribed to subtle differences in personality and general learning style, seem similar to those observed among the present disabled readers in the 3rd and 4th grades. However, when normally developing readers are in the 3rd and 4th grades, there is less evidence for strong individual differences in reading and spelling styles. Mitterer (1982) reported that his third-grade normal readers did not show the systematic style differences that were evident in his third-grade poor readers. A similar absence of significantly related reading and spelling style differences was observed in the youngest third of the normal readers in the present study.

Francis' (1982) interesting descriptions of reading and spelling style differences among normal first- and second-graders suggests that their expression may be at least partly a function of reading level. We are currently testing a normal reading-matched control sample for the present young disabled group. We will see if these normal readers in the first and second grades express the same dimensions and range of individual differences as disabled readers in the third and fourth grades.

The second factor that may contribute to developmental changes in the patterns of individual differences is the decline in phonetic coding and the increasing dominance of orthographic coding in reading and spelling for older readers. Reitsma (1984) has shown that the use of phonetic coding in lexical access falls off sharply in normal readers by the third grade. Also, during the early grades there is a corresponding increase in children's orthographic coding in reading (Ehri 1980; Reitsma 1983). Frith (1984) has described a similar developmental shift from phonetic to orthographic codes in spelling, although she believes that most disabled readers never reach the orthographic stage in spelling. For the present group of older disabled readers, the positive direction of the correlation between orthographic coding and the similarity of spelling errors to the target word ($r = .15$ for phonetic rating, $r = .14$ for visual rating) suggests that orthographic codes may have begun to play a dominant role in spelling for some of these disabled readers. We are currently testing this hypothesis with more sensitive measures of the subjects' orthographic coding and spelling. A decline in the dependence on phonetic processes for spelling in the older disabled readers was suggested by the nonsignificant correlations between phonetic coding and the spelling error ratings (phonetic rating $r = .09$, visual rating $r = -.05$). However, these declines in the spelling correlations with phonetic coding between the youngest and oldest groups of disabled readers were not strong enough to be significant by Fishers' z test.

The older disabled readers' increased automaticity and the dominance of orthographic coding in the later grades may diminish the expression of individual differences in word decoding and spelling process profiles. However, there were highly significant correlations between the eye movement variables and verbal intelligence in the older disabled group. For example, the correlation between the plodder-explorer dimension and verbal intelligence was $r = .58$. This correlation was not significant for the reading-level matched group of younger normal readers ($r = -.08$), and the respective correlations were significantly different by Fishers' z test ($p < .01$). The variance in verbal IQ was similar within the two groups, but it may play a more important compensatory role for inadequate word decoding skills in disabled readers who are higher in verbal intelligence.

Distribution and Etiology of Individual Differences in Reading Processes

Subtypes versus Dimensions. One source of information about the origins of individual differences in reading and spelling styles is the distribution of these differences. The distinct subtype view holds that there are discontinuities in the distribution of individual differences. Boder (1973) described her dyseidetic and dysphonetic subtypes as distinctly separate syndromes with distinctly different constitutional origins. This suggests that we should see bimodal distributions in reading, spelling, and cognitive process profiles for disabled readers. In fact, none of the relevant distributions showed significant deviations from univariate normality. For the present subjects, it seems more appropriate to speak of dimensions of individual differences rather than subtypes. The normally distributed dimensions suggest that there are many factors working to influence these individual differences. Some of the possible candidates are discussed below.

Teaching Method. Several researchers have speculated that one reason for individual differences in reading and spelling styles among disabled readers is the type of instruction given to the child (Baron 1979; Kinsbourne 1982; Mitterer 1982; Vellutino 1984). Phonics approaches to teaching reading, such as the Orton-Gillingham method, tend to emphasize both GPC rules in reading and PGC rules in spelling. Whole-word approaches tend to pay less attention to these rules in reading and spelling. Unfortunately, we were not able to obtain reliable data on the approach used with each child, and there does not seem to be any evidence on the influence of teaching method in other studies of individual differences among disabled readers. Interviews with several remedial reading teachers in the Boulder area revealed a variety of approaches. Some teachers said that they tailored the balance of phonics training to the aptitudes of the child, while others favored a phonics or whole word approach. It is clear that different disabled subjects were exposed to a wide variety of teaching methods, but the specific influence of these different methods on their reading and spelling processes is unknown.

Perceptual deficits. A popular view among researchers who have described subtypes in reading disability is that there is a distinct group with perceptual deficiencies that cause their reading problem (Boder 1973; Johnson and Myklebust 1967; Lyon and Watson 1981; Pirozzolo 1979). For example, Boder has argued that deficits in visual-gestalt processes limit orthographic coding for a subtype of disabled readers (dyseidetics), who must rely on their relatively intact phonetic processes in reading. Subjects in the other subtype (dysphonetics) were presumed to be deficient in verbal skills, but intact in their perceptual processes. Boder predicted that the dyseidetic subjects would be relatively low in the performance subscale of the WISC-R, and the dysphonetic subjects would be relatively low in the verbal subscale. If Boder's (1973) hypothesis for the dyseidetic subjects is correct, we would expect to see a significant positive correlation between orthographic coding and the combined scores for perceptual tasks on the WISC-R that compromise Kaufman's (1975) perceptual factor (Picture Completion, Picture Arrangement, Block Design, and Object Assembly). There should be significant negative correlations between the subjects' perceptual scores and their phonetic coding and phonetic spelling ratings. The correlation with the plodder-explorer dimension should be positive with the WISC-R perceptual tasks. However, none of the correlations approached significance.

Two other studies have also found that there was no significant relation between Boder's diagnostic categories and different measures of perceptual processes (Hooper and Hind Note 8; van den Bos 1984). There are some disabled readers who can be distinguished by their relatively poor performance in perceptual tasks when cluster analyses are applied to the distributions (cf. Lyon and Watson 1981), but these deficits apparently have no relation to their reading or spelling styles, and they may have no direct relation to their reading disability (Benton 1984; Liberman 1984; Vellutino, 1979).

Verbal Intelligence. In contrast to perceptual intelligence, we have seen that verbal intelligence was significantly related to phonetic coding, phonetic spelling, and the plodder-explorer dimension. The pattern of correlations indicated that the more verbally intelligent disabled readers were slightly less skilled in phonetic coding, and they were much less likely to use a small-unit phonetic coding strategy when reading text, as indicated by their eye movements.

What is the reason for the trade-off between phonetic skills and verbal intelligence? One possibility is that the more verbally intelligent disabled readers paid less attention to the development of phonetic coding skills because they could rely on their higher-level verbal skills in reading. Another possibility is that verbally intelligent disabled readers tend to be more constitutionally deficient in the low-level language skills that are important for phonetic coding in reading. If we think of reading as involving several different but interacting verbal processes (Carr, Vavrus, and Brown Note 9), phonetic coding and verbal intelligence could contribute independent variance to each subject's reading ability, resulting in a trade-off between the different levels of verbal skill when reading ability is controlled. Carr et al. have reported this type of trade-off in their sample of poor readers. Also, Denckla (1977) has described several subtypes of disabled readers based on their profiles of different verbal skills.

Phonetic deficits in language processes. Mitterer (1982) has speculated that subtle differences in phonetic language skills could influence the reading styles of young disabled readers. The younger disabled readers in the present study showed a deficit in phonetic memory compared to normal readers (Olson, Davidson, Kliegl, and Davies 1984), but the memory measure was not reliable enough to provide a stable estimate of within-group differences. There does seem to be some consensus that as a group, disabled readers are deficient in their ability to deal analytically with language (see Vellutino this volume), and these deficiencies in prereaders are predictive of later reading problems (cf. Bradley and Bryant 1983). Therefore, it is important that we understand the etiology of individual differences in phonetic language skills.

Individual differences within many areas of behavior are based on an interaction between environmental and genetic influences. This is certainly true of verbal intelligence. It may also be true of the basic language skills that seem to underlie individual differences in phonetic coding. On the environmental side, several recent studies have indicated that these basic language skills may be improved by training in prereaders, resulting in their more rapid progress in learning to read (Bradley and Bryant 1983; Treiman and Baron 1983). This may be a particularly valuable aid to children at risk for reading disability.

To determine the influence of genetic factors, we are currently testing monozygotic (identical) and dyzygotic (fraternal) twins in a variety of language skills and reading processes. Preliminary analyses of the twin data show greater similarity between monozygotic twins, not only for general reading ability (see Decker and Vandenberg this volume), but also for individual differences in reading and language profiles *among* disabled readers. For example, in a phoneme segmentation task, the monozygotic twin correlation was $r = .78$ (N = 12 pairs), while the dyzygotic twin correlation was $r = .24$ (N = 17 pairs). Twin correlations for several eye-movement variables also suggested the influence of genetic factors. The proportion of forward saccades correlated at $r = .72$ (N = 23 pairs) for monozygotic twins and $r = .39$ (N = 22 pairs) for dyzygotic twins. These are partial correlations, with twin differences in word recognition being controlled. The samples are still too small to make reliable heritability estimates, but the preliminary results indicate that genetic factors have a significant influence on reading and language profiles within the disabled group.

Summary and Conclusions

Evaluation of the component processes in reading and spelling revealed that as a group, disabled readers were deficient in phonetic coding and phonetic spelling. These deficits were significant even when older disabled and younger normal groups were matched in word recognition. In contrast, orthographic coding in reading and the visual or orthographic aspects of spelling were not significantly different for normal and disabled groups matched in word recognition. This result indicates that most disabled readers in the present large sample suffered from a qualitative phonetic deficit in reading and spelling, rather than a general developmental lag in all component reading and spelling processes.

The componential analyses of reading and spelling processes also revealed significant differences within the disabled sample when word recognition was statistically controlled. The primary dimension of within-group differences was based on processing-unit size and the use of phonetic codes in reading and spelling. These individual differences were most salient among the younger disabled readers.

Analyses of the disabled readers' eye movements in text revealed patterns that were consistent with individual differences in the other reading and spelling tasks. In addition, there was a strong and independent relation between eye-movement patterns and verbal intelligence. The more verbally intelligent disabled readers displayed eye-movement patterns indicating their use of larger processing units and less phonetic coding. Also, there appeared to be a trade off between phonetic skills and the high-level language skills measured in four of the WISC-R verbal subtests.

Several factors were considered regarding the etiology of the group and within-group differences for disabled readers. A number of studies have pointed to underlying linguistic deficits in disabled readers and in pre-readers who are likely to become reading disabled. The relative contribution of environmental and genetic influences on these language deficits is not known. In the second phase of our research program, we are currently testing twins and families in a variety of language processes, in addition to the reading processes described in this chapter. Heritability analyses will reveal the balance of genetic and environmental influences in these reading and language processes.

The present findings of developmental and individual differences in reading and spelling processes raise important questions about the appropriate remediation and long term prognosis for individual disabled readers. We have seen that phonetic coding deficits place severe constraints on reading level in the younger subjects, but some of the older subjects achieved relatively high levels of word recognition, even though their phonetic coding skills remained quite low. Conversely, some of the older subjects with relatively good phonetic coding were relatively low in word recognition. We need to learn much more about the factors that lead to success in some disabled readers and continued failure in others. Longitudinal follow up studies are needed to obtain this information (see Satz this volume). In our current research, we are retesting the younger subjects who were tested in the first phase of the project. It will be interesting to see how their reading process and cognitive profiles relate to improvement in reading ability with age.

The bottom line for basic research on reading disability is its ultimate contribution to prediction and remediation efforts. Initial attempts at training disabled readers in analytic language processes have shown beneficial effects on reading skills. But reading skills must also be taught, and there is no clear consensus on the optimal methods. To the extent that disabled readers' phonetic coding and related language skills are uniquely deficient, simply intensifying or extending the approaches used with normal readers may not be optimal. Current remediation approaches for disabled readers seem to break down into intensive training in the deficit (usually phonics), versus an emphasis on the stronger process (usually orthographic coding). We have seen several disabled readers whose intense training in phonics seemed to have led to little improvement in their reading. But other disabled readers may show significant gains from phonics instruction. A major conclusion from the present study is that disabled readers vary in their reading and language process profiles. Choices of the optimal teaching method for each disabled reader should be guided by a better understanding of these individual differences.

Reference Notes

1. Davidson, B. J., Olson, R. K., and Kliegl, R. Reading-process profiles in disabled and normal readers: Group and within-group differences. Manuscript in preparation for publication.

2. Siegel, L. S., and Ryan, E. B. Development of grammatical sensitivity and phonological skills in normally achieving and learning disabled children. Manuscript submitted for publication, 1984.
3. Seidenberg, M. S., Bruck, M., Fornarlo, G., and Backman, J. Word recognition skills of poor and disabled readers: Do they differ? Manuscript submitted for publication, 1984.
4. Treiman, R., and Hirsh-Pasek, K. Are there qualitative differences in reading behavior between dyslexics and normal readers? Manuscript submitted for publication, 1984.
5. Camp, B. W., and McCabe, L. Denver reading and spelling test. Unpublished manuscript, University of Colorado Medical Center, 1977.
6. Pennington, B. F., McCabe, L. L., Smith, S. D., Lefly, D. L., Bookman, M. O., Kimberling, W. J., and Lubs, H. A. Spelling errors in adults with a form of familial dyslexia. Manuscript submitted for publication, 1984.
7. Kliegl, R., Olson, R. K., and Davidson, B. J. Eye movements in disabled and normal readers: Group and within-group differences. Manuscript in preparation for publication.
8. Hooper, S. R., and Hynd, G. W. Differential diagnosis of developmental dyslexia with the Kaufman assessment battery for children (K-ABC). Manuscript submitted for publication, 1984.
9. Carr, T. H., Vavrus, L. G., and Brown, T. L. Cognitive skill maps of reading ability. Paper presented at the AERA meeting, Montreal, Quebec, 1983.

References

Backman, J., Bruck, M., Hebert, M., and Seidenberg, M. S. (in press). Acquisition and use of spelling-sound correspondences in reading. *Journal of Experimental Child Psychology.*

Baddeley, A. D., Ellis, N. C., Miles, T. R., and Lewis, V. J. 1982. Developmental and acquired dyslexia: A comparison. *Cognition* 11:185–199.

Baron, J. 1977. Mechanisms for pronouncing printed words: Use and acquisition. *In* D. LaBerge and S. J. Samuels. *Basic Processes in Reading: Perception and Comprehension.* Hillsdale, NJ: Lawrence Erlbaum Associates.

Baron, J. 1979. Orthographic and word specific mechanisms in childrens' reading of words. *Child Development* 50:60–72.

Barr, R. 1974. The effect of instruction on pupil reading strategies. *Reading Research Quarterly* 10:552–582.

Beech, J. R., and Harding, L. M. 1984. Phonemic processing and the poor reader from a developmental lag viewpoint. *Reading Research Quarterly* 19:357–366.

Benton, A. L. 1984. Dyslexia and spatial thinking. *Annals of Dyslexia* 34:69–85.

Boder, E. 1973. Developmental dyslexia: A diagnostic approach based on three atypical reading-spelling patterns. *Developmental Medicine and Child Neurology* 15:663–687.

Boder E., and Jarrico, S. 1982. *The Boder Test of Reading-Spelling Patterns: A Diagnostic Screening Test for Subtypes of Reading Disability.* New York: Grune & Stratton.

Bradley, L., and Bryant, P. E. 1978. Difficulties in auditory organization as a possible cause of reading backwardness. *Nature* 271:746–747.

Bradley, L., and Bryant, P. 1981. Visual memory and phonological skills in reading and spelling backwardness. *Psychological Research* 43:193–199.

Bradley, L., and Bryant, P. 1983. Categorizing sounds and learning to read, a causal connection. *Nature* 301:419–421.

Carr, T. H. 1981. Building theories of reading ability: On the relation between individual differences in cognitive skills and reading comprehension. *Cognition* 9:73–114.

Coltheart, M. 1978. Lexical access in simple reading tasks. *In* G. Underwood (ed.). *Strategies in Information Processing.* London: Academic Press.

Crowder, R. G. 1982. *The Psychology of Reading.* New York: Oxford University Press.

Denckla, M. B. 1977. Minimal brain dysfunction and dyslexia: Beyond diagnosis by exclusion. *In* M. E. Blaw, I. Rapin, and M. Kinsbourne (eds.). *Topics in Child Neurology.* New York: Spectrum Publications.

Denckla, M. B. 1979. Childhood learning disabilities. *In* K. Heilman and E. Valenstein (eds.). *Clinical Neuropsychology.* New York: Oxford University Press.

Doehring, D. G. 1984. Subtyping of reading disorders: Implications for remediation. *Annals of Dyslexia* 34:205–216.

Ehri, L. C. 1980. The role of orthographic images in learning printed words. *In* J. F. Kavanagh and R. L. Venezky (eds.). *Orthography, Reading, and Dyslexia.* Baltimore: University Park Press.

Ellis, A. W. 1984. *Reading, Writing and Dyslexia: A Cognitive Analysis.* London: Lawrence Erlbaum Associates.

Ellis, N. C., and Miles, T. R. 1981. A lexical encoding deficiency I: Experimental evidence. *In* G. Th. Pavlidis and T. R. Miles (eds.). *Dyslexia Research and its Applications to Education.* London: John Wiley.

Finucci, J. M., Isaacs, S. D., Whitehouse, C. C., and Childs, B. 1983. Classification of spelling errors and their relationships to reading ability, sex, grade placement, and intelligence. *Brain and Language* 20:340–355.

Firth, I. 1972. *Components of reading disability.* Unpublished doctoral dissertation, University of New South Wales, Kensington, N.S.W., Australia.

Fox, B., and Routh, D. K. 1980. Phonemic analysis and severe reading disability in children. *Journal of Psycholinguistic Research* 9:115–119.

Frith, U. 1980. Unexpected spelling problems. *In* Frith, U. (ed.). *Cognitive Processes in Spelling.* London: Academic Press.

Frith, U. 1981. Experimental approaches to developmental dyslexia: An introduction. *Psychological Research* 43:97–109.

Frith, U. 1984. Beneath the surface of developmental dyslexia. *In* Patterson, K., Marshal, J., and Coltheart, M. (eds.). *Surface Dyslexia.* London: Lawrence Erlbaum Associates.

Glushko, R. J. 1979. The organization and activation of orthographic knowledge in reading aloud. *Journal of Experimental Psychology: Human Perception and Performance* 5:674–691.

Hanna, P. R., Hanna, J. S., Hodges, R. E., and Rudorf, E. H. 1966. *Phoneme-Grapheme Correspondences as Cues to Spelling Improvement.* Washington, DC: U.S. Department of Health, Education, and Welfare.

Henderson, L. 1982. *Orthography and Word Recognition in Reading.* New York: Academic Press.

Henderson, L., and Chard, M. J. 1980. The reader's implicit knowledge of orthographic structure. *In* U. Frith (ed.). *Cognitive Processes in Spelling* London: Academic Press.

Huey, E. B. 1908. *The Psychology and Pedagogy of Reading.* Reprinted 1968. Cambridge, MA: MIT Press.

Humphreys, G. W., and Evett, L. J. (in press) Are there independent lexical and nonlexical routes in word processing? An evaluation of the dual route theory of reading. *The Brain and Behavioral Sciences.*

Ingram, T. T. S., Mason, A. W., and Blackburn, I. 1970. A retrospective study of 82 children with reading disability. *Developmental Medicine and Child Neurology.* 12:271–281.

Johnson, D. J., and Myklebust, H. 1967. *Learning Disabilities: Educational Principles and Practices.* New York: Grune & Stratton.

Kaufman, A. S. 1975. Factor analysis of the WISC-R at eleven age levels between 6½ and 16½ years. *Journal of Consulting and Clinical Psychology* 43:135–147.

Kinsbourne, M. 1982. The role of selective attention in reading disability. *In* R. N. Malatesha and P. G. Aaron (eds.). *Reading Disorders: Varieties and Treatments.* New York: Academic Press.

Kleiman, G. M. 1975. Speech recoding in reading. *Journal of Verbal Learning and Verbal Behavior* 14:323–339.

Kochnower, J., Richardson, E., and DiBenedetto, B. 1983. A comparison of the phonic decoding ability of normal and learning disabled children. *Journal of Learning Disabilities* 16:348–351.

Liberman, I. Y. 1973. Segmentation of the spoken word and reading acquisition. *Bulletin of the Orton Society* 23:65–77.

Liberman, I. Y. 1984. Should so-called modality preferences determine the nature of instruction for children with reading disabilities? *In* F. Duffy and N. Geschwind (eds.). *Dyslexia: Current Status and Future Directions.* Boston: Little, Brown, & Company.

Liberman, I. Y. 1985. A language-oriented view of reading and its disabilities. *Thalamus* Journal of the International Academy of Research in Learning Disabilities.

Lyon, R. and Watson, B. 1981. Empirically derived subgroups of learning disabled readers: Diagnostic characteristics. *Journal of Learning Disabilities* 14:256–261.

Massaro, D. W. and Venezky, R. L. 1983. Orthography and word recognition in reading. *American Journal of Psychology* 4:584–587.

Mattis, S. 1978. Dyslexia syndromes: A working hypothesis that works. *In* A. L. Benton and D. Pearl (eds.). *Dyslexia: An Appraisal of Current Knowledge.* New York: Oxford University Press.

McCusker, L. X., Hillinger, M. L., and Bias, R. G. 1981. Phonological recoding and reading. *Psychological Bulletin* 89:217–245.

McKinney, J. D. 1984. The search for subtypes of specific learning disability. *Journal of Learning Disabilities* 17:43–50.

Miles, T. R. 1983. *Dyslexia: The Pattern of Difficulties.* London: Granada.

Mitterer, J. O. 1982. There are at least two kinds of poor readers: Whole-word poor readers and recoding poor readers. *Canadian Journal of Psychology* 36:445–461.

Olson, R. K., Kliegl, R., and Davidson, B. J. 1983a. Eye movements in reading disability. *In* K. Rayner (ed.). *Eye Movements in Reading: Perceptual and Language Processes.* New York: Academic Press.

Olson, R. K., Kliegl, R., and Davidson, B. J. 1983b. Dyslexic and normal readers' eye movements. *Journal of Experimental Psychology: Human Perception and Performance* 9:816–825.

Olson, R. K., Davidson, B. J., Kliegl, R., and Davies, S. E. 1984. Development of phonetic memory in disabled and normal readers. *Journal of Experimental Child Psychology* 37:187–206.

Olson, R. K., Kliegl, R., Davidson, B. J., and Foltz, G. 1985. Individual and developmental differences in reading disabilities. *In* G. E. MacKinnon and T. G. Waller (eds.). *Reading Research: Advances in Theory and Practice, Vol. 4.* New York: Academic Press.

Olson, R. K., and Keenan, J. M. (in press). Segmentation in models of reading. *The Behavioral and Brain Sciences.*

Pavlidis, G. Th. 1981. Do eye movements hold the key to dyslexia? *Neuropsychologia* 19:57–64.

Pavlidis, G. Th. 1985. Eye movements in dyslexia: Their diagnostic significance. *Journal of Learning Disabilities* 18:42–50.

Perfetti, C. A., and McCutchen, D. 1982. Speech processes in reading. *Speech and Language: Advances in Basic Research and Practice, Vol. 7.*

Perfetti, C. A., and Roth, S. 1981. Some of the interactive processes in reading and their role in reading skill. *In* A. M. Lesgold and C. Perfetti (eds.). *Interactive Processes in Reading.* Hillsdale, N.J.: Lawrence Erlbaum Associates.

Pirozzolo, F. J. 1979. *The Neuropsychology of Developmental Reading Disorders.* New York: Praeger.

Reitsma, P. 1983. Printed word learning in beginning readers. *Journal of Experimental Child Psychology* 36:321–339.

Reitsma, P. 1984. Sound priming in beginning readers. *Child Development* 55 (2):406–423.

Rudel, R. G. 1981. Residual effects of childhood reading disabilities. *Bulletin of the Orton Society* 31:89–102.

Satz, P., and Morris, R., 1981. Learning disability subtypes: A review. *In* F. J. Pirozzolo and M. C. Wittrock (eds.). *Neuropsychological and Cognitive Processes in Reading.* New York: Academic Press.

Seymour, P. H. K., and Porpodas, C. D., 1980. Lexical and nonlexical processing of spelling in dyslexia. *In* U. Frith (ed.). *Cognitive Processes in Spelling.* London: Academic Press.

Shallice, T., Warrington, E. K., and McCarthy, R. 1983. Reading without semantics. *Quarterly Journal of Experimental Psychology* 35A:111–138.

Simon, D. P., and Simon, H. A. 1973. Alternative uses of phonemic information in spelling. *Review of Educational Research* 43:115–137.

Singer, M. H. 1980. The primacy of visual information in the analysis on letter strings. *Perception and Psychophysics* 27:153–162.

Snowling, M. J. 1980. The development of grapheme-phoneme correspondence in normal and dyslexic readers. *Journal of Experimental Child Psychology* 29:294–305.

Snowling, M. J. 1981. Phonemic deficits in developmental dyslexia. *Psychological Research* 43:219–234.

Spache, G. D. 1963. *Diagnostic Reading Scales.* Monterey: McGraw Hill.

Stanovich, K. E. 1981. Attentional and automatic context effects in reading. *In* A. M. Lesgold and C. Perfetti (eds.). *Interactive Processes in Reading.* Hillsdale, N.J.: Lawrence Erlbaum Associates.

Tinker, M. A. 1958. Recent studies of eye movements in reading. *Psychological Bulletin* 55:215–231.

Treiman, R. 1984. Individual differences among children in spelling and reading styles. *Journal of Experimental Child Psychology.*

Treiman, R., and Baron, J. 1983. Phonemic-analysis training helps children benefit from spelling-sound rules. *Memory & Cognition* 11:382–389.

van den Bos, K. P. 1984. Letter span, scanning, and code matching in dyslexic subgroups. *Annals of Dyslexia* 34:179–193.

Vellutino, F. R. 1979. *Dyslexia: Theory and Research*. Cambridge, MA: M.I.T. Press.

Vellutino, F. R. 1984. Theoretical issues in the study of word recognition: The unit of perception controversy reexamined. *In* S. Rosenberg (ed.). *Handbook of Applied Psycholinguistics,* Hillsdale, N.J.: Lawrence Erlbaum Associates.

Venezky, R. L. 1970. *The Structure of English Orthography*. Mouton.

Venezky, R. L., and Massara, D. W. 1979. The Role of Orthographic Regularity in Word Recognition. *In* L. Resnick and P. Weaver (eds.). *Theory and Practice of Early Reading*. Hillsdale, N.J. Lawrence Erlbaum Associates.

15

Eye Movement Techniques in Studying Differences Among Developing Readers

George W. McConkie and David Zola

*R*esearch on reading tends to be divided between studies that directly investigate reading itself and studies that investigate the relationship between reading performance and other variables, such as characteristics of the readers or their performance on tasks thought to be related to reading in particular ways. The goal of research that directly investigates the reading process is to understand the nature of the perceptual and language processing taking place; the deployment of attention to the text; the information being acquired; and the way that information is being represented in the mind. In research that investigates these issues in real time where people are studied as they actually engage in reading, eye movement monitoring plays a critical role.

There are three different ways in which eye movement recording can be involved in studying reading. Many studies employ more than one of these techniques. First, monitoring the eyes yields an eye movement record that can be a rich source of data. The eyes pause longer on some words than on others, they move various distances and directions between pauses, and they exhibit patterns of movements that can indicate what is being attended at different moments, what kinds of processing are taking place, and when processing difficulties arise. Second, the eyes can be monitored as a basis for analyzing simultaneously collected data, such as brain wave records or oral reading protocols. Third, on-line eye movement information can be used to exert experimental control over aspects of the stimulus or of response recording devices. Our own work has focused primarily on this last use of eye movement

The research reported in this paper was supported by the National Institute of Child Health and Human Development under Grant No. HD18116 to the authors, and by the National Institute of Education under Contract No. 400-81-0030 to the Center for the Study of Reading. The authors wish to express appreciation to Nancy R. Bryant, Harry E. Blanchard, and Patricia Greenan for their research assistance, and Open Court Publishing Company (La Salle, Illinois), for permission to use passages for this research from their Headway reading series.

monitoring; much of it involves eye movement contingent display changes that are made during reading as a means of studying the perceptual processes. All of these techniques are useful in studying the nature of the processing that takes place during reading and the processing differences that exist among readers.

Eye Movement Records as a Source of Data

Eye movement behavior itself is a part of the act of reading. Furthermore, there is increasing evidence that characteristics of the eyes' behavior relate to characteristics of the mental processing taking place (see reviews by Levy-Schoen and O'Regan 1979; McConkie 1983; Rayner, 1978). Thus, eye movement records can be examined either in an attempt to understand the nature of eye movement control, or, by making assumptions about eye movement control, to understand the mental processes that were taking place. In so doing, it is possible to focus either on the discrete components of the eye movement record, that is, on individual eye fixations and saccadic movements, or on the patterns present in sequences of fixations and saccades.

Individual Components of the Eye Movement Record

Eye movement records taken during reading are usually reduced to two components, i.e., fixations and saccades. The record then indicates where in the text the eyes were directed during each fixation, how long they remained at that location, and where they were sent next. In early eye movement studies (Buswell 1937; Huey 1908), these data were further reduced to indicate the mean duration of fixations, the mean saccade length, and the frequency of regressive movements for different groups of readers. It was found that these measures differed by grade and ability levels. Typically, better readers showed shorter fixations, longer saccades, and fewer regressive movements (Taylor 1965). These same trends were also found when text difficulty was reduced (Patberg and Yonas 1978; Walker 1933).

While these trends have been documented for several decades, their significance for understanding reading is not yet understood. For this purpose, it is necessary to become more analytical in our description of the eye movement data. To accomplish this goal, we have collected eye movement data from nine third graders as they read an entire children's novel. The eye movement records contained between 12,000 and 25,000 fixations per child. Data from four of these children, whose independent reading test scores range from 11 months above grade level to 12 months below, according to the Woodcock Reading Mastery Tests (Woodcock 1973), will be used here to illustrate characteristics of children's eye movements during reading.

Durations of Fixations. The termination of a fixation is the result of a decision that it is time to move the eyes to a new location. Figure 1 presents the frequency distributions of fixation durations for four of our young readers. While there is a difference in the mean fixation duration for these students, and this varies directly with their reading ability level, the most impressive charac-

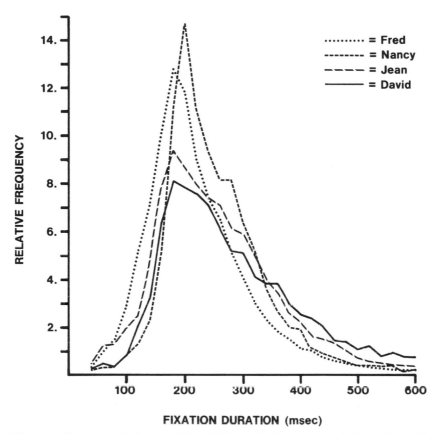

Figure 1.   Frequency distribution of four children's fixation durations during reading. All
fixations were preceded by a forward saccade.

teristics are the great amount of within-subject variability and the great amount
of overlap among the distributions. The small observed differences in the
means, while harmonious with previous findings, are not especially illuminat-
ing about the nature of these differences.

From a processing perspective, the duration of a fixation is the time that
passes from the beginning of that fixation until a decision to move the eyes is
executed. The distribution of fixation durations results from the differences in
the time when this decision is made and when it is executed for different
fixations. From this perspective, it is possible to describe these frequency
distributions in a rather different way. By dividing time into intervals, it is
possible to calculate for each interval the proportion of those fixations entering
the interval that terminated during that interval. The resulting curve is similar to
those used in survival analysis (Miller 1981). For each time period included,
the curve indicates the proportion of the surviving fixations which terminated
during that period. Figure 2 presents curves of this type for the four children
studied.

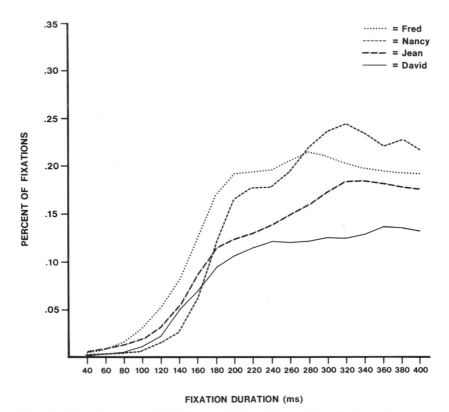

Figure 2.   Smoothed curves which indicate the likelihood that surviving fixations will terminate
            during different time intervals following the onset of the fixation. These four curves
            are derived from the same data used in Figure 1.

Figure 2 indicates that the likelihood of fixations terminating within the first 80 msec is very low; this likelihood then rises rather quickly and levels off to some degree about 180 msec after the onset of the fixation. While the distributions for these four children begin to rise and to decelerate at slightly different intervals, the primary difference among them is in the maximum level attained. That maximum is much lower for the poorest reader in our group, David, which results in more fixations continuing for longer periods of time, including many that last for 500 msec or more. Of course, the interesting question, and the one which we cannot answer at present, concerns what it is about the nature of the processing that leads one of these children to continue his fixations for so much more time than the others. Does this simply reflect the greater amount of time required by David to accomplish the mental processing that is required at most points in the text? And if so, what aspects of the processing are requiring this additional time? Equally intriguing is the question of why each of these children sometimes terminates a fixation after only 100 msec or less and sometimes continues it for 500 msec or more. Certainly this must be related to the nature of the processing taking place at different locations in the text. However, current evidence indicates that there is not a simple relationship between the duration of a fixation and the amount of time required to process the information acquired during that fixation (Hogaboam 1983; McConkie, Underwood, Zola, and Wolverton in press). Studies with adult readers do show longer fixations on unusual words (Just and Carpenter 1980; Kliegl, Olson, and Davidson 1983; Rayner 1977), words with spelling errors (Zola in press), and words for which there is less contextual constraint (Ehrlich and Rayner 1981; Zola in press). Similar studies have not yet been conducted with developing readers.

In research with adult readers we have found that fixations with a duration of less than 140 msec are too short to be affected by the information being perceived during those fixations. Thus, these fixations are being terminated by decisions based on previously acquired information. It is interesting that the number of short fixations of the four children studied are quite different, ranging from 5% to 25% of all fixations made. It seems likely that this is also an indicator of some not-yet-understood aspect of processing during reading.

Direction and Length of Saccades.   Every fixation is terminated by a saccadic eye movement that takes the eyes to some new location in the text. Figure 3 presents the frequency distributions of saccades of different directions and lengths for the four children studied.

These distributions are strikingly different from those of skilled adult readers in three ways. First, these children show many more regressive eye movements than adult readers do. In the data from Jean, Fred and David, 35% of all saccades are regressive, as compared to 20% for a group of college students recently studied. Second, there are many more short saccades in the children's data. For the same three children, nearly 40% of all saccades are less than 3.5 character positions in length. (In our eye movement monitoring system, four character positions occupy one degree of visual angle.) This could reflect a necessity for children to deal with smaller segments of text on each fixation, a difficulty in coordinating visual input and language processing aspects of reading, or some other factor.

The data presented in Figure 3 also indicates how children of the same age can differ in their eye movement characteristics. The saccade length distributions of one child, Nancy, are very different from those of the other three, and are quite similar to those of adults. Interestingly enough, this student is not particularly advanced in her reading ability, as indicated by the Woodcock test, on which she scores close to her grade level.

It is the nature of overall distributions of saccade lengths, such as those presented in Figure 3, that they cannot indicate the factors that lead to the variance observed. This requires a further breakdown of the data. One example of such a breakdown is shown in Figure 4. Figure 4a shows the distribution of saccade length and direction for two of the children, Jean and Fred, following all fixations in which the eyes were centered on the first letter of a six-letter word. The two curves are very similar, and differ greatly in shape from those in Figure 3. These curves seem to show three modes: one corresponding to a return to the prior word, another corresponding to refixations of the same word (with the 3rd letter of the word being the most probable location), and the third

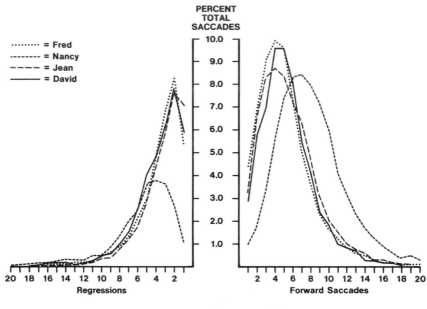

Figure 3.　Frequency distributions of the lengths of four children's forward and regressive saccades.

corresponding to fixations on the following word (with the eyes tending to go to one of the initial letters). This clearly suggests different mental states of the reader leading to the different alternative eye movement outcomes.

Figure 4b shows comparable distributions for a slightly different condition for two children, Jean and Nancy. In this case, their eyes were centered on the 3rd letter of a 6-letter word, rather than on the 1st letter. A comparison of Jean's data in Figures 4a and 4b shows a striking contrast. In Figure 4b, the likelihood of refixating the word is greatly reduced and the predominant tendency is to move the eyes to the following word. Fred, whose data are not shown here, again shows a very similar pattern. In contrast, Nancy's data are presented. This is the child who shows a more adult-like pattern. While she also shows the same preference for making a saccade to the next word, in other respects her distribution is quite different. Most notably, she is much less likely to refixate the same word. Apparently one of the differences between Nancy and the rest of the children lies in her ability to identify a word of this size on a single fixation.

These few examples serve to illustrate the fact that, buried in the saccade length data of children is a great deal of detail which is useful in detecting individual differences among readers and in suggesting some of the bases for these differences.

Eye Movement Patterns

The examples given so far deal with the eye movement data at a molecular level, that is, the analysis of individual fixations and saccades. The next level of

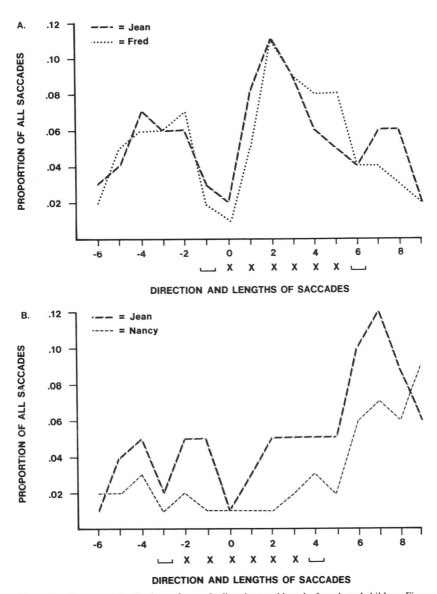

Figure 4.   Frequency distributions of saccade directions and lengths for selected children. Figure
4a compares the distributions for Jean and Fred for saccades which follow fixations
centered on the first letter of a 6-letter word. Figure 4b compares the distributions for
Jean and Nancy for saccades following fixations on the third letter of a 6-letter word.

complexity involves the examination of sequences of fixations and saccades in
terms of their pattern. This is more difficult because eye movement behavior
can be so variable. However, Frazier and Rayner (1982) were able to demonstrate that readers responded differently at different times when they encountered difficulties in reading garden path sentences (e.g., *The horse raced
past the barn fell*). Furthermore, no subjects exhibited one pattern that had been

expected. At a still more global level, Olson and his co-workers have found that when children are grouped by overall eye movement pattern, indexed as the ratio of regressive to forward saccades, the groups show differences on other tests as well, indicating differences in their general reading strategies (see Chapter 14 in this volume).

The fact that eye movement patterns are different at different places in the text, and for different subjects, is obvious as one peruses the data. So far, only minimal progress has been made in classifying these patterns and relating them to the mental processes that give rise to them. We do not know, for instance, what processing differences lead a reader to make multiple fixations on one difficult word prior to proceeding forward, and then to fixate another similar word only once before going on and later returning to the word for additional fixations.

Further Comments

It is our assumption that what children do with their eyes as they read, reflects the way they are attending to the text. This oculomotor behavior is, in turn, assumed to reflect both the nature of the processing of visual information and the child's ability to coordinate the controlling processes necessary to provide the information as it is needed. If these assumptions are accurate, then detailed explorations of eye movement patterns will give clues to processing differences that are taking place.

Eye movement data have been particularly useful in indicating whether experimental manipulations of the text, or of the manner of text presentation, are disruptive to on-going reading processes. A careful comparison of the eye movement data resulting from a control and an experimental condition can indicate whether the experimental manipulation involved caused a disruption in reading, and if so, just when this disruption occurred. The data can also suggest how the reader responded to the disruptive influence. Thus, eye movement data are useful both in studies in which the eye movements themselves are the primary focus of interest and in studies in which the eye movement record is used as an indicator of the effects of manipulations of other aspects of reading.

In almost all reading research involving eye movement monitoring, a single eye has been monitored. There are no studies in which highly accurate equipment has been used to monitor simultaneously the activities of both eyes during reading. This is important to note, since claims have been made that some reading disorders have at their base a failure to properly coordinate the movements of the two eyes during reading (Bedwell, Grant, and McKeown 1980; Taylor 1966). It is possible that our history of monocular eye monitoring is a critical limitation on current research in the field, blinding us to an important causative factor in reading disorders. On the other hand, it may be that with adequate equipment we would learn that lack of binocular coordination is an extremely rare source of reading difficulty. Clearly, research is needed on this issue, but it must be done with high precision equipment. Only by having two eyetrackers that have nearly identical dynamic characteristics can we be sure that coordination failures are true differences between what the eyes are doing, rather than differences in the characteristics of the eye movement monitors themselves. Considering the high cost of precision equipment and the added difficulty of adjusting, not one, but two eyetrackers, such research will be both expensive and painstaking.

Eye Movement Data as a Basis for Analyzing Other Data

A second use of eye movement records is as a basis for analyzing other, concurrently-collected data. Our laboratory is initiating a study which will use EEG data to investigate questions of processing at certain locations in the text. This research will involve the use of evoked potentials, that is, the Average Evoked Response technique. This technique requires that a subject encounter a particular situation a number of times, with brain waves being recorded during each. These EEG data from the different trials are then averaged by beginning at some known time, typically the onset of the stimulus, and then taking the average of the data samples across different trials at successive points in time, perhaps every 20 msec. The resulting averaged curve shows the characteristics of the brain signal that are common to the series of trials with transient characteristics of the individual trials removed. This is known as an Average Evoked Response, or sometimes referred to as an Event Related Potential. Such curves can be obtained from different conditions and then compared in order to study the characteristics of the brain processes in these conditions (Donchin 1984).

We plan to take a similar approach to studying ongoing processing during reading. EEG data will be recorded simultaneously with eye movements as the subject reads. It will then be possible to identify fixations that occur at particular locations in the text (for example, on particular words of interest) and the EEG data can be averaged as described above, beginning when the eye movement data indicate that the fixation began. In addition, the eye movement record can be used to select EEG data recorded during the execution of eye movements. This data can be similarly averaged in order to identify the brain signal that accompanies such eye movements. For some purposes, this signal can then be subtracted from the EEG data as a means of reducing artifacts produced by eye movements.

This technique may indicate how soon brain processes of different types are initiated after the visual stimulus is encountered. It may also indicate the areas of the brain that are involved in different processing.

Another example of the simultaneous collection of two types of ongoing data would be to monitor both eye movements and voice during oral reading. In this way, the time of vocalization of words can be related to the time the words are fixated. In addition, the eye movement data may clarify the mental activities and strategies that result in vocalizations as a beginning reader attempts to identify and say a novel word.

Thus, in any study in which recordings are made continuously of some aspect of the reader's behavior, and in which it is necessary to select those parts of the data record that correspond to the reading of a particular part of the text, eye movement records can provide a basis for this data selection. In addition, the eye movement record may also yield information about the nature of the reading processes taking place at the different points of interest in the text which can help specify how the data taken in parallel should be analyzed.

Use for Real-time Experimental Control

A third use of eye movement data is for real-time experimental control in studies of on-going reading. While there are other possible examples of potential research of this type, we will focus on research involving eye movement contingent display control.

In this research, the reader's eye movements are monitored while reading from computer-controlled text displays. Using this arrangement, it is possible to program the computer to make changes in the text display as it is being read, contingent upon the behavior of the eyes. Thus, the computer can change the display as the eyes are moving from one location to another so that the stimulus pattern present during one fixation is different than it was during the last. This ability to control the nature of the stimulus pattern that is present on any given fixation during reading provides a powerful technique for studying the perceptual processes that are taking place. We will illustrate this paradigm by describing two recent studies that have been conducted in our laboratory, and two other studies that are in progress.

The Perceptual Span of Children During Reading

In order to investigate the size of the region within which letter distinctions are being used during a fixation in reading, Underwood and Zola (1985) conducted a study using the technique originated by McConkie and Rayner (1975). Two versions of each line of text were stored in the computer's memory, one being the original line and the second being a line in which each letter had been replaced by a different letter. These will be referred to as the original line and the replacement line. The original line was initially displayed on the screen. However, on selected fixations as the child read, parts of it were replaced by parts of the replacement line. This manipulation was made in such a way that the text in the region where the eyes were centered on that fixation was from the original line, and text outside this region was from the replacement line, as shown in Figure 5. In one experiment, the region of normal text (referred to as the *window*) was made to be of different sizes in order to determine how large the region is within which young readers distinguish among letters while reading. It was assumed that if the window were smaller than the region within which letter information was used, then erroneous letters of the replacement text would be perceived during that fixation. Perceiving incorrect letters would interfere with normal word processing, resulting in disruptions which would be revealed in the eye movement pattern. Thus, the experiment was designed to see how small the window could be made without

Original Line

    One of the few stories about a cat saving someone happened

Replacement Line

    Zen ui hf n inx rhusbnr mluoh m vmh rmcbey ruanuen fmjjnent

Contingent Display Line

    Zen ui hf n inx rhusies about a cat sacbey ruanuen fmjjnent

Figure 5.   An example of a line of text showing how it might appear when parts of the Original
Line are replaced by parts of the Replacement Line contingent on the location of the
eyes on that fixation. The arrow (ˆ) indicates the letter where the eyes are centered.

causing a disruption in reading. This would give an estimate of the region within which letter distinctions were made during reading.

In our study, two groups of fifth-grade children were used: one group reading at or above grade level, and one group reading below, mostly at the third-grade level. The results indicated that there was no difference between the two groups on this measure. Thus, differences in their perceptual spans were not involved in their difference in reading ability.

Further research of this type needs to be carried out with younger and with more seriously disabled readers, examining individual differences in this aspect of reading.

Combining Information Across Fixation

In a second study using third-grade children, we investigated the visual images obtained on successive fixations during reading to see if they are integrated into a single image in the brain. This was done using a technique from an earlier study with adult readers (McConkie and Zola 1979). The text to be read was presented in AlTeRnAtInG cAsE, with every other letter capitalized. During certain eye movements, the case of every letter was changed, so that for the next fixation the shape of every letter and of every word would be different than it had been during the last fixation. An example is shown in Figure 6. We postulated that if the visual images from successive fixations are being integrated into a single image, the images from these two fixations would not fit together and, thus, the perceptual process would be disrupted. The results were similar to those found earlier with adults, in that the experimental manipulation produced no evidence of a disruption in their eye movement records. Thus, there was no evidence for a disruption of the ongoing reading process. However, whereas none of the adults were consciously aware of the change being made, a few of the children gave an indication that they had noticed that something was happening as they read. When they were interviewed after the experiment, some reported seeing flashes. One child was even able to describe the manipulation: "All the little letters changed to big letters, and all the big letters changed to little ones."

This study was originally conducted in order to investigate the possibility that, although people may integrate visual images across fixations while viewing non-textual stimuli, in learning to read they learn to deal with the stimulus pattern in a different way, using it as a source of linguistic information rather than as a picture to be perceived. One implication of this change, we thought, might be the elimination of the across-fixation integration. The fact that some children did seem to be aware of the changes in a way that the adults were not, indicates the need to study children at earlier grades to see if there is a point at which the hypothesized transition in style of processing takes place. If such a transition is found, this type of task may indicate whether one aspect of perceptual learning is progressing normally for a given child.

Other Studies Involving Eye Movement Contingent Techniques

The two studies just described represent only the beginning of the application of eye movement contingent display control techniques to the study of perceptual and cognitive processes taking place as children read, how these develop over time, and how children differ in their reading. Two other examples of studies currently underway illustrate further uses of this approach to studying reading.

As noted earlier, children frequently make multiple fixations on a word as they read. We would like to know whether, on these different fixations, they are seeing the entire configuration of the word, or are examining different parts of the word. To study this question, groups of words were identified that differ at two letter positions, for example, *cat, cap, mat,* and *map.* A sentence was written into which any of these four words fit appropriately, as shown in Figure 7. One of the words is in the text as the child begins to read. However, if the computer detects an eye movement that is taking the eyes to this word location a second time after initially encountering it, both critical letters of the word are changed. This manipulation places a new word at that location. If the entire word is being seen on each fixation, this type of change should be extremely disruptive to reading, showing up both through changes in the eye movement data and in the reader's conscious report. On the other hand, if different parts of the word are being examined on different fixations, the change will not disrupt reading but will produce an interesting perception on the part of the reader. For example, if the word *mat* is present on one fixation and *cap* on the next, the reader is likely to report having read the word *map* in the text, part of which was acquired during one fixation and part during the next. Of course, the results

It wAs tHe tImE Of tHe cIvIl wAr bEtWeEn tHe nOrThErN AnD SoUtHeRn

iT WaS ThE TiMe oF ThE CiViL WaR BeTwEeN ThE NoRtHeRn aNd sOuThErN

Figure 6.   Two versions of a line of text printed in alternating case. During selected saccades, one version was replaced by the other as children read.

may be different for different children, indicating differences in the types of perceptual units being used during reading.

It is also possible that when children make a second fixation on a word, the word was not identified on the first fixation. To investigate this possibility, a second study is being initiated. We are programming the computer to identify the initial fixation on certain words in the text. During the eye movement following such a fixation, the text will be removed and replaced by a patterned mask. Thus, no useful information will be obtained from the text during that or any following fixations. The subject's task will be to report the last words read. In addition to the children's reports, we will have eye movement data indicating whether the fixation following the first fixation on the word was to be on the same word or a different word. The hypothesis being tested predicts that when the following fixation is to be on the same word, the reader will not include that word in his or her report. On the other hand, when the following fixation is to be on some other word, the initially fixated word will be reported.

There are, of course, a number of other ways in which the eye movement contingent display control technique can be employed to investigate specific questions about the nature of the processing taking place during and across fixations as children read. However, these four examples illustrate the power of this approach to studying reading. Eye movement contingent display control actually makes it possible for the researcher to manipulate experimentally the stimulus pattern that is present during any particular fixation during reading, and, at the same time, to obtain a detailed eye movement record that can indicate when these manipulations are producing effects on reading and what the nature of the effects are. The use of these techniques to study the development of children's reading ability has only begun, and even less has been done in using them to study the nature of reading disorders.

Other Uses of Eye Movement Contingent Techniques

The use of eye movements to control the display is only one of a variety of eye movement contingent techniques that can be used. It would also be possible to study the "cognitive load" at certain points in the text by having a click sound a certain length of time after the fixation on which a particular word in the text was perceived, and by measuring the latency of a response to the sound. Another possible use would be to examine the interference in reading that is produced by having the computer "say" a word into the reader's earphones just at the time when some related word is fixated. In any research where it is

```
Mary said to Jim, "Did you see that ___ on the coffee table?"

                        cat
                        cap
                        mat
                        map
```

Figure 7.   An example of a sentence in which any of four words, differing at two letter positions, fits appropriately. Words are substituted during selected saccades as children read.

necessary to make an experimental manipulation in real time as the reader is encountering visually some specific part of the text, or is exhibiting some particular eye movement pattern, such as regressing to an earlier word, eye movement contingent experimental manipulation techniques become critical.

A Relation to Dyslexia

In this paper, we have attempted to show that various techniques involving the monitoring of readers' eye movements can play an important role in understanding the on-going processing taking place during reading. We assume that the study of dyslexia is essentially the study of individual differences among children learning to read. Research involving eye movement monitoring can help in understanding the nature of the mental processes involved in reading, how these develop as one learns to read, and what processing strategies or characteristics are more common in those children who fail to show normal progress in learning to read.

Thus, we suggest that one important branch of research on dyslexia will continue to investigate the nature of the perceptual and mental processes that are taking place as children are reading, or trying to read. Within this approach, eye movement monitoring will play a critical role. It may be that problems in the control of eye movements are a causative factor in the reading difficulties for occasional readers. However, of much greater importance is the fact that research techniques involving the monitoring of eye movements provide powerful new ways of studying, in detail, characteristics of the processing taking place during reading, even when eye movements themselves are not involved in the etiology of the reading disorder. Furthermore, it is likely that, at some point, eye movement monitoring techniques will play an essential role in the diagnosis of reading disorders.

References

Bedwell, C. H., Grant, R., and McKeown, J. R. 1980. Visual and ocular control anomalies in relation to reading difficulty. *The British Journal of Psychology* 50:61–70.

Buswell, G. T. 1937. How adults read. *Education Monographs (Supplement)* 45.

Donchin, E. 1984. *Cognitive Psychophysiology: Event-related Potentials and the Study of Cognition*. Hillsdale, NJ: Lawrence Erlbaum Associates.

Ehrlich, S., and Rayner, K. 1981. Contextual effects on word perception and eye movements during reading. *Journal of Verbal Learning and Verbal Behavior* 20:641–655.

Frazier, L., and Rayner, K. 1982. Making and correcting errors during sentence comprehension: Eye movements in the analysis of structurally ambiguous sentences. *Cognitive Psychology* 14:178–210.

Hogaboam, T. W. 1983. Reading patterns in eye movement data. *In* K. Rayner (ed.). *Eye Movements in Reading: Perceptual and Language Processes*. New York: Academic Press.

Huey, E. H. 1908. *The Psychology and Pedagogy of Reading*. New York: Macmillan.

Just, M. A., and Carpenter, P. A. 1980. A theory of reading: From eye fixations to comprehension. *Psychological Review* 87:329–354.

Kliegl, R., Olson, R. K., and Davidson, B. J. 1983. On problems of unconfounding perceptual and language processes. *In* K. Rayner (ed.). *Eye Movements in Reading: Perceptual and Language Processes.* New York: Academic Press.

Levy-Schoen, A., and O'Regan, K. 1979. The control of eye movements in reading. *In* P. A. Kolers, M. E. Wrolstad, and H. Bouma (eds.). *Processing of Visible Language.* New York: Plenum Press.

McConkie, G. W. 1983. Eye movements and perception during reading. *In* K. Rayner (ed.). *Eye Movements in Reading: Perceptual and Language Processes.* New York: Academic Press.

McConkie, G. W., and Rayner, K. 1975. The span of the effective stimulus during a fixation in reading. *Perception and Psychophysics* 17:578–586.

McConkie, G. W., Underwood, N. R., Zola, D., and Wolverton, G. S. (in press). Some temporal characteristics of processing during reading. *Journal of Experimental Psychology: Human Perception and Performance.*

McConkie, G. W., and Zola, D. 1979. Is visual information integrated across successive fixations in reading? *Perception and Psychophysics* 25:221–224.

Miller, R. G. 1981. *Survival Analysis.* New York: Wiley.

Patberg, J. P., and Yonas, A. 1978. The effects of the reader's skill and the difficulty of the text on the perceptual span in reading. *Journal of Experimental Psychology: Human Perception and Performance* 4:545–552.

Rayner, K. 1977. Visual attention in reading: Eye movements reflect cognitive processing. *Memory and Cognition* 4:443–448.

Rayner, K. 1978. Eye movements in reading and information processing. *Psychological Bulletin* 85:616–660.

Taylor, E. A. 1966. *The Fundamental Reading Skill (2nd ed.).* Springfield, Illinois: Charles C Thomas.

Taylor, S. E. 1965. Eye movements in reading: Facts and fallacies. *American Educational Research Journal* 2:187–202.

Underwood, N. R., and Zola, D. (in press). The span of letter recognition of good and poor readers. *Reading Research Quarterly* 20.

Walker, R. Y. 1933. The eye movements of good readers. *Psychological Monographs* 44:95–117.

Woodcock, R. W. 1973. *Woodcock Reading Mastery Tests.* Circle Pines, MN: American Guidance Service.

Zola, D. (in press). Redundancy and word perception during reading. *Perception and Psychophysics.*

16

A Word Is A Word—Or Is It?

Marion Blank

A consistent finding in dyslexia research over the past few decades is the presence of oral language difficulties in children who display problems in written language acquisition (see Benton and Pearl 1978). Given the numerous leads that have often led only to blind alleys, this result can and should be seen to represent a major advance in our understanding of dyslexia. By itself, however, it is far from sufficient. Language is a vast and complex area. If the individuals suffering from this syndrome are to be helped, it is essential to define precisely which components of their linguistic systems are awry.

A number of linguistically-based factors have thus far been implicated in the disorder. They include naming, sequencing, and phonological analysis (see Doehring and Hoshko 1977; Dochring, Hoshko, and Bryans 1979; Liberman, this volume; Rudel, Denckla, and Spalten 1976; Wolf 1982). Interestingly, and not surprisingly, the language deficiencies that have been identified are consonant with the emphasis that has long dominated the study of reading. That emphasis places great, if not total, reliance on the importance of decoding in mastering the reading process. This view is summarized by Gough (1972) in his statement that the child "comes to school equipped with a lexicon, a comprehension device and a phonological system . . . None of these is as elaborate or as extensive as they will be when he reaches adulthood . . . But at the same time, none of these shortcomings precludes the assembly of (at least) a primitive reading machine, for the child can readily make use of what he has. What is lacking is a character recognition device and the device which will

The research reported here was supported by National Institute of Child Health and Human Development HD 12278.

convert the characters it yields into a systematic phonemic representation (the Decoder)'' (p. 346).

It can readily be seen that the identified difficulties of dyslexics in naming, sequencing, and phonological analysis will all interfere with acquisition of ''the decoder'' (e.g., if one has a naming difficulty which causes problems in attaching labels to stimuli, it is highly likely that there will be difficulties in learning to attach sound correspondences to letters). Thus although language research has brought a new focus to studies of dyslexia, it has served primarily to elucidate ways in which the decoding process may be interfered with. In general, it has not been able to help us move beyond the widespread assumption that other components of the child's language system are present in sufficient amounts to allow ''the assembly of at least a primitive reading machine.'' Consequently, the current research focus has not served, and possibly has even blocked, efforts to identify other aspects of language that may be central to reading failure.

In this paper I would like to explore a dimension of language which may represent one of these other aspects of language. A focus of decoding is almost by definition a focus on individual sounds and words. By contrast, the unit that I wish to emphasize here is that of the sentence. In doing so, I am following a view put forth many years ago by Edward Sapir in his classic book entitled *Language* (1921). In that book, he talks about the fact that although sentences are always composed of words, different languages have different methods for ''binding'' the words. He notes that ''the more synthetic the language, in other words, the more clearly the status of each word in the sentence is indicated by its own resources, the less need is there for looking beyond the word to the sentence as a whole.'' Using the highly inflected Latin language as an example of a synthetic language, he goes on to state, ''The Latin *agit* '(he) acts,' needs no outside help to establish itself in a proposition. Whether I say *agit dominus,* 'the master acts' or *sic femina agit,* 'thus the woman acts,' the net result to the syntactic feel of the *agit* is practically the same. It can only be a verb, the predicate of a proposition and it can only be conceived as a statement or activity carried out by a person (or thing) other than you or me. It is not so with such a word as the English *act*. *Act* is a syntactic waif until we have defined its status in a proposition—one thing in 'they act abominably,' quite another in 'that was a kindly act.' The Latin sentence speaks with the assurance of its individual members, the English word needs the prompting of its fellows'' (pp. 109–110).

There are a number of ways in which the ''fellows'' that Sapir refers to may exert their role in creating the meaning of an English sentence. One primary technique is word order. This allows a sentence such as *John hit Mary* to have a quite different meaning from the sentence *Mary hit John* even though the words in both sentences are identical. (In this context, the sequencing difficulties of dyslexics take on new meaning. Generally, they have been seen as a major handicap in their handling of the flow of sounds in words. These difficulties should also play a major role in their understanding of the sequences of words that are necessary to the creation of sentences.)

While word order is a basic factor, another major component of sentences exists in the domain of relational terms—terms that are either words (e.g., *the, is*) or parts of words (e.g., *ing, ed*). These relational terms have no clear concrete referents but they nevertheless convey important information that modulates the meaning of sentences. Like most components of language, the terms are elusive and do not readily lend themselves to a definition. There is not even a single, agreed-upon label for these words which have been variously termed "functors," "grammatical morphemes," "noncontent words," and the "closed class of words." This range of labels is designed to contrast these words with the open class of content words which refer to particular ideas, events, or experiences (e.g., *house, car, drive, beautiful,* etc.). While the multiple terminology is confusing, in general it can be said that the categories of content, open, and contentive refer to words that are nouns, verbs, and adjectives—words that carry most of the representational meaning. By contrast, the categories of noncontent, closed-class, and functor include the grammatical categories of prepositions, conjunctions, and auxiliary verbs—words that primarily serve the syntactic function of organizing the content words into meaningful sentences (see Brown 1973; Quirk, Greenbaum, Leech, and Svartik 1972 and Thorne, Bratley, and Dewar 1968 for an elaboration of these issues).

Several lines of evidence exist to suggest the fruitfulness of exploring the content/noncontent distinction in the acquisition of the reading process. Although studies in this area are few, those that do exist indicate that the noncontent words are more difficult and/or less readily accessible. The greater difficulty has long been recognized in abnormal language functioning (see Bartolucci, Pierce, and Streiner 1980 for a discussion of autistic children's deficits in this area and Bradley, Garrett, and Zurif 1980 and Marin, Saffran, and Schwartz 1976 for similar discussions of aphasic language). The greater difficulty is also clearly reflected in normal language development where the earliest utterances of the young child consist mainly of content words (e.g., Brown 1973; Bloom and Lahey 1978; deVilliers and deVilliers 1973). Brown describes the first stage of language acquisition in the following terms: Content words "(chiefly nouns, verbs and adjectives) are always used frequently in Stage I speech while 'noncontent words' (chiefly inflections, auxiliaries, propositions, articles, and the copula) are used seldom or not at all" (p. 249). In the second stage the picture changes dramatically; " . . . a set of little words and inflections begins to appear. . . . All these, like an intricate sort of ivy, begin to grow up between and upon the major construction blocks, the nouns and verbs, to which Stage I is largely limited" (p. 249). The selective concentration of effort that the child engages in, that is, the child's focus on content words in Stage I and noncontent words in Stage II, suggests that even at a very young age, humans sense and respond to the differences between the two groups of words.

The distinction between the categories continues with development. For example, Ehri (1976) orally presented noncontent words (which she termed context-dependent words) and content words (which she termed context-independent words) to kindergarten and first grade children. Their task was to learn the words as paired associates to nonsense figures. The results indicated that the noncontent words were much more difficult for the first graders to learn than were the content words; for the kindergarten children, there was no indication of any measurable success with the noncontent words.

There is also evidence that some of the most frequent noncontent words (e.g., *is, the, a,* etc.) are not even recognized as individual lexical units prior to the development of reading. Holden and MacGinitie (1972) required kindergarten children to tap on poker chips to indicate each word in orally presented sentences. Their results suggest that, while a sentence such as *Children like chocolate candy* would be segmented accurately by a majority of the children, a sentence such as *Buy a pair of gloves* would be segmented as *buy/apair/ofgloves*. Similar results were obtained by Ehri (1975) even though her sentences were presented in a monotone to avoid the effects of intonational stress on the children's performance.

Egido (1981) tested whether the differences between content and non-content words in child language could be attributed to the oft-cited issues of concreteness or imageability (i.e., since content words tend to be more concrete or imageable, they would seem to be more readily available to the children). Using a lexical decision task with preschool children, she presented a set of content words which varied in abstraction and a set of noncontent words which also varied in degree of abstraction. She found that noncontent words, despite being highly frequent (e.g., *this* and *these*), are often not identified as words, while less frequent abstract content words (e.g., *smart* and *try*) are identified accurately by young children. These results must be interpreted with caution since degree of concreteness or imageability could not be equated in content and noncontent words. Further, lexical decision and reading may represent different processes since the performance of deep dyslexics on lexical decisions about noncontent words differs from their reading of the same words (Patterson 1979). Nevertheless, Egido's results are intriguing and cannot easily be dismissed.

In general, the above studies have been concerned with oral language. Similar findings have also been reported in the written language domain. The most striking have been with atypical populations (see Coltheart, Patterson, and Marshall 1980 and Patterson 1981 for a discussion of the distinction between content and noncontent words in deep dyslexics), but there are also interesting findings related to the normal reading process. First, there are a number of anecdotal reports which indicate that, in the process of learning to read, children find noncontent words particularly problematic (e.g., see Jolly 1981; Cunningham 1980). In fact, these words are often termed as "demons" in recognition of the fact that " . . . some of the most troublesome words for the beginning and disabled readers are the three-, four-, and five- letter words that make up the bulk of English prose" (Jolly 1981, p. 136). This differential performance seems to be maintained into adulthood. For instance, in written language tasks such as letter cancellation and spelling error detection, greater response accuracy has been shown for content than for noncontent words (e.g., Drewnowski and Healy 1977; Drewnowski 1978, 1981; Haber and Schindler 1981).

Before proceeding, it seems useful to summarize the line of reasoning that has led to the work that is to be presented below. It starts from the premise that while decoding is a vital operation in the acquisition of reading, a near-exclusive focus on this component has not allowed us to see the role of other potentially significant factors. One such factor revolves about the notion that the basic unit of meaning in a language is the sentence, not the word. In turn, in English, sentences critically depend upon the presence of noncontent words. Although the evidence is not extensive, all that does exist suggests that such words are perceived as different from content words. Furthermore, despite the fact that they are relatively few in number and very frequent in use, they are not as readily accessible as are the content words. In order to begin to evaluate their role in the reading process, a series of studies were undertaken and the section of the paper that follows will be concerned with reporting the results that were obtained.

In one study, a group of 40 third grade and a group of 40 fifth grade children were tested on their reading and spelling of content and noncontent words (see Bruskin and Blank 1984 for a full description of the study). In this study, as assessed by the Gilmore Oral Reading Test, all the children were normal readers, but they varied in proficiency from being highly skilled (i.e., scoring 1½ years or more above grade level on both accuracy and comprehension) to average (i.e., scoring 1½ years or more above grade level on either accuracy or comprehension) to relatively low readers (i.e., scoring below grade level on either comprehension or accuracy).

The children in each grade were presented with a list of words: 16 nouns (e.g., newspaper, house, fence), 16 verbs (e.g., bounce, walk, disappear) and 16 noncontent words (e.g., however, because, since). The three groups of words were equated for number of syllables and frequency in print for children's texts (Carroll, Davies, and Richman 1971). The words are shown in Table I. Half the list was identical for the two grades and half was different (i.e., the "different" list given to the third graders consisted of words with generally higher frequency while the "different" list given to fifth graders consisted of lower frequency words). This arrangement permitted us to see the comparability of performance of the third and fifth graders on the same set of words while also allowing us to see their responses to material that was more suited to their grade level. Within each grade, the same words were used for spelling and reading. The two tasks (i.e., spelling and reading) were presented in separate sessions with intervals of one week between each session. The order of task presentation was counterbalanced. Finally, to avoid the contaminating effects of context of word identification (Fredericksen 1981), the words were presented individually.

The results for the reading of the words are shown in Table II. They indicate that word class was a significant factor in both third and fifth grades ($F(2,72) = 58.95$, $p<.001$ for the third grade children and $F(2,72) = 43.80$,

Table I
Words Read and Spelled

Grade	Nouns	Verbs	Noncontent
3rd	children	happen	because
	window	carry	without
	man	make	these
	sound	walk	could
	boy	went	than
	bird	play	why
	house	put	has
	mother	follow	very
3rd	newspaper	remember	however
5th	worm	bounce	whose
	finger	compare	during
	fence	climb	since
	blanket	forget	rather
	grandfather	disappear	possible
	river	begin	also
	bath	yell	thus
5th	neighbor	receive	although
	cotton	listen	often
	baseball	produce	therefore
	piano	disappoint	heretofore
	forest	protect	toward
	station	threaten	throughout
	breakfast	arrive	neither
	table	divide	perhaps

$p < .001$ for the fifth grade children) with the noncontent words taking longer to identify than the nouns and verbs. An analysis was also carried out on the common set of words that was presented to both third and fifth graders. The findings indicated no effect of grade on the children's performance ($F(1,72) = .00, p > .95$.). In other words, the latencies for the third and fifth graders were equivalent when the same set of words was presented.

The latencies were also examined to determine if level of reading ability (high, average, or low) affected performance. The results indicated a significant interaction between ability and word class in that the content-noncontent differential increased with a decrease in reading level. For example, there was no difference between nouns and noncontent words for the high readers; the mean difference between the nouns and the noncontent words for the average readers was .1 sec. while the lowest readers exhibited a mean difference of .3 sec.

Reading ability was also shown to interact with other components of the task. Specifically, because of the importance of word frequency on response latency, correlations were computed for each category of words (i.e., nouns,

Table II
Reading Latencies by Grade: Normal Readers

Grade	Word Class		
	Nouns	Verbs	Noncontent
3	1.1*	1.1	1.3
	.2	.3	.5
5	1.2	1.2	1.4
	.3	.4	.5
3†	1.2	1.2	1.3
	.2	.4	.5
5†	1.2	1.2	1.2
	.4	.3	.6

*Upper number = mean, lower number = standard deviation (in seconds)
†These latencies are on the words identical for the two grades

verbs, and noncontent words). It was found that the correlations between frequency and latency were highest for the low readers ($-.46$, $-.61$ and $-.29$ for the nouns, verbs, and noncontent words respectively). For the average readers, the comparable figures were .09, .49 and $-.46$. By contrast, the correlations for the high readers were considerably lower (i.e., the median correlations were $-.12$, $-.04$ and $-.15$ for the nouns, verbs, and noncontent words respectively). These results suggest that the highest group of readers are less affected by the frequency of a word. They seem to have a readier accessibility for all words, while the less skilled, albeit still normal, readers find the more frequent words to be easier to read than the less frequent words.

The results until this point have been concerned with latency of word identification. The children's reading and spelling performance was also examined for accuracy. While the errors in reading were few (a total of 49 or less than 1 per child), the pattern exhibited was consistent with the children's latencies. More errors were made in the reading of noncontent words than in the reading of nouns and verbs. Thus, in third grade, a total of 23 noncontent words, 1 verb and 1 noun were misread by the children; in fifth grade the children misread 20 noncontent words, 3 verbs and 1 noun.

The spelling errors, as one might expect, were far more numerous than were those in the reading of the same words. Nevertheless, the pattern was quite similar and it served to reinforce the content-noncontent performance differential. For example, the third grade children misspelled a total of 115 noncontent words while they only misspelled a total of 20 nouns and 90 verbs. For the fifth grade children, the misspellings were 147 noncontent words, 31 nouns and 115 verbs.

When an analysis of the errors was carried out, taking into account the number of syllables, an interesting pattern was found to exist. Thus, among the third graders, of the 95 single-syllable words that were misspelled, 67% were noncontent words and only 33% were content words. (This result occurred in spite of the fact that the content words outnumbered the noncontent words by a factor of 2 to 1). By contrast, of the 130 multisyllable words that were misspelled, only 39% were noncontent words and 61% were content words. In fact, the absolute number of errors was greater on the single syllable noncontent than on the multisyllable noncontent words (i.e., 64 versus 51) even though the number of single and multisyllable noncontent words administered to the third graders was equal. Thus, despite being shorter and more frequent, the single-syllable noncontent words are a greater source of difficulty for the children.

The pattern for the fifth graders was similar. Of the 68 single syllable words misspelled, 82% were noncontent and 18% were content words, while for the 208 errors on the multisyllable words, 58% were noncontent words and 42% were content words. The greater number of multisyllable misspellings in the fifth grade reflected the fact that the older group was given many more multisyllable words. Overall, the results suggest that, while single syllable content words posed little difficulty for the children, noncontent words of the same length were a source of failure. Further, (a) the content words become as problematic as the noncontent words only when the number of syllables increased and (b) increasing the number of syllables in the noncontent words did not appear to increase their difficulty relative to single syllable noncontent words.

In the next study to be reported here, the content-noncontent issue was explored in a group of dyslexic children. The sample was composed of 16 boys, all of whom had a reading quotient of less than .85. Their mean chronological age was 11.2, their mean full scale I.Q. was 108, their mean grade placement was 5.7 and their mean reading age was 2.0. (See Blank and Bruskin 1985 for a full description of the study.)

The task given to these children was similar to that described above, but it was expanded to include an important feature which was not studied in the previous work. Specifically, the stimuli presented to the normal readers in the research cited above involved only the reading aloud of words in isolation. While this task yielded interesting effects of word class, the phenomenon is truly relevant only if it can be shown to exist in the actual reading process; that is, in the reading of connected text. In order to assess this, the children were given two tasks: (1) they were asked to read aloud words in isolation (the same words read by the third graders in the previous study were used since this list was most appropriate given their reading level); and (2) they were asked to read words in context. The Gilmore Oral Reading Test was used for this purpose. In this test, a child is given a number of passages of increasing levels of difficulty and is required to read aloud until reaching a passage in which he makes ten or more errors.

The pattern of response times for the words read in isolation is shown in Table III. As in the previous study, word class was shown to be significant ($F(2,15) = 20.35, p<.001$). Further, the noncontent words took longer to read than either the nouns or verbs, while the latter two categories did not differ from each other. Not surprisingly, the children took longer to read the multisyllable words than the single syllable words ($F(1,15); p<.001$). There was, however, no interaction between word class and number of syllables.

The error rate for the reading of words in isolation was quite low. (The

Table III
Responses to Words in Isolation and in Context: Dyslexic Readers

(a) Latencies to Words in Isolation

	Nouns	Verbs	Noncontent
Single Syllable Words	1.3*	1.3	1.5
	.2	.2	.3
Multisyllable Words	1.4	1.4	1.5
	.2	.2	.4

(b) Total Number of Errors to Words in Isolation

	Nouns	Verbs	Noncontent Words
Single Syllable Words	8	7	22
Multisyllable Words	10	5	2

(c) Total Number of Errors to Words in Context

	Content	Noncontent
Single Syllable Words	28	79/13†
Multisyllable Words	66	14/19

* The upper number represents the mean, the lower number the standard deviation.

† The first number represents errors on whole words, the second on bound morphemes (e.g. noncontent morphemes attached to content words such as wash*ing*)

words had been selected to be those which are common in third grade and hence, they were appropriate for the children's reading level.) In terms of the single syllable words, there were a greater number of errors on the noncontent words than on the nouns or verbs. In a total of 37 errors, 22 were made on the noncontent words, 8 were made on the nouns and 7 on the verbs. Thus, even though only 33 percent of the words were in the noncontent category, 59% of the errors were made on these words.

The analysis of errors in the multisyllable words yielded somewhat different results. First, there were fewer errors in the reading of the multisyllable words than in the single syllable words. This rather surprising result may be due to the children attending more fully to the longer words and being more careful in reading them. The pattern of errors was also different from the single syllable words. Of a total of 16 errors, 10 were made on the verbs, 5 on the noncontent words and only 1 noun was misread. This would suggest that, for some reason, the noncontent multisyllable words did not cause as much difficulty in terms of error, although they clearly did in terms of latency.

The Gilmore Oral Reading Test, which served as the material for the reading of connected text, is scored for a wide variety of errors, including repetitions, hesitations, and self-corrections. For the present purpose of studying the reading of connected text, we were interested only in the words that the children misread, failed to read, or inserted into the text. The results indicated that, in terms of rate, there were fewer such errors in the reading of contextual material than in the reading of isolated words. It could not be determined whether this result was due to the differential difficulty of the words in the two tasks or whether contextual reading leads to fewer errors than does the reading of words in isolation, as reported by Krieger (1981). Nevertheless, the results still revealed more errors on noncontent words and bound morphemes than on content words. A total of 120 errors were made on the single syllable words in the first six passages. Of these, 92 errors were on the noncontent words and bound morphemes, but only 28 were on the content words. Given that there is a differential frequency for the two words classes (973 content words vs. 1619 noncontent words read by the children), one might attribute the results to that factor alone. However, a chi-square analysis taking this factor into account indicated that the error difference was significant ($\chi^2 = 10.02$, $p<01$).

The error pattern is even more striking when one considers the issue of differential frequency in print. It is well-established that frequency affects readability, in that greater frequency is associated with better performance (Gibson and Levin 1975). This factor was controlled for in the words presented in isolation in that the words were matched for frequency across word class. In normal text, however, the noncontent words are generally of much higher frequency than the content words and hence, should have an advantage vis-a-vis word recognition. Nevertheless, the noncontent words still proved more difficult.

The pattern of errors on multisyllable words is somewhat harder to discern since there were relatively few multisyllable noncontent words in the text. Nevertheless, the results mirror those of the single syllable words read in text: of the 204 instances of noncontent words and bound morphemes, there was a total of 33 errors, for an error rate of 16%. By contrast, of the 735 instances of multisyllable content words, there was a total of only 66 errors, for an error rate of 9%. As tested by chi-square, this difference is significant ($\chi^2 = 8.02$, $p<.01$).

The research was not designed at this point to explore the children's performance on tests which they themselves create. Figure 1, however, does provide a sample of a text written by an 11-year-old dyslexic girl in response to a request to describe a story she had read. The typed material below the writing represents the way in which she read the text she had created.

A striking feature of the work is the extent to which it supports the results obtained in the research reported above. Not only is there a high percentage of errors in the high frequency noncontent words and bound morphemes, but the errors are of a quite different type from those made on the content words. In general, the errors on the latter words involved the omission of and/or minor misspelling of vowel sounds (e.g., the omission of the second vowel in the unstressed second syllable of the word *jewels* and spelling of *begin* in such a way as to make it accord with the rules for long vowel sounds). In all cases, however, the spelling of the content words is such as to preserve the sounds that they contain. By contrast, the spelling of the noncontent words and bound morphemes involves the omission of major elements (*the* for *there, lock* for *locked*, etc.) and numerous rewritings (e.g., note the corrections on the words *upon, always* and *they*). Thus, as in the reading and spelling tasks, this child's performance supports the findings that there are patterns of response different for the content and noncontent words of our language.

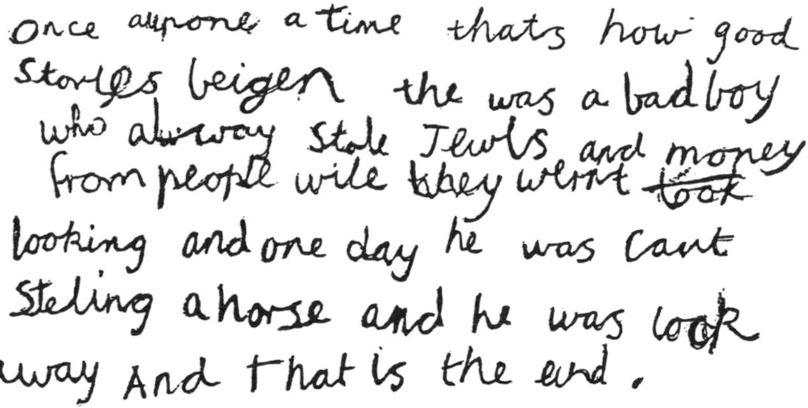

Once aupone a time thats how good Storyes beigen the was a bad boy who alwway stole Jewls and money from people wile thay wernt took looking and one day he was cant Steling a horse and he was look away And that is the end.

Once upon a time that's how good stories begin there was a bad boy who always stole jewels and
  money from people while they weren't looking and one day he was caught stealing a horse and he
  was locked away and that is the end.
Figure 1.

While the effects of word class are clearly discernible, the source of these effects is little understood. One promising explanation for the results has been offered from studies using the visual hemifield paradigm (Bradley and Garrett 1981). In that research, it was found that presentation of both classes of words to the left visual field (right hemisphere) resulted in poor, but equal, levels of accuracy in word identification. By contrast, when the words were presented to the right visual field (left hemisphere), accuracy increased—but not in a uniform manner. Performance on the content words was significantly better than performance on the noncontent words. These results led the investigators to suggest that there may be a differential access for content and noncontent words in the left hemisphere, whereas the same mechanism serves to access both word classes in the right hemisphere.

Some support for this hypothesis is available in studies of "deep dyslexics." These are a subgroup of adult alexics who have left hemisphere damage and show a complex set of symptoms in reading, including particular difficulties in identifying noncontent words (Coltheart 1980; Patterson 1981; Shallice and Warrington 1975). Their difficulties are aptly illustrated in the performance of a French dyslexic. In French, the orthographically identical word CAR can serve different semantic/syntactic roles. When it serves as a noun it means "vehicle" or "bus"; when it serves as a conjunction it means "because." A sentence was created in which the word was used in its two different roles: *le car ralentit car le moteur chauffe* which translates into: *the bus stops because the motor overheats*. Strikingly, the patient was able to read the word when it functioned as a noun (*bus*) but not when it functioned as a noncontent word (*because*).

Although it has not yet been considered, any discussion of the content-noncontent distinction clearly has bearing on the teaching of reading; in particular, the teaching of decoding. In line with the near exclusive emphasis on phonics discussed at the beginning of the paper, the teaching of word identification has concentrated on leading the child to achieve grapheme-phoneme correspondences. As has been commonly noted, many of the noncontent words do not lend themselves to the grapheme-phoneme correspondences which the children are taught (e.g., *are, be, whose, could, have,* etc.) But the implications of this fact of language life have not been pursued. Instead, clinging to the idea that our language can be taught as if consistent grapheme-phoneme correspondences existed, the noncontent words are taught as "sight" words that are "exceptions" to a system that is represented as being otherwise clearly patterned. Then, to allow the "exceptions" to hold the secondary place that they must hold if they are to remain exceptions, the noncontent words are given minimal analysis and attention. As a result, the teaching process does little, and probably even works against, the children gaining access to this vital, but subtle, component of language.

This analysis clearly suggests the importance, in the teaching of reading, of separating the content and noncontent words of our language. A program based on these principles has been outlined by the present investigator (Blank and Bruskin 1982) and it has shown promising results in the teaching of reading to children with oral and written language problems. While space limitations prevent a description of the program here, it seems worthwhile to discuss some of its features.

As implied in the discussion till now, the teaching is structured so that the two classes of words are taught separately. For the content words, grapheme-phoneme correspondences are stressed, while other analytic procedures are used for the noncontent words. But of greatest importance is the emphasis placed on helping the children realize the role that the noncontent words play in structuring language into meaningful units. This latter concept is vital to the issue of chunking. Many investigators agree that fluent reading requires automaticity (see LaBerge and Samuels 1974). Further, automaticity is not seen to be word-by-word indentification, but rather the grouping of words into larger units such as phrases, clauses, and sentences. Chunking into these larger units automatically entails the meshing of content and noncontent words (e.g., reading phrases such as *the boy, into the room, was walking,* etc.)

This meshing occurs in both oral and written language. In oral language, however, a number of distinct cues exist to facilitate the process. They include supra-linguistic features which help to mark the phrasal structures (e.g., prosody, gestures, pauses, etc.). In written language, however, such cues are largely absent. As a result, acquisition of reading fluency requires the child to "... transfer from a system in which prosodic marking plays a major role in identifying syntactic phrases" (i.e., oral language) "to a system in which the phrases go largely unmarked graphically" (i.e., written language). "The child must learn to compensate somehow for the lack of overt graphic marking of many syntactic units" (Schreiber 1980, p. 11).

The child's task is even more difficult than the above quote would indicate. Not only are the supra-linguistic cues minimally marked for the reader, but the manner in which the words are presented on a printed page conflicts with the implicit knowledge which the child has learned from oral (everyday) language. For example, in a spoken phrase such the "the boy," the two words are not of equal weight: "boy" is stressed and thus stands out as more salient than "the." Further, temporal factors clearly indicate a single semantic unit. By contrast, in the silence of the printed page, both words occupy equal amounts of space (3 letters each) and are separated by equal intervals. They thereby might tend to be processed by early and disabled readers as if they are to receive equal "psychological" weight. In other words, written text requires children to set aside their expectations regarding syntactic chunking gained in oral language and learn a new set of rules.

In order to help the children in this process, the teaching program is designed at the outset to convey the idea that words are not isolated units, but rather elements that merge to form an idea. For example, the first word taught is the word *the*. The initial exercises will pair this word with pictures of objects and the child will then "read" the resulting phrase, e.g., "the boy," "the dogs," "the shoes" etc.

The role played by the noncontent words in connecting language goes far beyond the unit of the phrase. Indeed, they are critical not only to the construction of sentences, but also to the linkage between sentences. This idea is perhaps illustrated best by example. Imagine the following three content words: *Jeff see dog*. The importance of word order easily leads us to think of these words as a truncated form of a sentence in which a person named Jeff is looking at a dog. The introduction of two different sets of noncontent words makes it clear that the situation is far more complicated. Specifically, the first set of noncontent words to be introduced is *does, not* and *a*; the second set is *can, not* and *his*. With these words, the sentences become:

> Jeff does not see a dog
>
> and
>
> Jeff cannot see his dog.

The introduction of the noncontent words not only creates two distinct sentences, but they have an impact that goes beyond the sentences. The words are central to the way in which the text can be formulated so as to convey a reasonable and cohesive set of ideas. Again, to use an example, consider the first pairing sentence above with the new set of sentences *he is glad* and *he is afraid of them*. The result would be the following comprehensible text: *Jeff does not see a dog. He is glad. He is afraid of them*. By contrast, if the pairing was changed so that the new set was joined with the second sentence considerable confusion would be introduced: *Jeff cannot see his dog. He is glad. He is afraid of them*.

This example illustrates the critical role that the closed class of noncontent words plays not only in the construction of sentences, but also in the creation of connected text. When these words are present and comprehended, a connection is established among the disparate sentences and the text that follows becomes more predictable and reasonable. Conversely, when these words are either not present (as in many texts for beginning readers) or if present, not understood, then comprehension of the total text is far more difficult.

The following first grade passage (Makar 1977) is representative of the phenomenon under discussion. Accompanying the text are pictures of a cat (Tab) and a small rat (Mac). The text proceeds as follows:

> Tab is a sad cat.
> Tab has a pal.
> His pal is Mac.
> Mac is a rat.

Although some of the same words reappear (e.g., Tab, Mac) they generally do not serve to enhance coherence. The ideas of each sentence are so independent that the reading of one sentence does not sufficiently prepare the reader for the content of the next (e.g., if one were asked to predict the second sentence after reading the first, it seems highly unlikely that the theme 'Tab has a pal' would be offered). As a result, beginning texts leave children—particularly children with difficulties—to confront an almost unmanageable linguistic situation. The explicit cues for coherence are misleading (certain content words are repeated, but the words lack an intrinsic relationship to a theme) and the implicit cues for coherence are practically nonexistent (the subtle connectives are deleted because they are seen as violations of the grapheme-phoneme correspondences that are being stressed). As a result, there is no clear organization for relating one sentence to the next.

The solution to this problem is not simple. If "naturally" occurring sentences were to be introduced, they would contain so many visually unfamiliar words as to make the reading task unbearable for the child. But a promising approach to the problem is available in a theme that has long been recognized in teaching individual words to children. A salient feature of words is their enormous variability. The number of words used in even everyday conversation numbers into the thousands. In order not to inundate children with this variability, tight controls have been placed on the vocabulary in beginning texts. The number of words introduced in any story is limited and the words are carefully selected to accord with specific rules.

Interestingly, while sentences are also marked by great variability, little attention has been directed toward controlling sentence types. The need for such control becomes apparent when one considers only the following three sentence types:

1. Here is an X (e.g., Here is a boy)
2. The X can Y (e.g., The boy can jump)
3. The X is Ying (e.g., The boy is jumping)

Analysis of these sentences within the framework of reading must include the fact that in text, sentences link with one another and the linkages affect the words that can be used. For example, if Sentence 3 were to appear in a text following Sentence 2, it is likely to be in the form *he is jumping* (rather than *the boy is jumping*). Similarly, if the subject in Sentence 2 had been a girl, the subject in Sentence 3 would have been changed to *she*.

When one considers the possible variations created by only three factors—gender (he, she, it), plurality (he, they) and deixis (here, there, this, that, etc.), the result is that the three sentence types can appear in over 40 permutations (e.g., Boys can jump. Here is a boy. He is jumping. Here are some boys. Boys can jump. This boy is jumping. etc.). Interestingly, much of the variation is carried by the noncontent words.

Given their difficulties in mastering these words, it is not surprising that children, particularly those not skilled in reading, are drawn to the salient content words. Indeed, the poorer the reader, the greater the likelihood of mistakenly clinging to the content words as anchoring points in a sea of variability. Ironically, the predisposition to hold onto the content words reinforces the avoidance of the more subtle but absolutely essential components of text.

If the children are to be helped, the variability must be reduced to manageable proportions while simultaneously preserving the central features that govern sentence organization and sentence relationships. This goal has been accomplished in the program developed by the present investigator through the creation of a series of books at ten levels (with ten books at each level). A level is defined in terms of the sentence types it contains. Thus, the first level is restricted to the three sentence types outlined above (here is an X, the X can Y, the X is Ying). The second level introduces the past (*was, were*), the yes-no question form, and the concepts of *but* and *now*. These are interwoven with the sentence types of the first level so that a much richer, but nevertheless controlled text is available. For example, on a page where ducks are shown asleep, the text might read: *Here are some ducks. Ducks can run but are these ducks running? No, they are not. They were running but now they are sleeping.* Each of the ten levels in turn introduces and interweaves additional sentence types.

At this point, the actual design of the reading program is not of central interest. Of greater importance is the recognition of the range of possibilities that have been opened by acknowledging *the sentence* as a vital unit in the acquisition of reading. The possibilities extend out from the sentence in two directions. In one direction, they lead to a reconsideration of individual words and from that to a recognition of the importance and the distinctiveness of the noncontent words of our language. These words cannot and should not be seen as a set of 'exceptions', but rather as representing a system that has its own organization and demands.

In the other direction, consideration of the sentence as a key unit leads to an analysis of the relationships among sentences and thereby to a consideration of the way in which texts ought to be constructed. This latter aspect of language has been almost totally neglected in the design of reading programs, even though it is a factor that is of critical importance in the creation of meaningful texts. The components of language dealt with here are almost certainly not the only ones that ought to be considered if we are to begin to understand the demands that initial reading places on the inexperienced and/or disabled reader. They do serve, however, to illustrate the rich and complex linguistic terrain that exists over and above the grapheme-phoneme correspondences that have for so long dominated our conception of the reading acquisition process.

References

Bartolucci, G., Pierce, S. J. and Streiner, D. 1980. Cross-sectional studies of grammatical morphemes in autistic and mentally retarded children. *Journal of Autism and Developmental Disorders* 10:39–49.

Benton, A. L., and Pearl, D. (eds.) 1978. *Dyslexia: An Appraisal of Current Knowledge.* New York: Oxford University Press.

Blank, M., and Bruskin, C. 1982. Sentences and non-content words: Missing ingredients in reading instruction. *Annals of Dyslexia* 32:103–121.

Blank, M., and Bruskin, C. 1985. The reading of content and non-content words by dyslexics. *Discourses in Reading and Linguistics.* New York Academy of Sciences, 433:59–69.

Bloom, L., and Lahey, M. 1978. *Language Development and Language Disorders.* New York: Wiley.

Bradley, D. C., and Garrett, M. F. 1981. Hemispheric Differences in Recognition of Function and Content Words. Unpublished Manuscript. Cambridge, MA.: MIT.

Bradley, D. C., Garrett, M. F. and Zurif, E. B. 1980. Syntactic deficits in Broca's aphasia. *In* D. Caplan (ed.). *Biological Studies of Mental Processes.* Cambridge, MA.: MIT Press.

Brown, R. 1973. *A First Language.* Cambridge, MA.: Harvard University Press.

Bruskin, C., and Blank, M. 1984. The effects of word class on children's reading and spelling. *Brain and Language* 21:219–232.

Carroll, J. B., Davies, P. and Richman, B. 1971. *Word Frequency Book.* New York: American Heritage.

Coltheart, M. 1980. Deep dyslexia: A right-hemisphere hypothesis. *In* M. Coltheart, K. Patterson, J. C. Marshall (eds.). *Deep Dyslexia.* London: Routledge and Kegan Paul.

Coltheart, M., Patterson, K., and Marshall, J. C. (eds.) 1980. *Deep Dyslexia.* London: Routledge and Kegan Paul.

Cunningham, P. M. 1980. Teaching were, with, what and other four letter words. *Reading Teacher* 34:163–169.

deVilliers, J. G., and deVilliers, P. M. 1973. A cross-sectional study of the development of grammatical morphemes in child speech. *Journal of Psycholinguistic Research* 2:267–278.

Doehring, D. G., and Hoshko, I. M. 1977. Classification of reading problems by the Q technique of factor analysis. *Cortex* 13:281–294.

Doehring, D. G., Hoshko, I. M. and Bryans, B. N. 1979. Statistical classification of children with reading problems. *Journal of Clinical Neuropsychology* 1:5–16.

Drewnowski, A. 1978. Detection errors on the word THE: Evidence for the acquisition of reading levels. *Memory and Cognition* 6:403–409.

Drewnowski, A. 1981. Missing -ing in reading: Developmental changes in reading units. *Journal of Experimental Child Psychology* 31:154–168.

Drewnowski, A., and Healy, A. F. 1977. Detection errors on THE and AND: Evidence for reading units larger than the word. *Memory and Cognition* 5:636–647.

Egido, C. 1981. Invisibility of closed class words in children's word judgments. Unpublished manuscript. Cambridge, MA. MIT.

Ehri, L. C. 1975. Word consciousness in readers and pre-readers. *Journal of Educational Psychology* 67:204–212.

Ehri, L. C. 1976. Word learning in beginning readers. Effects of form class and defining contexts. *Journal of Educational Psychology* 68:832–842.

Fredericksen, J. R. 1981. Sources of process interaction in reading. *In* A. M. Lesgold, and C. A. Perfetti (eds.). *Interactive Processes in Reading.* Hillsdale, N.J.: Lawrence Erlbaum Associates.

Gibson, E. J., and Levin, H. 1975. *The Psychology of Reading.* Cambridge, MA.: MIT Press.

Gough, P. B. 1972. One second of reading. *In* J. F. Kavanagh and I. G. Mattingly (eds.). *Language by Ear and by Eye.* Cambridge, MA.: MIT Press.

Haber, R. N., and Schindler, R. M. 1981. Error in proof reading: Evidence for syntactic control of letter processing? *Journal of Experimental Psychology: Human Perception and Performance* 7:573–579.

Holden, M. H., and MacGinitie, W. H. 1972. Children's conceptions of word boundaries in speech and print. *Journal of Educational Psychology* 63:551–557.

Jolly, H. B., Jr. 1981. Teaching basic function words. *Reading Teacher* 35:136–140.

Krieger, V. K. 1981. A hierarchy of "confusable" high frequency words in isolation and context. *Learning Disability Quarterly* 4:131–138.

LaBerge, D., and Samuels, S. J. 1974. Toward a theory of automatic information processing in reading. *Cognitive Psychology* 6:293–323.

Makar, B. W. 1977. *Primary Phonics*. Cambridge, MA.: Educators Publishing Service.

Marin, O. S. M., Saffran, E. M. and Schwartz, M. F. 1976. Dissociations of language in aphasia: Implications for normal function. *Annals of the New York Academy of Sciences: Origins and Evolution of Language and Speech* 280:868–884.

Patterson, K. E. 1979. What is right with "deep" dyslexic patients? *Brain and Language* 8:111–129.

Patterson, K. E. 1981. Neuropsychological approaches to the study of reading. *British Journal of Psychology* 72:151–174.

Quirk, R., Greenbaum, S., Leech, G. and Svartik, J. 1972. *A Grammar of Contemporary English*. London: Longman.

Rudel, R. G., Denckla, M. B. and Spalten, E. 1976. Paired associate learning of Morse code and braille letter names by dyslexic and normal children. *Cortex* 12:61–70.

Sapir, E. 1921. *Language*. New York: Harcourt Brace.

Schreiber, P. A. 1980. On the acquisition of reading fluency. *Journal of Reading Behavior* 12:177–186.

Shallice, T., and Warrington, E. K. 1975. Word recognition in a phonemic dyslexic patient. *Quarterly Journal of Experimental Psychology* 27:187–199.

Thorne, J. P., Bratley, P. and Dewar, H. 1968. The syntactic analysis of English by machine. *In* D. Michie (ed.). *Machine Intelligence*. Vol 3. New York: American Elsevier.

Wolf, M. 1982. An approach to the combined study of acquired and developmental reading disorders. *In* R. N. Malatesha and P. G. Aaron (eds.). *Reading Disorders: Variabilities and Treatments*. New York: Academic Press.

17

The Reliability, Validity and Flexibility of the Decoding Skills Test for Reading Research

Ellis Richardson

The Decoding Skills Test (DST) (Richardson and DiBenedetto 1985) was developed under a contract with the National Institute of Child Health and Human Development (NICHD). The objective was to produce a research tool that would identify children with developmental dyslexia and yield a performance profile of decoding skills that could be used to test specific hypotheses about dyslexia. This chapter describes the DST, presents evidence for its reliability and validity, and demonstrates its flexibility in providing researchers with a variety of measurement options for hypothesis testing.

The DST is composed of three subtests. Subtest I (Basal Vocabulary) measures a child's ability to read aloud (decode) words that are representative of the reader levels of most basal reader programs. One of the more interesting Subtest I scores is a grade equivalent (GE) that approximates program placement with regard to word recognition. For example, a GE score of 2.3 indicates that the child can read most first grade readers with ease but needs instruction in beginning second grade vocabulary. Subtest II (Phonic Patterns) provides a profile of phonic skills by testing items in a carefully designed matrix of spelling patterns. The profile depicts the child's ability to use vowel, consonant, and syllabic patterns and to transfer these skills to the decoding of

This work was supported, in part, by a contract with the National Institute of Child Health and Human Development (#NO1-HD-7-2837).

There are many individuals who have made significant contributions to the development of the DST and the data reported here. Barbara DiBenedetto, who has been my closest collaborator for over a decade, is probably the most significant of these. Recently, Daniel Foss become interested in this work, and he has spent countless hours of his own personal time dusting off our four-year-old data set and generating all of the analyses reported in this chapter. I am also indebted to the staff at NICHD. James Kavanagh, who served as project officer, has maintained an active interest in the DST over the years and has provided us with more encouragement than he may realize. Finally, Grace Yeni-Komshian had a great deal to do with the initial contract and design of the test and deserves no small measure of credit for her part in this effort.

unknown words. Subtest III (Contextual Decoding) measures both aspects of decoding (basal vocabulary and phonic skills) in contextual reading and it provides a variety of other measures of oral fluency.

Criterion-Referenced Scores

The DST is designed to provide criterion-referenced (CR) scores that reflect skill development with regard to the reading curriculum. It is important to distinguish CR scores from norm-referenced (NR) scores. NR scores measure performance with reference to a group used to "norm" the test while CR scores measure performance with reference to a specified skill domain (Alkin 1974; Hambleton and Novick 1973).

NR scores on reading tests include percentile ranks, scale scores, and the well known GE. These can only be used to compare the performance of individual children or groups of children to the performance of the children in the norm sample. They are not intended to represent how a child might actually perform on actual reading program materials. For example, a GE score of 3.2 on such a test gives no specific information as to where a child obtaining that score should be placed in a given reading program. The range of appropriate placements might conceivably vary by one or more years in either direction from the NR score obtained. In contrast, CR scores are designed for the express purpose of describing how a child might be expected to perform on specific curriculum materials. Thus, a GE score of 3.2 on such a test indicates that the child earning this score is appropriately placed at a beginning third grade level, that second grade material has been mastered, and that fourth grade material would be too difficult.

NR scores are extremely useful for research and clinical diagnosis, but given that they are comparative rather than descriptive, more information is required—especially when a child's score appears to fall at the extreme low end of the normal distribution. In both clinical practice and research, it is important to know how well children read words at a given grade level, how well they use phonic information, and how well these skills are applied in contextual reading. CR scores that are obtained from the DST provide this type of descriptive information.

The DST measures decoding in two primary domains: recognition of basal vocabulary words and use of letter-sound patterns. CR scores in the domain of basal vocabulary (Subtests I and III) reflect the child's ability to recognize words taught up to any specified level in any standard reading program. For example, an Instructional Level GE score of 3.8 on DST Subtest I indicates that the child reliably recognizes nearly all of the words taught in most reading programs through a mid-third grade level but needs instruction in high third grade vocabulary. Similarly, a GE of 3.8 on Subtest III indicates that the child can read text at this level in most basal reading programs. Scores on phonic development (Subtest II) reflect the child's ability to use letter-sound correspondence and spelling patterns in decoding words. Since the DST items were derived by collating words from many standard reading programs, they permit cross-program comparisons. That is, individual children or groups of children from different schools and environments may be compared on measures of skill mastery. This information has obvious value for cross-study inferences and it serves a variety of applied purposes: teacher feedback, initial program placement, special education evaluations, and program evaluation.

Subtest I: Basal Vocabulary

The Basal Vocabulary subtest is composed of 11 lists of words systematically selected from ten widely used reading programs. This approach was used in order to make the test as program-fair as possible. The selection procedures involved analyses of phonic/linguistic type programs as well as conventional basal vocabulary programs. Thus, a child's score will be determined by his mastery of the general reading curriculum at a given level rather than the curriculum of any particular program. This is an important feature of the test when one wishes to compare groups of children who have received different reading programs.

Each of the standard reader level divisions (preprimer, primer, first reader, two-one reader, two-two reader, etc.) are represented by individual lists of ten words. The test presents words only up through the fifth grade level, since decoding skills are well developed at a sixth grade reading level and language development (word meaning and comprehension) becomes a much more critical determinant of basal vocabulary development in the upper grades.

Table I shows the first 3 words in each of the 11 Subtest I lists and the reader level that each list represents. The elaborate procedures followed in selecting the most representative words for Subtest I are described in the final project report (Richardson, DiBenedetto, Adler and Kochnower 1981) to NICHD.

Subtest II: Phonic Patterns

The Phonic Patterns Subtest is composed of words that conform to the most common orthographic patterns of phonetic regularity. Items represent a total of four dimensions: consonant arrangements (single or multiple), vowel patterns (short vowel, silent *e,* long vowel, and vowel digraph), syllable

Table I
First Three Items In Each of the 11 Graded Word Lists in Subtest I

Pre-Primer	Primer	First Reader	Two-One Reader	Two-Two Reader	Three-One Reader
to	so	sing	shop	strong	famous
yes	was	when	fine	able	daughter
the	went	next	end	almost	crowd

Three-Two Reader	Four-One Reader	Four-Two Reader	Five-One Reader	Five-Two Reader	
natural	stalk	instruction	frequent	continent	
mutter	project	contact	purchase	trudge	
coin	stern	glare	advertise	desperate	

Table II
Examples of Monosyllabic and Polysyllabic Forms of Real and Nonsense Words
Corresponding to Each of the Six Subtest II Spelling Patterns

Spelling Pattern	Monosyllabic		Polysyllabic	
	Real	Nonsense	Real	Nonsense
CVC	nut	dut	mitten	pitten
·CCVCC	stack	glack	publish	sublish
CVCé	doze	voze	confuse	monfuse
CCVCé	flake	grake	provide	drovide
CVVC	raw	taw	sausage	wausage
CCVVCC	choice	froice	creature	threature

patterns (monosyllabic and polysyllabic), and meaning (real and nonsense words). These four dimensions of Subtest II will be made clear by referring to the sample items listed in Table II. The real words were selected from Harris' and Jacobson's (1972) graded word lists and the nonsense words were formed by changing one or two letters in each of the real words (e.g., *dut* was created from the word *nut, threature* was formed from *creature*, etc.). Each of the items shown in Table II is representative of five such items.

The five words in each list are organized by grade level (using Harris-Jacobson designations). This aspect of Subtest II is illustrated in Table III for the monosyllabic items in the Real Word section. The first item in each list (*hit, shut, hide*, etc.) is a second grade word, the second item (*fed, path, cute*, etc.) is a third grade word, up to the fifth item in each list (*lag, prop, tone*, etc.) at the sixth grade level. The same grade level pattern is repeated for the 30 polysyllabic items. Notice that no first grade items are included since the test seeks to determine the degree to which children use the letter-sound patterns and first grade words (e.g., *man, cat, fish, home*) are often simply memorized by children.

Subtest III: Oral Reading

The Oral Reading subtest includes 11 passages corresponding to each of the Subtest I lists. The ten Subtest I words, together with six selected Subtest II words, are embedded in each passage. Figure 1 shows the DST record form for

Table III
Subtest II Monosyllabic Real Word Items and their Grade-Level Designations

Grade	Item Type					
	CVC	CCVCC	CVCé	CCVCé	CVVC	CCVVCC
Second	hit	shut	hide	brave	loud	threw
Third	fed	path	cute	drove	join	grain
Fourth	jog	stack	doze	flake	raw	choice
Fifth	nut	flesh	fake	globe	loaf	bound
Sixth	lag	prop	tone	crime	bail	preach

PASSAGE #7: THREE-TWO READER

A boy named Harold, who lived at the North Pole, caught a _creature_ and kept it in a small _shelter_ to _protect_ it. Every day Harold had to _provide_ his creature with _raw sausage_ for food and snow _flakes_ for water.

The other boys at Harold's school thought that Harold was a _square_ for saying he had a creature that ate raw sausage. One day Harold heard the boys _muttering_ about how square they thought Harold was. He jumped up and said, "I'll _prove_ it. If everyone brings me one _coin_ to help me pay for its food, I'll show it to you."

Naturally, it was an easy _choice_. All the boys _arrived_ at Harold's house. He took them to the shelter and the boys looked in through the windows. When the creature saw the boys watching it, it started to _bounce_ up and down. Then Harold and the boys took the coins to the store to buy raw sausage and they had a _pleasant_ day feeding the creature.

BASAL TARGET WORDS (# Correct _____)				PHONIC WORDS		COMPREHENSION	
1.	shelter _____	6.	coin _____	1.	creature _____	1.	_____
2.	protect _____	7.	naturally _____	2.	provide _____	2.	_____
3.	square _____	8.	arrived _____	3.	raw _____	3.	_____
4.	muttering _____	9.	bounce _____	4.	sausage _____	4.	_____
5.	prove _____	10.	pleasant _____	5.	flakes _____	5.	_____
				6.	choice _____		

Reading Time: _____ Min. _____ Sec.

PASSAGE SCORES			SCORE SUMMARY	
Nonsense Sub. _____	Word Order _____		Basal Target Words _____	
Real Word Sub. _____	Stumbling _____		Phonic Words _____	
Word Omission _____	Place Lost _____		Comprehension _____	
Word Addition _____	Punctuation _____		Reading Rate _____	
Word Ending _____	Total Errors _____		Error Rate _____	

Figure 1. Page from DST scoring booklet showing the Subtest III scoring sheet for the three-two passage with the complete passage text. Space for tallying target items and oral reading errors is provided at the bottom of the page.

the three-two passage. Words with single underlines (_shelter, protect, square_, etc.) are from the three-two list of Subtest I. That is, they are on grade level with respect to the passage. The double underlined words (_creature, provide, raw_, etc.) are from Subtest II and represent items that are above grade level, thus increasing the probability that letter-sound knowledge will be used in decoding them. All other words were selected from lists designated by Harris and Jacobson (1972) to be below grade level with respect to the passage.

During administration, errors are phonetically encoded and responses to target items (i.e., embedded Subtest I and II words) in each passage are later translated into scores that parallel those obtained for Subtests I and II. Thus, responses to these words are obtained twice during DST administration, once in isolation (in Subtests I or II) and once in context (in Subtest III). Using this feature of the DST, one can draw conclusions concerning the effects of context on decoding. In addition, other parameters of oral reading can be measured, such as reading rate and the traditional oral reading errors we are measuring (shown at the bottom of Figure 1). Finally, the test includes a set of five simple recall comprehension questions which may be asked following the reading of each passage.

Scores from Subtests I and II are being used to provide feedback to teachers and program staff, for program evaluation, and for the monitoring of the progress of individual children across years.[1] We are using all three subtests in a study of the effects of psychostimulant medication on reading achievement in hyperactive, reading disabled children (Winsberg, Richardson, and Kupietz 1983) and we have used it in several studies of the decoding skill deficits of poor readers (Kochnower, Richardson, and DiBenedetto 1983; Richardson, DiBenedetto, and Adler 1982).

Method
DST Scores

A variety of scores may be derived from DST data. The final project report (Richardson et al. 1981) presents analyses of over 40 scores, many of which were subsequently used in a comparison study of good and poor readers (Richardson et al. 1982). Those interested in a more complete description of the DST scores should refer to these two sources. The reliability and validity analyses presented in this chapter involve most of the basic scores (e.g., raw scores) and only one of the more interesting derived scores (the Phonic Transfer Index).

Subjects

The results presented are based on data collected during the three-year test development project. The complete DST was administered twice to the entire student body of a New York City school ($N = 238$); an abbreviated form was administered to a very large sample in Atlanta, GA ($N = 1,231$); and, three good and poor reader studies, involving a combined total of more than 300 children, were conducted. The data from the NYC sample are particularly interesting since these children were tested twice and the data set for these children includes standardized test scores and a variety of other measures as well.[2]

The NYC sample is composed of the entire population of first through fifth grade children in a single school that was participating in a much larger national study on the effects of various instructional models on the achievement of

[1]Since the DST was first introduced in the Interdependent Learning Model Follow Through classrooms (discussed later in this chapter) it has been administered regularly to provide data for teacher feedback and program evaluation. Indeed, participating schools have come to rely on the DST as an important source of information for the management of their reading program.
[2]We wish to thank Harold Freeman, Jr., Director of the Interdependent Learning Model at Fordham University for his assistance in providing these data and for his continued support.

children from economically depressed neighborhoods (Project Follow Through). The first through third grade children in this sample were being taught by procedures prescribed by the Interdependent Learning Model (sponsored by Fordham University) which includes a special approach to reading instruction. The children were tested on the DST in October of 1978 and again, five months later in April of 1979.

Measures

The Fordham project maintained an extensive data file on these children and provided selected data for reliability and validity analyses. Table IV shows the measures used in the analyses and the numbers of children for whom data were available at each of the five grade levels. It will be noted from the table that a total of 238 children took the DST in both October and April.

The Iowa Test of Basic Skills (ITBS) (Hieronymus and Lindquist 1975) was routinely administered by the Fordham staff to evaluate the effects of their intervention. The ITBS is a standardized achievement test that includes subtests of Vocabulary (word recognition), Reading (comprehension), Math Concepts (verbal problems), Math Problems (computation), and Language Usage (e.g., punctuation, use of capitalization, etc.). A total of 175 children in the DST sample took the ITBS in May 1978 (five months prior to the first DST administration). The first grade children in the sample were in kindergarten in 1978 and therefore did not take the ITBS that year. In June 1979 (two months after the final DST administration), a total of 232 of the 238 children who took the DST twice were also given the ITBS.

Finally, the Fordham project systematically collects reading program placement information from teachers each month. Children are assigned GE scores by their teachers depending upon where they are placed in the reading program. For example, a child who has read approximately 50 pages of the early second grade reader might be assigned a program placement value of 2.2 (a GE score representing the second month of second grade). We included placement data from June 1978 and 1979 in the analyses. These data are particularly important in establishing the validity of the criterion-referenced aspect of the DST with regard to basal vocabulary development. As previously noted, the special instructional model is only used in kindergarten through third

Table IV

Numbers of Children in Each Grade in NYC Sample with Scores on Various Achievement Measures Used in Validity Analyses

Measures	Grade					
	1	2	3	4	5	Total
DST: 10/78 & 4/79	36	46	54	50	52	238
ITBS: 5/78	—	35	49	44	47	175
ITBS: 6/79	35	46	54	46	51	232
Bas. Pla. 6/78	28	41	46	49	—	164
Bas. Pla. 6/79	35	46	54	—	—	135

grade classrooms, therefore, no teacher reports were available on fourth and fifth grade children from June 1979.

Results and Discussion

Reliability

It has been argued that conventional procedures for assessing reliability are not appropriate for CR scores (Hambleton and Novick 1973). However, Hayladnya (1974) presents arguments favoring the use of classical reliability assessment for tests that yield CR scores, and the DST satisfies many of the classical test construction conditions. Thus, several of the more conventional reliability coefficients were obtained. Split-half correlation coefficients (using an odd-even division of the items) were computed separately for the 110 Subtest I items and the 120 Subtest II items using the NYC data ($N = 238$) from both test administrations. None of these coefficients was less than 0.99. Moreover, when the coefficients were recomputed controlling for grade placement, none was less than 0.98.[3]

Next, both NYC data sets and the large Atlanta data set were subjected to the SPSS program package (Hull and Nie 1981) reliability procedures. This procedure yields an array of coefficients including Cronbach Alphas and Guttman Lambdas. Most of the resultant coefficients were .99 and none was less than .97.

Since Subtests I and III include the same 110 items administered according to the same basal and ceiling criteria, scores from these two subtests may be correlated to estimate immediate test-retest reliability. (This cannot be done for Subtest II items since they are administered in a different order in Subtest III.) The correlations computed for the total scores and two GE scores generated by these items were all greater than .97 for both NYC data sets and the Atlanta set. While these coefficients fail to assess factors which may influence reliability across time, they do show that these scores are highly reliable across contextual settings (i.e., in isolation versus in context).

Stability

Although the two DST administrations (October 1978 and April 1979) were separated by five months, pretest-posttest correlations provide an estimate of stability of the relative standing of the children across time. It should be stressed that these are not conventional test-retest reliability coefficients which are usually based on test administrations separated by two to four weeks.

---

[3]Reliability and validity coefficients are generally computed for separate samples in each grade. In order to avoid presenting large tables of correlations here, coefficients are reported for the total sample and control for grade level is achieved by computing partial correlation coefficients. Coefficients computed for each grade separately are presented in the final project report (Richardson et al. 1981) and do not differ substantially from the partial correlations presented in this chapter.

However, they certainly represent the lower limits of correlations that might be obtained from a more conventional test-retest time frame.

Table V shows the zero order and grade level partials resulting from this analysis. For the Subtest I Total Score (number correct of the 110 items), we obtained a coefficient of 0.96, indicating a high degree of stability in the relationship of the individual scores across five months and the grade partial is only .03 less. The two additional Subtest I scores, the Instructional Level Grade Equivalent (ILGE) and the Frustration Level Grade Equivalent (FLGE), are derived from the error patterns in individual children's performance. The ILGE is the highest reader level list on which the child demonstrates at least 80% mastery and the FLGE is the lowest reader level list on which the child fails more than 50% of the items. These scores are expressed in GEs by adding 0.3 to the grade level of the first semester lists (e.g., 2.3 for the two-one list, 3.3 for the three-one list, etc.) and by adding 0.8 to the second semester lists (e.g., 2.8 for two-two, 3.8 for three-two, etc.). The pretest-posttest correlations of these scores are both 0.94 and the effects of controlling for grade level are minimal.

Pretest-posttest correlations for Subtest II are only slightly lower than those for Subtest I and, as with the Subtest I coefficients, controlling for grade level has only a small effect. Finally, the Subtest III correlations are almost identical to those obtained with Subtest I. Correlations were also computed using the total scores of the three subtests obtained by children in each grade separately (Ns ranged from 37 to 52). The lowest coefficient to emerge was that for the first grade, Subtest II scores (0.79) and most of the coefficients were greater than 0.90.

These pretest-posttest correlations may be regarded as transitional between the concepts of test-retest reliability and content validity. They are at the lower limit of more conventional test-retest reliability coefficients which one might expect to be approaching 1.0 (as we observed in the correlations of Subtest I and III Total Scores). The fact that the relationship of individual scores remains relatively constant across five months in spite of the influence of other variables such as quality of instruction and individual ability, indicates that the same thing was being measured at both test points.

Table V
Pretest-Posttest Correlations of Representative DST Scores from October 1978 to May 1979

Score		Zero Order	Grade Part.
Subtest I	Total Score	.96	.93
	Instructional Level GE	.94	.91
	Frustration Level GE	.94	.91
Subtest II	Total Score	.90	.87
	Real Words	.88	.86
	Nonsense Words	.85	.84
Subtest III	Total Score	.95	.93
	Instructional Level GE	.92	.89
	Frustration Level GE	.93	.90

Validity

The demonstration of a convergent trend is one of the most important techniques for establishing the construct validity of a test. A convergent trend is observed in the degree to which the strength of a test's association with other measures increases as a function of the degree to which the external measures represent the construct that the test purports to measure. Thus, since the DST is criterion-referenced to the reading curriculum, one would expect it to relate best to the Program Placement measures. Since it measures decoding, it should also correlate highly with measures of vocabulary and word recognition. Since decoding is primary to reading comprehension, one expects correlations with comprehension to be high, but lower than those with curriculum placement or vocabulary. Finally, measures of less decoding-related academic skills (e.g., math) should correlate less well with DST scores. Thus, in examining the validity coefficients presented here, reference will be made to the tendency of the correlation coefficients to reflect a convergent trend on the construct of decoding development within the reading curriculum.

Table VI presents predictive validity coefficients relating DST scores from October 1978 to other achievement scores obtained in May 1979. These data display a strong convergent trend on program placement and word recognition (ITBS Vocabulary). After Vocabulary, the convergent trend is not apparent for the ITBS zero-order coefficients. That is, the correlations with Reading (comprehension), Math Concepts, Math Problems, and Language Usage are all about the same. However, the convergent trend is apparent throughout the data when grade level is controlled. The grade level control reduces the correlations with Math Problems more than those with Reading or Math Concepts (both measures which require decoding as well as comprehension) but it has little effect on the correlations with Language Usage. Thus, the convergent trend for the ITBS scores follows from Math Problems (the least decoding-related), up through Reading and Math Concepts (both of which require decoding *and* comprehension) to Vocabulary and Language Usage (presumably the two most decoding-related measures in the ITBS battery). Finally, the extremely high validity coefficients with Program Placement

Table VI

Predictive Validity Coefficients Relating DST Total Scores from October 1978 to Other Achievement Measures from May 1979

Achievement Measures	N	Subtest I		Subtest II		Subtest III	
		Zero Order	Grade Part.	Zero Order	Grade Part.	Zero Order	Grade Part.
Program Placement	135	.93	.90	.83	.80	.93	.90
ITBS Vocabulary	232	.80	.61	.76	.66	.82	.71
ITBS Reading	232	.71	.53	.66	.51	.71	.54
ITBS Math Concepts	232	.76	.44	.71	.55	.72	.57
ITBS Math Problems	232	.72	.35	.67	.49	.72	.49
ITBS Language Usage	85	.64	.62	.61	.61	.64	.62

provide powerful evidence for the validity of the criterion-referenced construct of the DST, while the convergent trend of increasing correlations with the degree of active involvement of decoding supports the validity of the decoding construct of the test.

One more point should be considered before leaving the Table VI data. The selective effects of the partialing procedure on the less decoding related measures noted above provides further evidence for construct validity. This pattern suggests that the zero order correlations for the less decoding related measures contain a strong developmental component and are substantially reduced by controlling for grade level. In contrast, the more decoding related measures are relatively unaffected. This tends to confirm the notion that the DST is measuring decoding independently of a child's development in other areas.

Flexibility

Up to this point, the reliability and validity of only the more conventional DST scores have been considered. However, the validity of scores derived from DST response patterns is fundamental to the assertion that the DST may be used for specific hypothesis testing. The relationships of many of the derived scores to developmental dyslexia have been assessed in a previous study (Richardson et al. 1982), and the final DST project report presents grade by sex ANOVAs and correlation matrices relating these scores to each other and to several external measures (Richardson et al. 1981). These analyses provide substantial support for the validity of many of the derived DST scores. We will now consider the validity of one of these scores, the Phonic Transfer Index (PTI), by assessing the degree to which it relates to academic gains. This is an extremely important issue when one wishes to test hypotheses about the relationship of decoding skill development to dyslexia.

The PTI is designed to measure the degree to which a child's working knowledge of letter-sound patterns, expressed in responses to real words, transfers to novel items (nonsense words). Recall that each nonsense word item parallels (i.e., is derived from) a corresponding real word item (e.g., *dut* is derived from *nut*). The PTI simply states the empirical probability that a nonsense word response is correct given that its corresponding real word response is correct. Stated mathmatically:

$$PTI = P\,(NWC:RWC) = \frac{\Sigma\,(NWC:RWC)}{\Sigma\,(RWC)}$$

Where P (NWC:RWC) is the probability that a nonsense-word response is correct given that its corresponding real word response is correct; Σ (NWC:RWC) is the number of nonsense words correct for which the corresponding real words are also correct; and Σ RWC is simply the total number of correct real-word responses (or the Real Word Total Score).

The PTI, therefore, assesses the likelihood that a child's correct responses to the real words are based on that child's knowledge of spelling patterns, independently of word meaning or prior exposure. The degree to which the PTI relates to gains on an academic measure reflects the degree to which that measure is dependent upon phonic transfer. Positive findings should support the validity of the PTI as a research tool for studying transfer of letter-sound knowledge. This issue is extremely important in studies of phonemic segmentation and other linguistic factors in developmental dyslexia (e.g., Mann, Liberman, and Shankweiler 1980; Treiman and Baron 1983; Vellutino, Steger, Harding, and Phillips 1975; and Zifcak 1981).

To assess the effects of PTI on academic gains, two separate regression equations were computed. In the first equation the dependent measure (i.e., posttest scores on ITBS, Program Placement, or DST) is predicted from three variables: (a) pretest measure (to generate an unbiased estimate of gain), (b) Grade Placement (to control for prior exposure to instruction), and (c) ITBS Math Problems (to control for general academic ability). The second equation includes all three predictor variables plus PTI. The change in the R^2 from the first equation (without PTI) to the second (with PTI) represents the effects of PTI on academic gains. This measure, called the R^2 increment (i.e., the semipartial squared), reflects the added unique variance accounted for by PTI independently of prior instruction and more general academic ability and it is assessed by t-test procedures (Cohen and Cohen 1975).

Table VII presents the results of the regression analysis. The first three rows of the table report results for the ITBS scores using pretest scores obtained in May 1978 to predict posttest scores in June 1979. The total R^2s (from the second equations which include PTI) range from .5953 to .6470, indicating that about 60% of the posttest variance in the ITBS scores is accounted for by the

Table VII
Results of Regression Analysis Predicting Achievement Gains from PTI
Controlling for Expected Grade Level and Math Problems

| Dep. Mea. | | R^2 Increment | | | | t-vals for Regres. Params | | | |
		Tot.	Inc.	F	df	Grade	Math	Pre.	PTI
ITBS	Voc.	.6470	.0008	0.37	165.1	−0.35	4.70**	7.78**	0.62
	Read.	.5580	.0045	1.67	164.1	−1.15	5.85**	4.20**	1.64
	Lang.	.5953	.0012	0.24	81.1	1.51	3.72**	6.27**	1.12
Prog. Place.		.8615	.0114	8.97**	109.1	−2.20	4.82**	8.84**	3.16*
DST I	Tot.	.9199	.0082	8.97**	227.1	0.10	0.00	23.63**	4.94**
	ILGE	.8919	.0149	31.29**	227.1	1.31	0.72	19.60**	5.70**
	FLGE	.8765	.0133	24.45**	227.1	−1.06	0.60	15.99**	5.25**
DST III	Tot.	.9229	.0131	38.57**	227.1	0.25	−0.05	23.78**	6.32**
	ILGE	.8709	.0216	34.63**	227.1	−2.18	0.24	18.09**	6.01**
	FLGE	.8749	.0105	17.37**	207.1	0.20	1.33	19.38**	4.29**
DST II	Tot.	.8504	.0341	23.24**	227.1	−2.15	0.53	14.60**	7.27**
	Real	.8308	.0110	14.76**	227.1	−2.23	0.46	14.96**	3.98**
	Nons.	.8449	.0841	123.09**	227.1	−1.61	1.11	12.72**	11.16**

$*p < .01$
$**p < .001$

four predictor variables. The unique variance in the ITBS scores that is accounted for by PTI (i.e., the R^2 increment) is negligible in every case (no more than 0.1%) and none is significant. Finally, among the t-values assessing the regression parameters that predict ITBS scores (shown in the last four columns of the table) only those for Math and Pretest are significant.

In contrast to results with the ITBS, the R^2s associated with Basal Placement and all of the DST scores are large, ranging from .8308 (for DST II, Real Words) to .9229 (for DST III, Total Score). The F-values assessing the R^2 increments associated with PTI are all significant ($p < .01$).

Special note should be made of the t-values associated with the regression parameters for Math (Problems) in Table VII. Reference to these results reveals that while Math contributes significantly to the prediction of ITBS and Program Placement gains, its contribution to the prediction of DST gains is negligible. This suggests that progress in decoding (i.e., basal vocabulary and letter sound decoding) is relatively independent of more general academic ability but highly dependent on PTI (i.e., the ability to transfer knowledge of spelling patterns to novel words).

Finally, it should be noted that this technique for assessing the effects of PTI is extremely rigorous. The pretest scores contain a large measure of variance associated with PTI, so that the R^2 increments for PTI represent the tip of the iceberg—PTI's effect on relatively short-term gains independent of its prior effects (in the pretest scores). The fact that the PTI passes this rigorous test, affirms its reliability and validity as a measure of transfer ability.

The demonstration of a significant transfer component in decoding skill development over five months is important in its own right. In fact, this particular score has been shown to have potential in research on the subtypes of dyslexia (Richardson 1984). However, the primary point here is that the PTI, derived from responses made to various DST items and based on the logical construction of the test, has obvious research value. A variety of such measures reflecting automaticity, use of context, error patterns, and various facets of oral reading may also be derived from the DST. Many of these measures may be used to further our understanding of developmental dyslexia in particular and of the more general development of reading skills in normal readers. Thus, the DST is not only a highly reliable and valid test of decoding skill development, it is also an extremely flexible tool for studying various aspects of how these skills are expressed in different groups (e.g., dyslexic versus normal children, girls versus boys).

Uses and Limitations of the DST

Research Uses

The good and poor reader study.   The objective of the NICHD contract for the DST was to develop a test with a standard item pool for accurate subject identification and hypothesis testing. The previously mentioned good and poor reader study (Richardson et al. 1982) adequately demonstrates both uses. In that study, standardized test scores were used to identify 15 good and 15 poor readers of normal IQ at each of four grade levels (second through fifth grades). As expected, all mastery level scores and several of the derived scores reliably discriminated between the two groups. There were large differences on PTI at all four grade levels and the poor readers were more likely to make errors with little phonological resemblance to the actual items than were the good readers.

The finding that good and poor readers, equated for grade level and IQ, differ in decoding skill development is hardly a startling discovery. The more interesting question of how the decoding skills of poor readers differ from those of good readers when they are equated for reading level is addressed in a second study based on the same data set. In that study, 17 younger, good readers were matched with older, poor readers on IQ and Subtest I ILGE (using the DST for subject identification) and the two groups were compared on various derived scores (using the DST for hypothesis testing). The important result of this study was that, given equivalent levels of basal vocabulary development, the older, poor readers displayed specific deficiencies in the use of the phonetic code in decoding relative to the younger, good readers. While the two groups did not differ on various measures with minimal phonemic involvement (e.g., oral reading rate, basal vocabulary response strength, certain oral reading error tendencies), they differed on nearly all of the measures that are dependent on the use of letter-sound patterns in decoding (e.g., PTI, incidence of sound-related errors, decoding of both Real and Nonsense Words). These findings were replicated in a later study (Kochnower et al. 1983) and further traced to specific difficulties in using vowel generalizations in decoding (DiBenedetto, Richardson, and Kochnower 1983).

Genetic research.   Now we will consider how the DST would be valuable in just one of the several areas of research that are currently making important contributions to the understanding of developmental dyslexia, the area of genetic research. There is an accumulation of evidence that reading disability is heterogeneous in nature (Decker and DeFries 1981; Finucci 1978; Lovett 1984; Mattis, French, and Rapin 1975). Some cases may be genetic in origin, others environmental, and others a combination of these factors. Even if it can be shown that some cases are primarily genetic in origin, in all likelihood these too will involve heterogeneous subtypes (Finucci and Childs 1983; Omenn and Weber 1978) and it is possible that different genetic mechanisms are involved in their transmission. Finucci and her associates at Johns Hopkins, in particular, have made use of Boder's (1971) classifications (dyseidetic, dysphonetic, and mixed) to isolate homogeneous groups and trace specific genetic mechanisms within families. This work has led them to point out the need for more refined behavioral instruments that can be used to further characterize the various subtypes (Finucci and Childs 1983). We think the DST is just such an instrument.

DST measures such as the PTI should help in the effort to characterize children and their families according to subtypes. It would be extremely interesting to know, for example, if in the Colorado Project (Decker and DeFries 1981) the Subtype 3 children (characterized by depressed scores in reading only), would demonstrate specific types of decoding deficits on the

DST as compared to the other three groups (which were weak in other areas as well). If this were the case, and if these specific deficits were also found in the siblings and parents of the affected children, a stronger case could be made for genetic transmission. And, had the DST been available to the Johns Hopkins group, we would know whether transfer deficits would characterize the children with a high proportion of dysphonetic spelling errors. It is very possible that this measure would help clarify the familial patterns reported by these investigators. Finally, had DST data been available for their efforts to define reading disabilities in adults through regression analysis (Finucci, Whitehouse, Isaacs, and Childs 1984), the DST scores might have helped in differentiating between the ''border line'' and ''severe'' groups.

We could continue to examine the potential research value of the DST. Throughout this chapter we have made reference to the literature on linguistic and phonemic processing deficits in dyslexia. Numerous studies have appeared in the past decade that document this phenomenon. We will not pursue this issue further here, but we refer the reader to the chapters by Liberman and by Vellutino and Scanlon in this volume and we invite the reader to consider how valuable it would have been to have had DST basal vocabulary and phonic pattern scores on the samples in these studies.

Limitations of the DST

The merits of the DST have been emphasized throughout this chapter. In order to maintain a realistic perspective, it is important to consider some of its limitations.

First, as with any test of its kind, the number of items used to represent each of the skill domains is smaller than one would wish. There are 30 first grade items (10 each in the preprimer, primer, and first reader lists), but most standard reading programs present between 600 and 1,000 words during first grade instruction. At successive grade levels, the DST includes only 20 items for each year. Yet, the actual vocabulary presented in most programs expands rapidly in the second through fifth grade curriculum. Most programs present between 2,000 and 3,000 new words in second grade alone. Clearly, it would be desirable to have more than 20 items at each grade level to represent this much larger pool. This same argument may be applied to Subtest II. Five items for each pattern is simply not enough to draw firm conclusions about a child's ability with each pattern. Furthermore, although Subtest II includes many of the common orthographic patterns in our language, there are several important patterns (e.g., controlling ''r'' as in ''bird'' and ''lord'') which are not represented. However, given that the item set spans five grade levels and that the test format is restricted to a linear sequence, we feel that the arduous search for the most discriminating words paid off with an item set that approaches the best possible, within the limits of time and the test format. Limitations of the DST's linear design may now be overcome with the branching procedures used in the type of computerized testing discussed by Inouye and Sorensen in this volume. With computers, it becomes feasible to use the DST as a surface upon which to discover where to explore a child's decoding skills in much greater depth.

Although the DST's range of measurement may be regarded as restricted to first through fifth grade levels, this limitation is necessary if we wish to restrict the instrument to decoding as opposed to more general language development issues. Instruments with a broader range (e.g., WRAT, PIAT) may be desirable for measuring dimensions of reading in older samples, but they must simultaneously measure both decoding *and* more general vocabulary development and therefore cannot be used to draw inferences specifically about decoding. We have found many of the DST scores clinically useful with dyslexic children and adults who score as high as seventh-grade level on standardized tests, because such persons often show continued deficiencies in decoding skill development. But, if one wishes to study decoding skill development per se, it is best to select samples within a first to fifth grade range.

A major problem with the DST is its failure to test phonemic processing as an auditory skill. A variety of techniques have been used to measure development in this domain (e.g., Rosner 1974; Liberman, Shankweiler, Liberman, Fowler, and Fischer 1976; Fox and Routh 1980, 1983). We had been interested in sound blending (Richardson, DiBenedetto and Bradley 1977) and we proposed a sound blending subtest for the DST. Unfortunately, the NICHD contract review committee felt that the sound blending task would be too partisan and recommended that this feature of the test be dropped. At this point I regret that some measure of phonemic processing, regardless of the particular task used, was not included in the test. It is important to note for future research with the DST that it is possible to construct phonemic processing tasks around existing DST items. Data of this type could be used to address questions concerning the degree to which decoding development is dependent on auditory/linguistic processing skills.

Finally, we will consider the limitations of Subtest III. We went to great lengths to establish semantic and vocabulary patterns in the passages that are representative of the material in most readers (see Richardson et al. 1981). To achieve this objective, rigid constraints were followed in writing the passages (e.g., sentence length, grammatical structure). In addition, each passage had to contain the 16 words from Subtests I and II assigned to it and the conceptual relationships among these words was minimal. Adherence to these constraints resulted in passages of varying conceptual complexity and this may produce some distortion of Subtest III measures such as reading rate, oral reading errors, and responses to the comprehension questions.

A second point regarding Subtest III concerns the oral reading error categories. The categories used (see Figure 1) are modeled after those in other tests (e.g., the Gilmore Oral Reading Test) and do not represent the full range of possible errors one might wish to measure. Also, the names assigned to these categories are somewhat arbitrary. For example, Transformations are grammatic derivatives of the actual words ("made" for "make") and Error Substitutions are nonsense word responses given for actual words in the text. Others might wish to give different labels to these categories. The important point to bear in mind when using the DST is that the particular oral reading errors one might choose to measure and the names one wishes to ascribe to them is up to the individual investigator.

Summary and Conclusions

NICHD sponsored a contract to develop a test that could be used effectively in research on developmental dyslexia. The final product of that effort, the DST, is a criterion-referenced test that measures in several domains of decoding skills. The results presented in this chapter support the conclusion that the DST fulfills this objective. It is reliable, displays a high degree of content and construct validity, and provides several scores which are relevant to specific aspects of developmental dyslexia. Since it was first developed, we have used the DST in our own research on dyslexia and on reading problems associated with other childhood disorders. We have shared the DST with a number of other investigators in its prototype form but until recently we have not had the resources to encourage wide dissemination.[4]

This chapter has focused on the DST as a research tool. We have made only brief reference to the fact that it also serves a variety of applied purposes. In the Atlanta Follow Through project it has been used for the past six years to provide information to teachers, to assist in program placement decisions, and for formative and summative evaluation. It is also being used for diagnosis and evaluation in a number of clinics with which we are currently affiliated. These uses of the DST have been very encouraging and we feel that it has considerable applied value. Although research with the DST to date offers more support for the validity of its clinical application than many of the instruments in common use, additional research will be necessary to further validate and extend its applied value.

References

Alkin, M. C. 1974. Criterion-referenced measurement and other such terms. *In* C. W. Harris, M. C. Alkin, and Popham, W. J. (eds.). *Problems in Criterion-Referenced Measurement.* Los Angeles: Center for Study of Evaluation, UCLA.

Boder, E. 1971. Developmental dyslexia: A diagnostic screening procedure based on three characteristic patterns of reading and spelling. *In* B. Bateman (ed.). *Learning Disorders,* Vol. IV, Reading. Seattle: Special Child Publications.

Cohen, J., and Cohen, P. 1975. *Applied Multiple Regression/Correlation Analysis for the Behavioral Sciences.* Hillsdale, NJ: Lawrence Erlbaum Associates.

Decker, S. N., and DeFries, J. C. 1981. Cognitive ability profiles in families of reading disabled children. *Developmental Medicine and Child Neurology* 23:217–227.

DiBenedetto, B., Richardson, E., and Kochnower, J. 1983. Vowel generalizations in normal and learning disabled readers. *Journal of Educational Psychology* 75:576–582.

---

[4]The DST is scheduled for publication by York Press, Inc. in the winter of 1985. Inquiries concerning obtaining copies of the test should be addressed to York Press, 2712 Mt. Carmel Rd.; Parkton, MD 21120.

Finucci, J. M. 1978. Genetic considerations in dyslexia. *In* H. R. Myklebust (ed). *Progress in Learning Disabilities,* Vol. IV. New York: Grune and Stratton.

Finucci, J. M., and Childs, B. 1983. Dyslexia: Family studies. *In* C. Ludlow and J. Cooper (eds). *Genetic Aspects of Speech and Language Disorders.* New York: Academic Press.

Finucci, J. M., Whitehouse, C. C., Isaacs, S. D., and Childs, B. 1984. Derivation and validation of a quantitative definition of specific reading disability for adults. *Developmental Medicine and Child Neurology* 26:143–153.

Fox, B., and Routh, D. K. 1980. Phonemic analysis and severe reading disability in children. *Journal of Psycholinguistic Research* 9:115–119.

Fox, B., and Routh, D. K. 1983. Reading disability, phonemic analysis and dysphonetic spelling: A follow-up study. *Journal of Clinical Child Psychology* 12:28–32.

Hayladnya, T. M. 1974. Effects of different samples on item and test characteristics of criterion-referenced tests. *Journal of Educational Measurement* 11:93–99.

Hambleton, R. K., and Novick, M. R. 1973. Toward an Integration of theory and method for criterion-referenced testing. *Journal of Educational Measurement* 10:159–169.

Harris, A. J., and Jacobson, M. D. 1972. *Basic Elementary Reading Vocabularies.* New York: MacMillan.

Hieronymus, A. N., and Lindquist, E. F. 1975. *Manual for Administrators—Iowa Test of Basic Skills.* Boston, MA: Houghton-Mifflin.

Hull, C. H., and Nie, N. H. 1981. *SPSS Update 7–9.* New York: McGraw-Hill.

Kochnower, J., Richardson, E., and DiBenedetto, B. 1983. A comparison of the phonic decoding ability of normal and learning disabled children. *Journal of Learning Disabilities* 16:348–351.

Liberman, I. Y., Shankweiler, D., Liberman, A. M., Fowler, C., and Fischer, F. W. 1976. Phonetic segmentation and recoding in the beginning reader. *In* A. S. Reber and D. Scarborough (eds.). *Toward a Psychology of Reading.* Hillsdale, NJ: Lawrence Erlbaum Associates.

Lovett, M. W. 1984. A developmental perspective on reading dysfunction: Accuracy and rate criteria in the subtyping of dyslexic children. *Brain and Language* 22:67–91.

Mann, V. A., Liberman, I. Y., and Shankweiler, D. 1980. Children's memory for sentences and word strings in relations to reading ability. *Memory and Cognition* 8:329–335.

Mattis, S., French, J. M., and Rapin, I. 1975. Dyslexia in children and adults: Three independent neuropsychological syndromes. *Developmental Medicine and Child Neurology* 17:150–163.

Omenn, G. S., and Weber, B. A. 1978. Dyslexia: Search for phenotypic and genetic heterogeneity. *American Journal of Medical Genetics* 1:333–342.

Richardson, E. 1984. The impact of phonemic processing instruction on the reading achievement of reading disabled children. *In* S. White (ed). *Annals of the New York Academy of Sciences,* 433:97–118.

Richardson, E., and DiBenedetto, B. 1985. *The Decoding Skills Test.* Parkton, MD: York Press.

Richardson, E., DiBenedetto, B., and Bradley, C. M. 1977. The relationship of sound blending to reading achievement. *Review of Educational Research* 47:319–334.

Richardson, E., DiBenedetto, B., and Adler, A. 1982. Use of the decoding skills test to study differences in good and poor readers. *In* K. Gadow and I. Bialer (eds.). *Advances in Learning and Behavioral Disabilities,* Vol. 1. Greenwich, Conn.: JAI Press.

Richardson, E., DiBenedetto, B., Adler, A., and Kochnower, J. 1981. *Final Report: The Decoding Skills Test (DST) Project.* NICHD Contract #NO1-HD-7-2837.

Rosner, J. 1974. Auditory analysis training with prereaders. *Reading Teacher* 27:379–384.

Treiman, R., and Baron, J. 1983. Phonemic analysis training helps children benefit from spelling-sound rules. *Memory and Cognition* 15:49–54.

Vellutino, F. R., Steger, J. A., Harding, C. J., and Phillips, F. 1975. Verbal vs. non verbal paired-associates learning in poor and normal readers. *Neuropsychologia* 13:75–82.

Winsberg, B. G., Richardson, E. and Kupietz, S. 1983. *Ritalin and Reading Achievement in Reading Disabled, Hyperactive Children.* Proposal Submitted to NIMH, Application #MRPRO727.

Zifcak, M. 1981. Phonological awareness and reading acquisition. *Contemporary Educational Psychology* 6:117–126.

18

Profiles of Dyslexia: The Computer as an Instrument of Vision

Dillon K. Inouye and Matthew R. Sorenson

*N*otwithstanding the progress that has been made by researchers like the contributors to this volume, research on dyslexia has been unsuccessful in the attainment of three important goals:

(1) Prediction—predicting reliably in advance who is at risk for dyslexia, or specific reading disability;

(2) Understanding—identifying the causal antecedents of specific instances of the disability; and

(3) Remediation—developing remedial measures that are geared to individual students.

The practical consequences of these failures are sobering. No empirically validated procedures are widely available to help teachers and parents discover whether a preschool child will have difficulty learning to read. If, later on, the child manifests specific reading disabilities, no certain etiological diagnosis can be offered. If an unspecific diagnosis of reading disability is made, no specific individualized remediation program can be prescribed.

Although there are many legitimate goals for research on reading retardation, it is difficult to disagree with Applebee's (1971) contention that the goals of advance prediction, etiological understanding, and individualized remediation are, for school children and their families, the most important motivations for research. In this final chapter, strategies will be suggested for drawing together some of the manifold and widely divergent "profiles" of dyslexia found in the literature into a smaller number of convergent representations. To effect this convergence, progress will be required on three fronts: first, greater conceptual clarity should be obtained about that for which investigators are looking; second, more efficient research designs and strategies should be used to gain more reliable information about relationships among profiles; and third, new developments in theory and technology of measurement should be exploited.

Before offering suggestions in these three areas, it will be helpful to present a summary of the current state of dyslexia research and the epistemic predicament in which it stands.

An Epistemic Predicament and Three Critical Problems

Dyslexia research is caught in an epistemic predicament. Attempts to contribute new knowledge or to understand are hedged in on three sides by problems that critically limit progress. On one side, researchers are working with definitions of dyslexia that seriously handicap the search for causes of reading retardation. On another side, they are faced with proliferating profiles of disability that nominate ever more loci of deficit. Because little study is devoted to logico-theoretical relationships among profiles, the number of factors to be considered is exploding. Although an obvious solution to this problem would be to use repeated-measures designs with multiple measures on the same set of subjects, this is practically impossible because, on a third side, investigators are faced with the practical and methodological requirements of sound measurement practice. Discussing each of these problems in turn will bring their contribution to the predicament into sharper focus.

The Problem of Definition

Many definitions of dyslexia in current use are not helpful to researchers. They obscure rather than enhance insight. In some cases, early clinical definitions have had behavioral, sociological, instructional, and neurological requirements added to them. In other cases, criterion-referenced, behavioral definitions have been supplemented with biological requirements. These eclectic definitions often mix assumptively different models of disability, having contrary, and sometimes contradictory, assumptions. The adoption of such definitions and their accompanying conceptual baggage makes it difficult, if not impossible, to translate the definitions into a coherent set of concrete operations.

Why this is so may be seen by referring to the difficulties of a typical example. Many of the more widely used definitions resemble that of Critchely (1970) who defines dyslexia as:

> A disorder manifested by difficulty in learning to read despite conventional instruction, adequate intelligence, and socio-cultural opportunity. It is dependent upon fundamental cognitive disabilities which are frequently of constitutional origin. (p. 11)

There are several problematic elements in this definition that are worthy of consideration:

First, the phrase "A disorder manifested by difficulty in learning to read," is difficult to operationalize in any non-arbitrary way. In some cases the phrase has meant "at least two years below grade level." In others it has been defined on a sliding scale, where a half year of retardation is added for every grade, e.g., 1 year retardation at grade 2, 1½ years at grade 3, 2 years at grade 4, etc. (Lyle and Goyen 1969). To still others it means a specified interval on an oral reading test, e.g., "between the 4th and 10th percentile" (Vellutino and Scanlon this volume). These behavioral definitions have a common weakness: they are normative definitions which impose arbitrary cut-off points upon data whose underlying structures may not justify them.

Second, the exclusion from dyslexia of all cases of retarded reading due to lack of "conventional instruction, adequate intelligence, and socio-cultural opportunity" is a case of definition *via negativa* that tells us what dyslexia is not rather than what it is. It assumes that for reading-retardation cases the variables of conventional instruction, intelligence, and socio-cultural opportunity may be successfully scaled and appropriate threshold points chosen below which retardation is dyslexic and above which retardation is simply poor reading. It assumes, furthermore, that the causes of dyslexia do not interact with any of these exclusionary variables. Dyslexia is therefore arbitrarily defined as a residual disorder, i.e., what is left after everything else is accounted for. As a consequence, a truly "dyslexic" reader who is also unfortunate enough to have had either a lack of instruction, or inadequate intelligence, or a lack of socio-cultural opportunity would not be diagnosed as dyslexic, implying paradoxically that other etiologies, whenever present, are the diagnoses of choice.

Third, the stipulation that dyslexia should be "dependent upon fundamental cognitive disabilities which are frequently of constitutional origin" opens the door to comparisons of the cognitive abilities of normal and dyslexic readers at any level of cognitive functioning instead of just those that are associated with reading. Also, although Critchely's definition states that deficiencies are frequently of constitutional origin, many other definitions require that dyslexic readers have an "intact neurology" or be "free from neurological impairment," thus seriously confusing the search for possible causes. In fairness, it should be noted that requirements like these are modified in some current definitions. Newer definitions use less constraining locutions like "free of 'gross' or 'obvious' neurological disorder" (Denckla this volume).

Fourth, it has been uncritically assumed by many investigators that to determine the etiology of dyslexia is to find a universal cognitive disability shared by all dyslexics. Both the seeking of the universal and the reifying of the "dyslexic" as a certain type of person, rather than seeing dyslexia as an aspect of the person's behavior, are intellectual mistakes against which we have been warned from classical times.

Fifth, it is obvious that an arbitrary setting of threshold points for exclusionary criteria in the definition governs the operationalization of definitions. This in turn governs the frequency of incidence of the disorder and the selection of subjects for research. Although the presumption is that dyslexia is a disorder of nature and not of nurture, the selecting, comparing, and defining cycle is based upon arbitrary normative procedures. As in the case of the dependent variable, to the extent that distribution assumptions of our statistical procedures are not being met for the independent variable (Applebee 1971), the research community is systematically misleading itself.

To the extent that the foregoing difficulties are also present in other definitions, they, too, must be considered problematic. A negative consequence of the use of definitions having these problems is an increase in error variance and a consequent reduction of acuity. The arbitrariness of definitions increases sampling error, lowers external validity, and systematically blurs profiles of dyslexia that appear in the literature. It is to a consideration of these profiles that we now turn.

Profiles of Dyslexia

Scientific studies of dyslexia have resulted in many profiles of the disorder. A ''profile'' may be defined as a collection of measurements of theory relevant variables. A profile is less complete than a definition, portraying only a selected facet of the disorder. An underlying assumption of research in the field is that some future juxtaposition of profiles will faithfully portray the disorder.

Unfortunately, the hoped for convergence of profiles has not yet occurred and does not appear to be immediately forthcoming. In fact, the total number of different profiles is increasing rather than decreasing. Table I presents a sample of profiles, adapted from Taylor and Taylor (1983) and others, where dyslexic, poor, and disabled readers were compared to normal controls. (An unfortunate limitation of this literature is the heterogeneity of its subjects. For purposes of the table, a poor reader is one who scores below the 27th percentile, or one standard deviation below the mean, on a standard reading test. A disabled reader is one who has ''an imperfect ability to listen, think, speak, read, write, spell, or to do mathematical calculation.'') An inspection of this rather lengthy table gives the reader a feeling for the complexity of the problem, a complexity actually underrepresented in the table.

An inspection of the profiles of Table I shows some properties of the profiles as well as their dimensions of proliferation. In general, profiles are snapshots of variables measured at some moment in time. The modal number of variables per profile is one, although some profiles do offer a more diversified picture. The types of variables nominated range widely from reading or linguistic dimensions on one hand to neurological or genetic dimensions on some others. So many sites of the system are nominated for the loci of deficit and the variability among subjects is so great that it seems unlikely that a single, simple dyslexic universal will be found. Indeed, the data show that few, if any, of the measures chosen by investigators discriminated perfectly between those subjects defined as dyslexic and their normal controls. These patterns of differential responding are consistent with the suggestion of Satz and others (Satz and Morris 1981; Satz, Morris and Fletcher this volume) that the question is not one of dyslexia, but rather of the dyslexias. However, until sampling procedures can be improved and patterns of responding stabilized across replications, the subject of subtypes will remain an open question.

Table I
Profiles of Dyslexia

Perceptual deficits

Eye movements

Some dyslexics showed difficulty in scanning lines of x's arranged in word-like patterns (Elterman, Abel, Daroff, Dell'Osso, and Bornstein 1980).

Auditory linguistic subtypes showed normal patterns; visual spatial subtypes showed faulty right to left scanning and inaccurate return sweeps (Pirozzolo 1979).

Unclassified dyslexics showed erratic eye movements in reading and in following sequentially illuminated light sources (Pavlidis 1981).

Severely disabled readers showed sharply reduced peripheral vision (Fisher 1979).

Unlike normal readers, 50 out of 80 dyslexics showed inconsistent patterns of eye dominance. All 50 were classified in a "visual" subtype which responded favorably to treatments with eyeglasses that blocked out the left eye (Stein and Fowler 1982)

Perceptual tests

Disabled readers, in studies too numerous to list, showed many different kinds of perceptual deficits. Although it has been argued by Vellutino (1979) and Vellutino and Scanlon (this volume) that findings of perceptual deficit are actually findings of verbal deficit (Vellutino, Steger, Harding, and Phillips 1975), there exist some studies where these variables are not confounded.

Some impaired readers showed the inability to discriminate the order of two rapidly presented auditory stimuli (Tallal 1980).

Dyslexics showed slower rates of processing in backward masking tasks and more difficulty in temporal integration tasks (Di Lollo, Hanson, and McIntyre 1983).

Sequencing and orientation errors

Dyslexics made a large number of orientation and sequencing errors in reading words aloud, i.e., "din-bin," "cod-cob," although they could generally copy them correctly (Vellutino, Steger, and Kandel 1972).

Dyslexics made proportionally fewer reversal and orientation errors (i.e., 15 and 10%, respectively), than sound confusion errors (75%) (Liberman, Shankweiler, Orlando, Harris, and Berti 1971).

Disabled readers who suffered left-right confusion also had difficulties discriminating body parts and object relations (Belmont and Birch 1963; Benon 1978; Corballis and Beale 1976; Ginsberg and Hartwick 1971).

Memory deficits

Short-term memory (STM)

Dyslexics had deficits of short-term memory and not long-term memory (Jorm 1979).

Disabled readers performed poorly on STM tasks (300 to 2000 msec.) when compared to normal readers, but did no worse on perceptual tasks (0–300 msec.). The STM tasks involved letters, geometric forms and abstract forms (Morrison, Giordani, and Nagy 1977).

Disabled readers were worse at matching temporal patterns of flashing lights with spatial

(continued)

Table I continued

representations of the same patterns. They were also unable to code the patterns verbally (Blank and Bridger 1966).

Poor readers used inefficient verbal codes (Bryden 1972).

Disabled readers scored worse in a serial recall task, but did just as well as normals when taught how to rehearse properly (Torgesen and Goldman 1977).

Poor readers showed poor memory for the order of digits and letters (Mason, Katz, and Wicklund 1975; Stanley, Kaplan, and Poole 1975).

Poor readers made more errors in retaining temporal sequences of figures and letters when materials were meaningful (Bakker 1972).

Poor second grade readers (40th percentile) were worse than good readers (80th percentile) in their ability to order a five-item series that could be recoded as words (Katz, Shankweiler, and Liberman 1981).

Specific memory deficit

Poor readers were worse than normal readers in word storage and retrieval, possibly due to a deficiency in coding the structural and purely linguistic attributes of spoken and printed words (Vellutino and Scanlon this volume).

Decoding and comprehension deficits

Word decoding

Dyslexic readers showed little understanding of sound-symbol correspondence (Boder 1971; Vernon 1957).

Dyslexic readers showed difficulty at recalling or reading aloud visually presented words, but not orally presented words (Fisher 1980; Shankweiler and Liberman 1972).

Dyslexic readers were poorer at decoding words (Calfee 1982; Mackworth and Mackworth 1974).

Dyslexic readers were slower to identify embedded letters ('xcx' and 'xfx') and words (Bouma and Legein 1980).

Dyslexic readers were worse at phonemic segmentation tasks (Vellutino and Scanlon 1984).

Dyslexic readers suffered from a qualitative phonetic deficit in reading and spelling (Olsen this volume).

Phonetic spelling and word knowledge

Dyslexics were poor spellers, but not all poor spellers were dyslexics (Naidoo 1972).

Poor readers were less fluent and knew fewer words than good readers. Their definitions were less mature (Fry, Johnson, and Muehl 1970).

Dyslexic readers seemed to be slower at retrieving words they knew on rapid naming tasks (Denckla and Ruel 1976). Learning disabled readers behaved similarly (Wiig and Semel 1975).

Comprehension and integration deficits

Reading units

Poor readers tended to read in smaller reading units (Cromer 1970; Gioffi 1982; Isakson and Miller 1976).

Table I continued

Use of context

Poor readers showed less efficient use of context (Guthrie 1973).

Syntax, Sentence, and Text

Dyslexics showed poorer syntactic skills (Vogel 1974; Wiig and Semel 1975).

Disabled readers showed comparable ability in learning individual ideographs, but were poorer at reading and producing them (Fisher 1980).

Learning disabled readers of grades 2, 4, and 6 did not comprehend text as well as average readers and bottom-quartile poor readers. Their comprehension was much worse in reading than in listening (Calfee 1982).

Poor readers recalled fewer idea units, especially important ones (Smiley, Oakley, Worthen, Campione and Brown 1977).

Neurological and constitutional factors

Abnormal neurological factors

One male dyslexic who died in an accident showed anatomical evidence of slowed development in the planum temporale of the left hemisphere (Galaburda and Kemper 1979; Geschwind 1979).

10 of 24 adolescent and adult dyslexics had brains that were wider in the right parieto-occipital region than in the left. The group also had lower verbal IQ (Hier, LeMay, Rosenberger, and Perlo 1978).

Minimal brain dysfunction

Phonemic dyslexics, whose disorder is acquired, apparently made reading errors similar to those of developmental dyslexics, e.g., decoding letters into sounds, recognizing function words, and deciphering complete syntax (Holmes 1978).

Dyslexic readers showed linguistic, perceptual, and cognitive skills scores like those of adults who had an alexia (acquired dyslexia), although one third of the college students and one quarter of the third and fourth grade children subjects did not match any of the 3 alexic types (Aaron, Baker, and Hickox 1982).

Electrophysiological studies

Dyslexics showed a higher number of abnormal electrophysiological patterns. These patterns may be related to different patterns of reading abnormality, but great care should be taken in the evaluation of this literature (Hughes 1982, this volume).

Disabled readers measured at the left parietal showed smaller word-flash differences in evoked response than normals, thus indicating problems in verbal processing (Preston, Guthrie, Kirsch, Gertman, and Childs 1977).

Phonetic dyslexics showed smaller left hemisphere/right hemisphere differences in evoked potential to words and musical phrases (Fried 1979; Fried, Tanguay, Boder, Doubleday, and Greensite 1981; Wood, Goff, and Day 1971).

Psychological tests of laterality

Disabled reader's assymmetries in brain activity (left hemisphere greater than right hemisphere), in relation to controls, were greater in 3 studies, equal in 21, and less in 15 (Naylor 1980).

(continued)

Table I continued

Twelve-year-old auditory linguistic dyslexics showed the expected superiority of left visual hemifield processing for faces, but did not show the expected superiority of right visual hemifield processing for words (Pirozzolo and Rayner 1979).

Eleven of 15 phonetic dyslexics evidenced right lateralization of verbal material (Dalby and Gibson 1981).

Disabled readers showed lower right visual hemifield advantage for processing words (Kerschner 1977).

Genetic factors

Dyslexics' families

Reading disabled children had male relatives who showed deficits in reading, spelling, auditory memory, perceptual speed, and verbal reasoning. Their mothers and sisters appeared to be less severely affected (Foch, DeFries, McLean, and Singer 1977; DeFries 1985).

Dyslexic pedigrees of 86 boys and 27 girls showed 47% brothers, 35% sisters, 47% fathers, and 38% mothers affected. Dyslexia could be observed in families for three successive generations (Hallgren 1950).

Dyslexic children in Israel showed consistently better performance on tests of right hemispheric function than on tests of left hemispheric function. 90% of first degree family members performed similarly even though most claimed never to have had reading problems (Gorden 1980).

Monozygotic twins who manifested dyslexia had higher rates of concordance (84% versus 24%) for dyslexia than their dizygotic counterparts (Bakwin 1973). Similar findings have been reported by Zerbin-Rudin (1967) and Decker and Vandenberg (this volume).

Sons of fathers who reported reading problems had a 40% risk of developing a reading disability. Sons of mothers who reported reading problems had a 35% risk. For daughters of parents with a positive history, the risk was 17–18% (DeFries this volume).

But even if one assumes that the question is about dyslexic subtypes rather than a unitary disorder, the question of the logico-theoretical relationship among different profiles remains. What are the relationships among profiles? For a given subtype in the dyslexic population, which profiles would be shared in common? Since profiles are collections of measurements, questions about common properties are questions about convergent measurements. Let us now review some of the problems of measurement that obscure our ability to see these possible convergences.

Problems of Measurement

The conventional strategy for answering questions about the relationship among profiles would be to use repeated-measures designs where repeated measures would measure variables of different profiles. In these designs, measurements would be made on a common set of subjects, each subject being his own control. Another important element of conventional strategy would be to use standardized tests under standard conditions of administration. Unfortunately there are a number of practical obstacles to the adoption of these strategies:

First, concurrent measurement requires cooperation among those making the measurements and there are difficulties associated with obtaining cooperation among investigators from different fields. These include establishing a common language of discourse, solving the logistical problems associated with bringing researchers together, arriving at a consensus about which variables should be measured, developing and validating the measures, etc.

Second, there are problems of work and time. The scope of nominated profiles is so wide that the work and time necessary to measure variables becomes very great. This difficulty is compounded by the fact that classical theories of measurement require administration of many items to arrive at stable estimates of ability, e.g., subjects try all items even though only a few are appropriate for their ability level.

Third, subjects may be difficult to find and their availability for research may be limited. Despite estimates of high incidence, investigators report difficulty in finding adequate numbers of dyslexic subjects who are willing to participate in long-term research projects.

Fourth, measurements made in research may be difficult to replicate. They may require special conditions, expert knowledge, specialized equipment, or novel techniques. Also, they may have been made with samples which were taken from an extreme end of the distribution, e.g., Vellutino and Scanlon (this volume).

Empirically defensible answers to questions about relationships among profiles will wait on satisfactory solutions to problems like these. To summarize the argument thus far, research on dyslexia, or specific reading disability, is currently locked in a three-sided predicament. The problems of definition, of proliferation of profiles, and of difficulties in measurement threaten to impede progress of research. Until such problems are solved, efforts to predict, understand, and remediate dyslexic disorders will be frustrated. It is to suggested strategies for solution that we now turn.

Three Suggested Strategies

Toward Defining the Disorder

Separating dependent and independent variables. Efforts to define the disorder should be distinguished from efforts to find its causes. The disorder should not be defined by its causes; it is the *effect* of its causes! As Table I shows, attempts to define dyslexia often indiscriminately mix profiles of reading and language performance with profiles of cognitive and constitutional disability, and although the profiles are intimately connected, they are also profoundly different. They belong to different categories. Reading and language performance are dependent variables and cognitive and constitutional factors are independent variables. They belong to the general reading equation:

reading behavior $= f$ (age, instruction, motivation, intelligence, cognitive abilities, constitution, etc.). To the extent that a general equation like this holds, dyslexia will be a special case where inadequate reading behavior $= f$ (cognitive disabilities, constitutional factors) or, alternatively put in the language of this chapter: reading disability profiles $= f$ (cognitive profiles, constitutional profiles).

Equations like these partition variables into separate but related classes, thus providing a way to avoid some of the dilemmas of definition that have plagued the field and to circumvent some of the persistent controversies in the literature, e.g., the perception versus reading dispute. The description of inadequate reading components by itself would constitute an excellent foundation for a descriptive definition of dyslexic reading. After more evidence is collected, this definition may later be elaborated for types and subtypes. Definitions generated after etiological classification will be less heterogeneously mixed and therefore less conceptually confused.

Another benefit of classifying variables according to categories of cause and effect is that specification of the cognitive and constitutional factors and the function relating them to reading *and* to each other will contribute to our functional understanding. One way of summarizing this suggestion is to use the analogy of the etiological tree. Many of the problems of definition may be avoided if leaves (small reading units), branches (larger reading units), limbs (largest reading units), trunk (cognitive capabilities), and roots (constitutional factors) are separated from each other, but their functional interdependency acknowledged.

Mapping the dependent variables.   After the variables are categorized, one of the most important tasks would be to map the different categories of reading performance. There would, of course, be many possible ways to represent the different aspects of reading performance and there are a number of excellent models in use. Almost any criterion-referenced method would be better than the norm-referenced methods in current use. The use of normative scores, i.e., "reading ability in the 27th percentile," "reading ability two years below grade level," has sometimes erroneously conveyed the impression that reading can be summarized along a single dimension. Obviously, it cannot. Mapping the many dimensions of reading performance would significantly enrich our understanding of ways in which the dependent variables of reading may vary. Whether it be phenotypes as a function of genotypes or whether it be reading performance as a function of cognitive competencies, only when we obtain specificity of dependency will it be possible to search for specificity of causation.

Mapping the independent variables.   The elaborated profiles of reading and language behavior will help us find and further define the etiological profiles of cognitive performance and constitutional causation. When the profiles are in place, what will be predicted will not be some vague grade or ranking of general reading ability, but rather a more carefully quantified measure of specific components of general reading performance.

Settling the question of individual profiles and profile types.   When the dimensions of dependent and independent variables are mapped, then an individual reader's reading performance and its underlying causes may also be inventoried. Resulting scores on the reading dimensions will constitute an individual's reading ability profile. The profile might consist of a series of digits, like a postal zip code where each digit has a special meaning. Each digit might represent performance along a specific dimension, indicating the level of competence along that dimension. For example, the digits of the reading profile 86453792 might represent one of nine levels of performance along eight dimensions. In the first dimension that represents, for example, the ability to read individual words, the subject is in the 8th level; in the eighth dimension which represents the ability to use context, the subject is in the 2nd, etc.

After many individuals have been inventoried, then answers to the question of typicality and subtypes may be raised. The use of standard multivariate techniques like cluster analysis and multi-dimensional scaling will help answer the question of whether individual profiles tend to form constellations and what the dimensions of difference might be. Canonical correlation and multivariate linear regression procedures might then be used as preliminary screening devices to determine the degree of relationship between constellations of reading profiles and etiological profiles of cognitive ability and constitutional factors.

Dyslexic universals.   Inherent in the suggestions given above is the recommendation to abandon the search for dyslexic universals, or defining properties which must be present in all cases. A philosophically more satisfying approach might be that of searching for "family resemblances" of the type suggested by Wittgenstein (Bambrough 1966). For Wittgenstein, the common property of all games was that they were games, not that there was a universal property shared by all of them. Games are related to each other by their family resemblances in the same way that family members are related to each other. For example, a member of the Orton family might have the Orton nose and the Orton chin, but not the Orton eyes; another member might have the Orton chin and the Orton eyes, but not the Orton nose; still another might only have the Orton eyes. In this example, the first and last Orton had no properties in common, but were related through the chain of family resemblances. Adopting a similar approach to the definition of dyslexia might be more fruitful than continuing the search for universal defining properties. If universals are eventually found, so much the better, but until they are found, let the search be for dimensions of similarity. How these similarities might be sought is the object of the second set of strategic suggestions.

Toward Understanding the Profiles

Repeated-measures designs and standardization.   In order to improve understanding of the relationships among profiles, repeated-measures designs should be used. Where possible, measures of relevant variables should be made for each subject. If the number of variables is too large, then appropriate sampling procedures should be used. Where possible, measures should be standardized and standard procedures of administration should be observed.

After measurements have been made, multivariate procedures may be used to explore relationships that might exist among the resulting profiles, or collections of measurements. Among the obvious models to be explored are the following: reading inadequacy $= f$ (cognitive disabilities) and cognitive disabilities $= f$ (constitutional factors), where f is a function and "cognitive disabilities" and "constitutional factors" are classes of variables. One of the potentially important contributions of such modeling is that it allows stratification of profile categories according to the level of their causal influences. Continuing the analogy of the tree, some variables operate at the level of the roots and some others operate at the level of the branches.

Cooperation among investigators. The difficulty, scope, and complexity of dyslexia research demand greater cooperation among investigators. Few investigators have the necessary resources to mount systematic studies across such a wide front. Interdisciplinary cooperations like The Colorado Project (DeFries, Decker and Vandenberg, Olson, and Schucard, all in this volume) should receive continued support. Frequent teleconferences of investigators interested in the subject should be encouraged. A central database drawing together research literature on dyslexia from different disciplines should be established under the auspices of the National Institutes of Health and made generally available through one or more of the database services. The NIH or agencies like it should support development of standardized tests of reading and linguistic performance. Design and dissemination of computer administered measurement systems should be supported. Indeed, the word "measures" in the title of this volume is aptly chosen, for the success of dyslexia research will depend upon improving measurement. Without such improvements, problems of definition and etiology will be difficult to solve.

Toward Improved Measurement

Measurement in the study of dyslexia could be dramatically improved by adopting new technologies of measurement and the theoretical foundations upon which they stand. Historically, technological innovations like the microscope, telescope, and electron cloud chamber have made visible the previously invisible, opening new doors to fundamental breakthroughs of understanding. Today, the computer can serve as an instrument of vision to enhance powers of observation and improve practices of measurement (Inouye and Bunderson, in press).

The value of using computers in the study of dyslexia has already been aptly demonstrated in this volume. Vital contributions of computers in the measurement of eye movements, evoked potentials, and internal states of the brain have already been noted. In addition to these, this chapter suggests the use of computers in profiling dyslexia and its etiological antecedents. Computerized testing systems operating at extremely high speeds can provide the work, distribute the measurement knowledge and expertise, and provide the standardization needed to create, administer, score, store, and compare measurements upon which the profiling of dyslexia depends.

The profiles resulting from improved practices of definition and measurement will serve more usefully as diagnostic instruments. To the extent that they do, they will be more useful as guides for remedial prescription. Because of the importance of measurement technology and theory to the profiling of dyslexia, a review of current developments in this rapidly changing field may be helpful. Although limitations of space will permit only a cursory outline, additional details may be found in Inouye and Bunderson (in press) or in Bunderson, Inouye, and Olsen (in press).

The Four Generations of Computerized Test Administration

The degree to which measurement practices have tapped technology's power to do work at light speeds varies widely in the measurement industry. As one might expect, there are variations in psychometric sophistication. Despite many differences, there are at least four qualitatively different degrees of observational enhancement that differ in the extent to which they capitalize on computer technologies as instruments of vision. These represent four generations of psychometric sophistication whose names, characteristics, and examples are discussed below.

Computerized Testing (CT): The First Generation

Computerized testing is defined as the translation of both paper and pencil tests and individually administered tests to computer administered format. When paper and pencil tests are translated to computer, the subject responds to the same test items as before, although computerization makes it possible to. (1) present these items in n different random orders and thus control for order effects; (2) standardize conditions of test administration; (3) reduce measurement error through simplification of responses; (4) immediately score and report test results; (5) produce profiles with immediate remediative prescriptions; (6) use more complex items to test for more complex responses; (7) reduce testing time by 20–50%; and (8) collect response latency data. These rather significant advantages make the CT generation much more than just electronic page turning. These advantages, in themselves, could significantly improve the profiling of dyslexia.

When individually administered tests, such as the Stanford-Binet, Kaufmann, and Luria-Nebraska are translated to computer format, the need for one-to-one administration by an expert examiner may sometimes be avoided. Computer software can replicate some of the skills of the expert examiner, thus allowing paraprofessional examiners to substitute. Many of the items can be presented by computer and subjects can respond by pointing, pressing a key, or, in the case of older students, typing a few words. When responses are vocalizations or movements that must be rated by a trained observer, the observer can use the computer to enter the results of the evaluations. The remaining scoring and reporting tasks may be done by the computer. Computerizing the individually administered test promises to reduce training time of test administrators while increasing the degree of standardization. Because so many measures of dyslexia are the results of individual administration, computerized testing may be a labor saving boon.

An additional advantage of the CT generation is the use of the computer to create tests and test items. The computer can create customized tests and test items to meet objectives of the dyslexia researcher. With the use of commercially available "testware," or test creation software, and a bank of item generation algorithms and item forms, heretofore arduous tasks of test development become comparatively easy. The developer is assisted in this process by a series of interactive screen displays that allow him to guide the test creation process, specifying item content, format, and scoring options.

The improvements mentioned thus far have enhanced traditional procedures, doing better what has been done in the past, but the CT generation also provides for measurement practices that are new, that would not be possible without the computer. An example of these is the use of the computer to present simulation items as part of an examination. Through the use of a computer controlled videodisc, the computer can administer test items that present the subjects with, for instance, a patient in a medical examination, a piece of equipment needing repair, or images of fruitflies in a genetic experiment. The student might be asked to respond to these situations by making a series of decisions. Scoring is accomplished by evaluating the outcomes reached by the student and evaluating the strategies and sophistication of the path followed.

Presently, 90% of all computer administered testing belongs to the computerized testing (CT) generation. As illustrated above, the first generation promises to enhance the observation power of the dyslexia researcher in many ways, but additional equating and linking research must be done to establish relationships between CT tests and their non-computerized versions.

Computerized Adaptive Testing (CAT): The Second Generation

Computerized adaptive tests are different from conventional paper and pencil tests not only in differences of presentation media, but also because CAT tests are designed to adapt to the subjects and deliver only those items that are appropriate for their ability levels. There are four major steps in an adaptive test:

(1) A preliminary estimate is made of the subject's ability level.

(2) A test item is administered. This item is chosen to provide maximum information at the estimated ability level. The information value of the item is either calculated on-line or stored in a pre-computed information matrix. Generally, if the subject answers the item correctly, a more difficult item is presented; if the subject misses an item, an easier item is administered. Of all the items available, the one selected is calculated to maximize new information about the subject.

(3) The ability estimate is revised after each item. There are three methods proposed for updating ability estimates: Bayesian Sequential Ability Estimation (Owen 1969, 1975), Maximum Likelihood Ability Estimation (Birnbaum 1968; Lord 1977, 1980; Samejima 1977), and Expected A Posteriori Algorithm or Biweighted Bayesian Estimation (Bock and Aitkin 1981; Mislevy and Bock 1982).

(4) The testing process is terminated when a certain exit criterion has been met. Typical exit criteria are administration of a predetermined number of test items, reduction in variance below a minimum standard error, or reaching a maximum information value.

As noted previously, in conventional tests the majority of items are either too easy or too hard for a given subject. The subject would probably answer all easy items correctly and would miss the items that were too difficult. The items that were too difficult or too easy would contribute little information for measurement of the individual's true ability level. For most subjects, and especially for the handicapped or disabled, conventional tests based on classical test theory are inefficient, time consuming, and wasteful. In the judgment of many psychometricians, tests of the second generation of computer-administered testing offer a more practical, more efficient, and theoretically stronger alternative.

Item response theory. At the heart of computer adaptive testing is Item Response Theory (IRT), a theory of measurement developed and promulgated by Rasch (1960), Birnbaum (1968), Lord (1970, 1980), Novick (Lord and Novick 1968), Hulin, Drasgow, and Parsons (1983), Hambleton and Swaminathan (1985), and others. The fundamental postulate of the theory is that subjects differ on a unidimensional continuum of ability. The estimated ability of each subject is designated "theta" and is compared to all other subjects in the continuum. For each subject the probability of answering an item correctly is dependent on the current ability estimate of the subject and the item response curve for the item.

As Figure 1 shows, item response curves may be specified by three parameters: their location ("b"), their slope ("a"), and their lower asymptote ("c"). The "b," or location, parameter is a function of the item difficulty: higher difficulty items shift the response curve to the right while lower difficulty items shift it to the left on the theta continuum. The "a," or slope, parameter is an index of discrimination: higher values make the item response curve steeper; lower values make it flatter. The steeper the curve, the better the discrimination between subjects of high and low ability and, conversely, the flatter the curve, the poorer the discrimination. The "c," or pseudo-chance, parameter indexes the probability of a correct response from guessing by a subject of very low ability.

This three parameter model is a general model for dichotomously scored items. Special cases of the model are also possible. If the pseudo-chance parameter is assumed to be zero, a two parameter model dependent on only difficulty and discrimination results. If the pseduo-chance parameter is as-

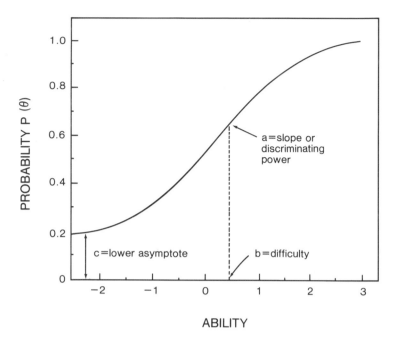

Figure 1. A Typical Three-Parameter Model Item Characteristic Curve

sumed to be zero and the discrimination parameters are assumed to be constant, the model reduces to the one parameter Rasch model. Since empirical evidence provides little support for the assumption that the pseudo-chance parameter is zero and that items have the same discrimination parameters, the three parameter model would seem to be the model of choice (Koch and Reckase 1978; Patience and Reckase 1979; Green, Bock, Humphries, Linn, and Reckase 1982). Yen (1981) found that the three parameter model provided a better fit for multiple choice items than its one or two parameter alternatives.

A thought experiment applying IRT models to items of current dyslexia screening tests is instructive because it points to an area of needed improvement in dyslexia testing. For each dichotomously scored item administered to readers of high and low ability on a unidimensional continuum, such as the ability to decode phonemes, there would be a three parameter item response curve. Examination of any single item response curve would show a "b" parameter indexing the probability of a correct response or relative difficulty, an "a" parameter indicating the steepness of the item response curve slope and the degree to which the item discriminates between the dyslexic and the normal reader, and a "c" parameter indicating the probability of a correct answer by a subject of very low ability. This information about the three parameters, especially for parameters "a" and "c," is virtually unknown for items currently used in screening tests. Because of the meaning of the different parameters, it is clear that this gap in knowledge could greatly increase the probability of misclassifications. For example, students might be screened on the basis of items with a flat "a," or discrimination, parameter. Their passing would be a matter of chance and not of ability.

Calibrated item banks. CAT tests require careful development and calibration of relatively large item pools—usually over 100. The large number of items allows the test developer to draw randomly from several items at each different ability level. These items are administered to a large number of subjects from the target population and reponse vectors are obtained for each subject. Calibration programs then estimate the three parameters of the response curve based on the response vectors of large numbers (i.e., hundreds and even thousands) of subjects. Item curves are inspected and items with poor characteristics are discarded. A special advantage of computerized adaptive testing is that item calibration may be continually updated as CAT tests are scored and subjects added.

As one might surmise, item calibration programs are extremely useful to the CAT test developer. The most widely used include LOGIST (Wingersky, Barton, and Lord 1982), BILOG (Mislevy and Bock 1982), ASCALE (Assessment Systems Corporation 1985), MICROSCALE (Linacre and Wright 1984) and M-SCALE (Wright, Rossner and Congdon 1984).

Advantages of CAT. Since CAT tests are administered by computer, the advantages of the first generation of computerized testing are also advantages of the CAT generation. Those advantages include increased standardization, reduced measurement error, immediate scoring and reporting, the ability to measure more complex items, the ability to measure response latencies, and the ability to create items and tests by computer. The following additional advantages accrue in the second generation:

(1) increased precision of measurement, including higher precision at high and low ability levels;

(2) equivalent precision with as high as 60–70% reduction in testing time (Olsen, Maynes, Ho, and Slawson, in press; Moreno, Wetzel, McBride and Weiss 1983; McKinley and Reckase 1984; McKinley and Reckase 1980);

(3) conditions under which individuals can work at their own pace and where speed of response can be used as additional information in assessing ability;

(4) conditions under which subjects stay productively engaged—all are challenged and none are discouraged.

These last four advantages may be particularly helpful to dyslexia researchers. When more precision is needed, an adaptive test can offer many more items in the immediate vicinity of the subject's level. When a reduction in time is needed, a 60–70% savings can be obtained with precision equivalent to that of conventional paper and pencil tests. The ability to work at one's own pace is especially important to disabled populations. The ability to measure response time adds a new and sensitive measure of temporal processes, particularly for tests of cognitive ability. Finally, the ability to administer only those items appropriate for subjects prevents discouragement and loss of self-esteem.

Continuous Measurement (CM): The Third Generation

In the continuous measurement generation, units of the curriculum are calibrated so that the student's ability may be estimated by observing performance within a given unit. The unit as a whole may serve as the ''item'' or individual test items may be embedded in the curriculum at appropriate intervals. Hallmarks of this generation are the unobtrusiveness of the testing process, the obliteration of the distinction between instruction and curriculum, and the continuous monitoring of the student's position and velocity within a growth space.

A necessary condition of the calibration of the curriculum units is that presentation of the units be standardized. Computer-aided educational (CAE) delivery systems are among the best ways to standardize instruction. At present, the system would involve either a set of microcomputers in a network or a time-shared or multi-tasking central computer with multiple workstations. Most stand-alone microcomputers with only floppy disk storage would not be suitable because experience has shown the logistics of central scoring to be formidable. The instruction might be either individually paced or group administered.

Although most readers of this chapter will be familiar with procedures of individually based computer-aided education, group procedures are less well known and a brief outline of typical procedures may be helpful. Group administration uses a computer-controlled videodisc system where curriculum modules are stored on discs. Presentation of modules is controlled by the teacher. Modules include visual displays with audio, simulations, quizzes, and a variety of interactive learning exercises. Students communicate with the computer through either a wired or wireless response terminal. From time to time the teacher directs the computer to display items that require responses from the students. These responses are collected and scored. Depending on the nature of the items, these scores may be used to construct achievement, ability, or preference profiles of the student. (For additional detail regarding group computer-aided instruction, see Bunderson and Inouye, in press.)

The benefits of applying continuous measurement procedures to the problems of poor and dyslexic readers are prospectively large and significant. These benefits stem from the potential ability of the third generation to provide for widespread delivery of both assessment and remediation, two key concerns of researchers in the area. Delivery of these two services through technology promises to partly ameliorate the critical shortage of trained diagnosticians and special education instructors. Packaging of instruction in either individually paced or group administered formats promises to alleviate one of the most important problems of specialized instruction: the preservation of distinctive character of the educational treatment through one or more generations of trainees. All too often, curative properties are lost because training procedures do not faithfully communicate all key attributes of the remedy. Technology's ability to replicate instruction of the expert or master, although far from perfect, is a significant advantage in this regard.

Intelligent Curriculum and Continuous Measurement (ICCM):
The Fourth Generation

The fourth generation adds the word ''intelligent'' to curriculum and continuous measurement. It thus differs from the third generation to the extent that it makes uses of artificial intelligence strategies to improve both. The ICCM generation draws upon four bases: (1) learner profiles; (2) curricular units; (3) calibration data for the curricular units; and (4) a knowledge base of prescriptive rules for adaptively improving the students' strategies and enhancing their trajectories through the curriculum. Because these bases serve as the foundation for the computer adaptive calibrated curriculum system, they should be discussed in greater detail.

Learner profiles are stored in a database containing information about each individual student's abilities, achievement, preferences, and trajectory through the curricular units. Information about the student's trajectory is updated after each module has been passed or failed. When a profile of a student's trajectory though the curriculum is brought together with the calibrations of the curriculum, a continuous estimate of growth of the student's ability results. It is from these estimates that the student's relative position and velocity, i.e., rate of growth toward the curriculum's objectives, are calculated.

Curricular units of the ICCM generation are contained in "intelligent" knowledge bases. These knowledge bases contain summarized knowledge of experts in a form accessible to other computer programs called "inference engines." Inference engines provide ways of searching the knowledge of experts through the use of predicate calculus. When a student queries the knowledge base about the implications of a proposition or set of propositions, the inference engine can rapidly search the knowledge base for appropriate answers. The answers are presented via graphic displays, interactive instruction, videodisc simulations, etc., which are indexed and referenced through the internal logic of the curriculum in the knowledge base.

Calibration data about curricular units is stored in a separate database. Calibrated parameters for each curricular unit are stored in much the same way as in the CM generation. These calibrations are updated when the units are recalibrated or new units added.

The final knowledge base used in the system contains a set of prescriptive rules for improving student trajectories through the curriculum. Development of such knowledge may be the most important contribution of the ICCM generation. Although current expert systems have attempted to summarize the knowledge of an expert or group of experts, few experts are to be found who can prescribe optimal strategies for students passing through a specific curriculum. Therefore, the knowledge base of prescriptive rules must be developed from the ground up. Instruments of this development would be computer programs that allow the entry of data on the observation of empirical regularities and an inference engine that would assist teachers and students to organize logical implications of their growing knowledge. In this enterprise, for those areas where the required distinctions, discriminations, and actions overrun the capabilities of human information processing, the inference engine could be programmed to assist in developing a body of logically consistent inferences and prescriptions about optimizing student growth.

Although development of a fully operational ICCM system has yet to be demonstrated, such demonstrations will be forthcoming shortly. It is instructive to consider how a prospective ICCM system might be used to test for dyslexia, prescribe needed instruction, and deliver needed remediation. It is to features of such a future system that we now turn.

An example of an ICCM reading system. As defined above, a hypothetical ICCM system for reading would have at least four major parts:

(1) Learner profiles. These would include reading, cognitive, and constitutional profiles. The reading profiles would contain measurements of specific reading and linguistic abilities and disabilities, e.g., knowledge of letter-sound correspondences, spelling ability, etc. The cognitive profiles would contain measurements of cognitive abilities and disabilities, e.g., ability to perceive or to sequence sounds, etc. The constitutional profiles would contain data regarding constitutional abilities and disabilities, e.g., genetic pedigrees, the results of neurological examinations, etc.

(2) A reading curriculum. This would be composed of units designed to build specific reading abilities measured by the reader's profile. In the case of dyslexic readers, the "normal" effect of the instruction would be mediated by cognitive and constitutional disabilities. Special therapy units would be necessary. The units would draw upon the body of practices that can be empirically certified as efficacious in remediation of specific reading disabilities.

(3) Calibration data. The data would contain difficulty estimates for curricular units for typical and special populations.

(4) An intelligent knowledge base mapping the curriculum to the reader's profiles. For students with one of the dyslexias, the prescriptions would be modified by information found in their cognitive and constitutional profiles. Prescriptions would be generated from the knowledge base in accordance with the best generalizations that could be made for students with their peculiar patterns of reading, cognitive, and constitutional profiles.

Although a system like this is only hypothetical, it is easy to see how it would benefit research on dyslexia. If those building it were properly qualified, it could qualitatively accelerate the rate of investigation. Building such a system would force the investigators to model diagnoses and remediation of dyslexia with an unusual degree of explicitness. Because outcomes would be continually monitored, the measurement, prescription, and remediation cycle could be iteratively tested and refined. The efficiency and pace of the refinement process would be difficult to duplicate without the power of high speed electronic computers.

Conclusion

Like Janus, this final chapter tries to look backward and forward at the same time. In the past, attempts at predicting, understanding, and remedying dyslexia have foundered on three closely related problems: the problem of defining dyslexia; the problem of understanding the meaning of its many profiles; and the problem of improving the theory and practice of measurement. In the future, these problems may be ameliorated by:

(1) Taking a new approach to the definition of the phenomenon, one which looks for family resemblances instead of universals and which recognizes the different levels of causal operation of the various profiles. The suggested approach would categorize the profiles into three broad classes: reading and language profiles, cognitive ability profiles, and constitutional profiles. Reading and language profiles would contain detailed measures of specific linguistic and reading abilities and disabilities. Cognitive profiles would contain detailed measures of non-linguistic cognitive variables. Constitutional profiles would contain detailed measures of physiological, neurological, and genetic variables. As a first cut, it was suggested that dyslexia be defined in terms of specific patterns found in linguistic and reading profiles and the causes of these profiles be sought in related cognitive and constitution profiles. One practical consequence of adopting these suggestions would be that normative dependent variables of retardation like "two years below grade level," which imply only one dimension of variation, would be replaced by profiles consisting of matrices of specific reading ability measures for which multiple causes may be sought.

(2) Adopting new strategies to study relationships among the profiles of dyslexia. Repeated-measures designs and multivariate-statistical techniques were suggested as ways of studying the strength and nature of the relationship between profiles. Cognitive and constitutional profiles might be regressed against reading performance profiles and constitutional profiles might be regressed against cognitive profiles. These procedures, if properly performed, could not help but add to our knowledge.

(3) Exploiting new technologies of computerized measurement and the theories that make them possible. In addition to the uses of computers mentioned in previous chapters, four generations of computerized measurement were introduced. Each generation was examined for the prospective contribution it might make to defining profiles of dyslexia. Advantages of the first two generations included increases in precision, savings of time, standardization of administration, measurements of greater complexity, use of response latency information, immediate scoring and reporting, and use of the computer to develop items and tests. Advantages of the third generation included unobtrusive measurement, obliteration of the distinction between instruction and curriculum, and continuous monitoring of the position and velocity of the student in a growth space. Advantages of the fourth generation included the application of artificial intelligence to problems of measurement and curriculum, with its consequent enhancement of our abilities to predict, understand, and remediate.

The advantages of the four generations suggest ways in which the computer can serve as an instrument of vision, enhancing the ability of scientists to see, understand, and use the many profiles of dyslexia. Although a chapter that looks into the future must, of necessity, remain somewhat speculative, if it stimulates imagination and engenders understanding about how computerized biobehavioral measures might contribute to the prediction, understanding, and remediation of dyslexia, its immediate aims are met.

References

Aaron, P. G., Baker, C., and Hickox, G. L. 1982. In search of the third dyslexia. *Neuropsychologia* 20:203–208.

Applebee, A. N. 1971. Research in reading retardation: Two critical problems. *Journal of Child Psychology and Psychiatry* 12:91–113.

Assessment Systems Corporation. 1985. *User's Manual for the MicroCAT Testing System*. St. Paul, Minn.: Assessment Systems Corporation.

Bakker, D. J. 1972. *Temporal Order in Disturbed Reading*. Rotterdam: University Press.

Bakwin, H. 1973. Reading disability in twins. *Developmental Medicine and Child Neurology* 15:184–187.

Bambrough, J. R. 1966. Family resemblances. *In* G. Pitcher (ed.). *Wittgenstein: The Philosophical Investigations*. Garden City, N.Y.: Anchor Books.

Belmont, L., and Birch, H. G. 1963. Lateral dominance and right-left awareness in normal children. *Child Development* 34:257–270.

Benton, A. L. 1978. Neurological aspects of developmental dyslexia and reading disorders. *In* A. L. Benton and D. Pearl (eds.). *Dyslexia: An Appraisal of Current Knowledge*. New York: Oxford University Press.

Birnbaum, A. 1968. Some latent trait models and their uses in inferring an examinee's ability. *In* F. M. Lord and M. R. Novick (eds.). *Statistical Theories of Mental Test Scores*. Reading, Mass.: Addison, Wesley.

Blank, M., and Bridger, W. H. 1966. Deficiencies in verbal labeling in retarded readers. *American Journal of Orthopsychiatry* 36:840–847.

Bock, R. D., and Aitkin, M. 1981. Marginal maximum likelihood estimation of item parameters: Application of an EM algorithm. *Psychometrika* 46:443–459.

Boder, E. 1971. Developmental dyslexia: Prevailing diagnostic concepts and a new diagnostic approach. *In* H. R. Myklebust (ed.). *Progress in Learning Disabilities*, Vol. II. New York: Grune and Stratton.

Bouma, H. Y., and Legein, Ch. P. 1980. Dyslexia: A specific recoding deficit? An analysis of response latencies for letters and words in dyslectics and in average readers. *Neuropsychologia* 18:285–298.

Bryden, M. P. 1972. Auditory-visual and sequential-spatial matching in relation to reading ability. *Child Development* 43:824–832.

Bunderson, C. V., and Inouye, D. K. In press. Computer-aided educational delivery systems. *In* R. Gagne (ed.). *Instructional Technology*.

Bunderson, C. V., Inouye, D. K., and Olsen, J. B. In press. *In* R. Linn (ed.). *Educational Measurement*, 3rd. Edition. Washington, D.C.: American Council on Education and National Council of Measurement in Education.

Calfee, R. C. 1982. Cognitive models of reading: Implications for assessment and treatment of reading disability. *In* R. N. Malatesha and P. G. Aaron (eds.). *Reading Disorder: Varieties and Treatments*. New York: Academic Press.

Corballis, M. C., and Beale, I. L. 1976. *The Psychology of Left and Right*. Hillsdale, N.J.: Lawrence Erlbaum Associates.

Critchley, M. 1970. *The Dyslexic Child*. London: William Heinemann Medical Books.

Cromer, W. 1970. The difference model: A new explanation for some reading difficulties. *Journal of Educational Psychology* 61:471–483.

Dalby, J. T., and Gibson, D. 1981. Functional cerebral lateralization in subtypes of disabled readers. *Brain and Language* 14:34–48.

Denckla, M. B., and Rudel, R. 1976. Naming of pictured objects by dyslexic and other learning disabled children. *Brain and Language* 3:1–15.

Di Lollo, V., Hanson, D., and McIntyre, J. S. 1983. Initial stages of visual information processing in dyslexia. Unpublished manuscript, University of Alberta.

Duffy, F. H., Denckla, M. B., Bartels, P. H., and Sandini, G. 1980. Dyslexia: Regional differences in the brain electrical activity by topographic mapping. *Annals of Neurology* 7(5):412–420.

Duffy, F. H., Denckla, M. B., Bartels, P. H., Sandini, G., and Kiessling, L. S. 1980. Dyslexia: Automated diagnosis by computerized classification of brain electrical activity. *Annals of Neurology* 7(5):421–428.

Elterman, R. D., Abel, L. A., Daroff, R. B., Dell'Osso, L. F., and Bornstein, J. L. 1980. Eye movement patterns in dyslexic children. *Journal of Learning Disabilities* 13:11–16.

Fisher, D. F. 1979. Dysfunctions in reading disability: There's more than meets the eye. *In* L. B. Resnick and P. A. Weavers (eds.). *Theory and Practice of Early Learning,* Vol. I. Hillsdale, N.J.: Lawrence Erlbaum Associates.

Fisher, D. F. 1980. Compensatory training for disabled readers: Research to practice. *Journal of Learning Disabilities* 13:134–140.

Foch, T. T., DeFries, J. C., McLearn, G. E., and Singer, S. M. 1977. Familial patterns of impairment in reading disability. *Journal of Educational Psychology* 69:316–329.

Fried, I. 1979. Cerebral dominance and subtypes of developmental dyslexia. *Bulletin of the Orton Society* 29:101–112.

Fried, I., Tanguay, P. E., Boder, E., Doubleday, C., and Greensite, M. 1981. Developmental dyslexia: Electrophysiological evidence of subtypes. *Brain and Language* 12:14–22.

Fry, M. A., Johnson, C. S., and Muehl, S. 1970. Oral language production in relation to reading achievement among select second graders. *In* D. J. Bakker and P. Satz (eds.). *Specific Reading Disability: Advances in Theory and Method.* Rotterdam: Rotterdam University Press.

Galaburda, A. M., and Kemper, T. L. 1979. Cytoarchitectonic abnormalities in developmental dyslexia: A case study. *Annals of Neurology* 6:94–100.

Geschwind, N. 1979. Specialization of the human brain. *Scientific American* 241:180–199.

Ginsberg, G. P., and Hartwick, A. 1971. Directional confusion as a sign of dyslexia. *Perceptual and Motor Skills* 32:535–543.

Gioffi, G. 1982. Recognition of sentence structure in meaningful prose by good comprehenders and skilled decoders. *Journal of Reading Behavior* 14.86–92.

Gorden, H. W. 1980. Cognitive asymmetry in dyslexic families. *Neuropsychologia* 18:645–655.

Green, B. F., Bock, R. D., Humphries, L. G., Linn, R. L., and Reckase, M. D. 1982. *Evaluation Plan for the Computerized Adaptive Vocational Aptitude Battery.* Baltimore, Md.: Johns Hopkins University Department of Psychology.

Guthrie, J. T. 1973. Reading comprehension and syntactic responses in good and poor readers. *Journal of Educational Psychology* 65:294–299.

Hallgren, B. 1950. Specific dyslexia ("congenital word blindness"): A clinical and genetic study. *Acta Psychiatrica et Neurologica Scandinavica* Supplement No. 65.

Hambleton, R. K., and Swaminathan, H. 1985. *Item Response Theory: Principles and Applications.* Boston, Mass.: Kluwer Nijhoff Publishing.

Hier, D. B., LeMay, M., Rosenberger, P. B., and Perlo, V. P. 1978. Developmental dyslexia: Evidence for a subgroup with a reversal of cerebral asymmetry. *Archives of Neurology* 35:90–92.

Holmes, J. M. 1978. "Regression" and reading breakdown. *In* A. Caramazza and E. B. Zurif (eds.). *Language Acquisition and Breakdown.* Baltimore, Md.: The Johns Hopkins University Press.

Hughes, J. R. 1982. The electroencephalogram and reading disorders. *In* R. N. Malatesha and P. G. Aaron (eds.). *Reading Disorders: Varieties and Treatments.* New York: Academic Press.

Hulin, C. L., Drasgow, F., and Parsons, C. K. 1983. *Item Response Theory: Application to Psychological Measurement.* Homewood, Ill.: Dow Jones-Irwin.

Hynd, G. W., and Cohen, M. 1983. *Dyslexia: Neuropsychological Theory, Research, and Clinical Differentiation.* New York: Grune and Stratton.

Inouye, D. K., and Bunderson, C. V. In press. The four generations of computer administered testing. *Journal of Man and Machine.*

Isakson, R., and Miller, J. 1976. Sensitivity to the syntactic and semantic cues in good and poor comprehenders. *Journal of Educational Psychology* 9:12–20.

John, E. R. 1977. *Functional Neuroscience: Clinical Application of Quantitative Electrophysiology.* Hillsdale, N.J.: Lawrence Erlbaum Associates.

Jorm, A. F. 1979. The cognitive and neurological basis for developmental dyslexia: A theoretical framework and review. *Cognition* 7:19–33.

Katz, R. B., Shankweiler, D., and Liberman, I. Y. 1981. Memory for item order and phonetic recoding in the beginning reader. Status Report on Speech Research SR-66, Haskins Laboratories.

Kerschner, J. R. 1977. Cerebral dominance in disabled readers, good readers, and gifted children: Search for a valid model. *Child Development* 48:61–67.

Koch, W. R., and Reckase, M. D. 1978. A line tailored testing comparison study of the one- and three-parameter logistic models. Research Report 78-1, Tailored Testing Research Laboratory, Educational Psychology Department, University of Missouri, Columbia, Mo., June 1978.

Liberman, I. Y., and Shankweiler, D. 1978. Speech, the alphabet and teaching to read. *In* L. Resnick and P. Weaver (eds.). *Theory and Practice of Early Reading.* New York: Wiley.

Liberman, I. Y., Shankweiler, D., Orlando, C., Harris, K. S., and Berti, F. B. 1971. Letter confusion and reversals of sequence in the beginning reader: Implications for Orton's theory of developmental dyslexia. *Cortex* 7:127–142.

Linacre, M., and Wright, B. D. 1984. *MICROSCALE*. Chicago, Ill.: MESA Press.

Lord, F. M. 1970. Some test theory for tailored testing. *In* W. H. Holtzman (ed.). *Computer-Assisted Instruction, Testing, and Guidance*. New York: Harper and Row.

Lord, F. M. 1977. Practical applications of item characteristic curve theory. *Journal of Educational Measurement* 14:117–138.

Lord, F. M. 1980. *Applications of Item Response Theory to Practical Testing Problems*. Hillsdale, N.J.: Lawrence Erlbaum Associates.

Lord, F. M., and Novick, M. R. 1968. *Statistical Theories of Mental Test Scores*. Reading, Mass.: Addison-Wesley Publishing.

Lyle, J. G., and Goyen, J. 1969. Performance of retarded readers on the WISC and educational tests. *Journal of Abnormal Psychology* 74:105–112.

McKinley, R. L., and Reckase, M. D. 1980. Computer applications to ability testing. *Association for Educational Data Systems Journal* 13(3):193–203.

McKinley, R. L., and Reckase, M. D. 1984. Implementing an adaptive testing program in an instructional program environment. Paper presented at the American Educational Research Association Annual Meeting, April 1984, New Orleans.

Mackworth, J. F., and Mackworth, N. H. 1974. How children read: Matching by sight and sound. *Journal and Reading Behavior* 6:295–303.

Mason, M., Katz, L., and Wicklund, D. A. 1975. Immediate spatial order memory and item memory in sixth-grade children as a function of reader ability. *Journal of Educational Psychology* 67:610–616.

Mislevy, R. J., and Bock, R. D. 1982. *Maximum Likelihood Item Analysis and Test Scoring with Binary Logistic Models*. Mooresville, Ind.: Scientific Software, Inc.

Moreno, K., Wetzel, C. D., McBride, J. R., and Weiss, D. J. 1983. Relationship between corresponding Armed Services Vocational Aptitude Battery (ASVAB) and computerized adaptive testing (CAT) subtests. (NPRDC TR 83-27). San Diego, Calif.: Navy Personnel Research and Development Center, August, 1983.

Morrison, F. J., Giordani, B., and Nagy, J. 1977. Reading disability: An information-processing analysis. *Science* 196:77–79.

Naidoo, S. 1972. *Specific Dyslexia*. New York: Wiley.

Naylor, H. 1980. Reading disability and lateral assymetry: An information-processing analysis. *Psychological Bulletin* 87:531–545.

Olsen, J. B., Maynes, D. D., Ho, K., and Slawson, D. A. In press. The development and pilot testing of a comprehensive assessment system, phase I. Report submitted to the California Assessment Program, Department of Education. Provo, Utah: Waterford Testing Center.

Owen, R. J. 1969. A Bayesian approach to tailored testing. Research Bulletin 69-92, Educational Testing Service, Princeton, N.J.

Owen, R. J. 1975. A Bayesian sequential procedure for quantal response in the context of adaptive mental testing. *Journal of the American Statistical Association* 70:351–356.

Patience, W. M., and Reckase, M. D. 1979. Operational characteristics of a one-parameter tailored testing procedure. Research Report 79-2, Tailored Testing Research Laboratory, Educational Psychology Department, University of Missouri, Columbia, Mo., October 1979.

Pavlidis, G. Th. 1981. Do eye movements hold the key to dyslexia? *Neuropsychologia* 19:57–64.

Pirozzolo, F. J. 1979. *The Neuropsychology of Developmental Reading Disorder*. New York: Praeger Publishers.

Pirozzolo, F. J., and Rayner, K. 1979. Cerebral organization and reading disability. *Neuropsychologia* 17:485–491.

Preston, M. S., Guthrie, J. T., Kirsch, I., Gertman, D., and Childs, B. 1977. VERs in normal and disabled adult readers. *Psychophysiology* 14:8–14.

Rasch, G. 1960. *Probabilistic Models for Some Intelligence and Attainment Tests*. Copenhagen: Nielsen and Lydiche.

Samejima, F. 1977. A comment on Birnbaum's three-parameter logistic model in the latent trait theory. *Psychometrika* 38(2):221–233.

Satz, P., and Morris, R. 1981. Learning disability subtypes: A review. *In* F. J. Pirozzolo and M. C. Wittrock (eds.). *Neuropsychological and Cognitive Processes in Reading*. New York: Academic Press.

Shankweiler, D., and Liberman, I. Y. 1972. Misreading: A search for causes. *In* J. K. Kavanagh and I. G. Mattingly (eds.). *Language by Ear and by Eye*. Cambridge, Mass.: MIT Press.

Smiley, S. S., Oakley, D. D., Worthen, D., Campione, J. C., and Brown, A. 1977. Recall of thematically relevant material by adolescent good and poor readers as a function of written versus oral presentation. *Journal of Educational Psychology* 69:381–387.

Stanley, G., Kaplan, I., and Poole, C. 1975. Cognitive and nonverbal perceptual processing in dyslexics. *Journal of General Psychology* 93:67–72.

Stein, J. F., and Fowler, S. 1982. Towards the physiology of visual dyslexia. *In* Y. Zotterman (ed.). *Dyslexia: Neuronal, Cognitive and Linguistic Aspects.* Wenner-Gren Symposium Series, Vol. XXXV, New York: Pergamon.

Tallal, P. 1980. Auditory temporal perception, phonics, and reading disabilities in children. *Brain and Language* 9:182–198.

Taylor, I., and Taylor, M. M. 1983. *The Psychology of Reading.* New York: Academic Press.

Torgesen, J. K., and Goldman, T. 1977. Rehearsal and short-term memory in reading disabled children. *Child Development* 48:56–60.

Vellutino, F. R. 1979. *Dyslexia: Theory and Research.* Cambridge, Mass.: MIT Press.

Vellutino, F. R., Steger, J. A., and Kandel, G. 1972. Reading disability: An investigation of the perceptual deficit hypothesis. *Cortex* 8:106–118.

Vellutino, F. R., Steger, J. A., Harding, C. J., and Phillips, F. 1975. Verbal vs non-verbal paired-associates learning in poor and normal readers. *Neuropsychologia* 13:75–82.

Vernon, M. D. 1957. *Backwardness in Reading.* Cambridge: Cambridge University Press.

Vogel, S. A. 1974. Syntactic abilities in normal and dyslexic children. *Journal of Learning Disabilities* 7:103–109.

Wiig, E. H., and Semel, E. M. 1975. Productive language abilities in learning disabled adolescents. *Journal of Learning Disabilities* 8:578–586.

Wingersky, M. S., Barton, M. A., and Lord, F. M. 1982. *LOGIST User's Guide.* Princeton, N.J.: Educational Testing Service.

Wood, C. C., Goff, W. R., and Day, R. S. 1971. Auditory evoked potentials during speech perception. *Science* 173:1248–1251.

Wright, B. D., Rossner, M., and Congdon, R. 1984. *M-SCALE.* Chicago, Ill.: MESA Press.

Yen, W. M. 1981. Using simulation results to choose a latent trait model. *Applied Psychological Measurement* 5(2):245–262.

Zerbin-Rudin, E. 1967. Congenital word blindness. *Bulletin of the Orton Society* 17:47–54.

Index